LYMPHOKINES

A FORUM FOR IMMUNOREGULATORY CELL PRODUCTS

VOLUME 13

Lymphokines

A Forum for Immunoregulatory Cell Products

EDGAR PICK
Laboratory of Immunopharmacology
Department of Human Microbiology
Sackler School of Medicine
Tel-Aviv University
Ramat-Aviv, Tel Aviv, Israel

ADVISORY EDITOR
MAURICE LANDY
P.O. Box 2423
La Jolla, California

VOLUME 13

Molecular Cloning and Analysis of Lymphokines

EDITED BY

DAVID R. WEBB
Roche Institute of Molecular Biology
Roche Research Center
Nutley, New Jersey

DAVID V. GOEDDEL
Molecular Biology Department
Genentech, Inc.
South San Francisco, California

1987

Harcourt Brace Jovanovich, Publishers
Orlando   San Diego   New York   Austin
Boston   London   Sydney   Tokyo   Toronto

ACADEMIC PRESS, INC.
Orlando, Florida 32887

United Kingdom Edition published by
ACADEMIC PRESS INC. (LONDON) LTD.
24–28 Oval Road, London NW1 7DX

LIBRARY OF CONGRESS CATALOG CARD NUMBER: 0197-596X

ISBN 0–12–432013-9 (alk. paper)

PRINTED IN THE UNITED STATES OF AMERICA

87 88 89 90   9 8 7 6 5 4 3 2 1

Contents

Strategies for Cloning Mouse and Human Lymphokine Genes Using a Mammalian cDNA Expression Vector

TAKASHI YOKOTA, FRANK LEE, NAOKO ARAI, DONNA RENNICK, ALBERT ZLOTNIK, TIM MOSMANN, ATSUSHI MIYAJIMA, YUTAKA TAKEBE, ROBERT KASTELEIN, GERARD ZURAWSKI, AND KEN-ICHI ARAI

Identification and Expression of cDNA Plasmids Corresponding to Human Interferon-Gamma (IFN-γ) and Interleukin 2 (IL-2)

RENE DEVOS, HILDE CHEROUTRE, GEERT PLAETINCK, AND WALTER FIERS

T Cell Growth Factor (Interleukin 2) Gene: Organization and Expression in Human T Lymphotropic Virus-Infected Cells in Leukemia and AIDS

SURESH K. ARYA AND ROBERT C. GALLO

Regulation of Human Interleukin 2 Gene Expression

RAYMOND KAEMPFER, SHIMON EFRAT, AND SUSAN MARSH

Expression Patterns of Lymphokines and Related Genes

VERNER PAETKAU, JENNIFER SHAW, JOHN F. ELLIOTT, CALLIOPI HAVELE, BILL POHAJDAK, AND R. CHRIS BLEACKLEY

Molecular Cloning of the Human Interleukin 2 Receptor

WARREN J. LEONARD

Cloning and Expression of Human and Mouse IL-2 Receptor cDNAs

DAVID COSMAN, JANIS WIGNALL, ANDREW LEWIS, ALAN ALPERT,
KATE MCKEREGHAN, DOUGLAS PAT CERRETTI, STEVEN GILLIS,
STEVEN DOWER, AND DAVID URDAL

Molecular Analysis of the Murine Interleukin 2 Receptor

JIM MILLER, THOMAS R. MALEK, ETHAN M. SHEVACH,
AND RONALD N. GERMAIN

Cloning and Expression of Murine, Human, and Rabbit Interleukin 1 Genes

PETER T. LOMEDICO, UELI GUBLER, AND STEVEN B. MIZEL

Molecular Biology of Interferon-Gamma

PATRICK W. GRAY AND DAVID V. GOEDDEL

Cloning and Characterization of the Genes for Human and Murine Tumor Necrosis Factors

DIANE PENNICA AND DAVID V. GOEDDEL

Isolation and Expression of the Genes Coding for Mouse and Human Tumor Necrosis Factor (TNF) and Biological Properties of Recombinant TNF

JAN TAVERNIER, LUCIE FRANSEN, ANNE MARMENOUT,
JOSE VAN DER HEYDEN, RITA MUELLER, MARIE-ROSE RUYSSCHAERT,
ADRI VAN VLIET, RITA BAUDEN, AND WALTER FIERS

Molecular Characterization of Human Lymphotoxin

PATRICK W. GRAY

Expression of Hemopoietic Growth Factor Genes in Murine T Lymphocytes

ANNE KELSO AND NICHOLAS GOUGH

Cloning and Expression of the Murine Interleukin 3 Gene

H. D. CAMPBELL, M.-C. FUNG, A. J. HAPEL, AND I. G. YOUNG

Organization of Chromosomal Genes for Interleukin 3 and Granulocyte–Macrophage Colony Stimulating Factor and Their Expression in Activated T Cells

TAKESHI OTSUKA, SHOICHIRO MIYATAKE, TAKASHI YOKOTA, JOAN CONAWAY, RON CONAWAY, NAOKO ARAI, FRANK LEE, AND KEN-ICHI ARAI

Glucocorticoid Regulation of Lymphokine Production by Murine T Lymphocytes

JANICE CULPEPPER AND FRANK LEE

And Now for Something Completely Differential

C. G. LOBE, V. H. PAETKAU, AND R. C. BLEACKLEY

Preface

It is safe to say that ten years ago few molecular biologists had any interest in cellular immunology with its plethora of cells and factors. As is amply evident from the contents of this volume, the situation has changed, and the advances in technology that took place during this period contributed enormously to that change. Developments in molecular biology as well as in microanalytical protein chemistry are by now well chronicled. Equally important was the formation of small, highly focused companies whose primary goals were to use the new biotechnology to develop a new generation of pharmaceuticals and drug therapies based on the newly discovered growth regulators, including, especially, the lymphokines. Many cellular immunologists who watched these developments were somewhat less than enthusiastic about the intrusion into "their field" by outsiders—and molecular biologists at that! They felt overwhelmed by talk of introns and exons and restriction enzyme polymorphisms, and not a few expressed the opinion that knowing what a lymphokine gene looked like would not explain its role in immune regulation. To many others, however, the availability of pure lymphokines in large amounts with uniform activity represented a garden of delights. By 1985 it was clear that cellular immunologists were truly entering a "golden age" with well-defined growth regulatory and effector molecules to be used in carefully defined systems, and questions that had long been unanswerable became experimentally approachable. This volume represents, in a way, a celebration of the coming of age of cellular immunology in that it focuses attention on cloning and molecular analysis of both growth regulatory and effector lymphokines. The various chapters demonstrate the tremendous range of questions that are now being addressed by biochemists and immunologists about how the immune system operates at its most fundamental level. It is also clear from these works that there is much more undone than done, a point that should not be lost on both students and legislators the world over.

The eighteen chapters presented are a good representation of the areas of lymphokine research that have seen the successful application of molecular biology. Chapters 1 and 2, by Yokota *et al.* and Devos *et al.*, present an excellent sampling of the general strategies to be used in the cloning of lymphokine genes.

Several authors deal with interleukin 2 and the interleukin 2 receptor, reflecting the enormous amount of attention which this lymphokine has attracted in the past few years. Arya and Gallo present an interesting

analysis of the regulation of IL-2 gene expression, with particular emphasis on its expression in HTLV-infected cells. Of particular note is the
observation that the IL-2 gene is repressed in HTLV-I-infected cells,
whereas in HTLV-III-infected cells the gene remains active. Kaempfer
and colleagues have analyzed IL-2 gene expression in mitogen-stimulated human T cells. They present evidence suggesting that a labile repressor exists which regulates the flow of IL-2 mRNA processing as well
as a nonlabile element that controls IL-2 mRNA degradation. The apparently rigid control exerted by the labile repressor on IL-2 mRNA processing underscores the utility of studying transcriptional and
translational control in lymphokine genes and may have broad implications for control of cell growth in general. In contrast, Paetkau and
colleagues offer a somewhat different interpretation of the effects of
cycloheximide on the superinduction of IL-2 mRNA to that presented by
Kaempfer *et al.* They show that addition of cycloheximide induces RNase
L which may control mRNA stability. These authors also present an
instructive description of the strategy that may be employed to clone a
set of inducible genes in activated lymphocytes. It is of interest that one
of the genes identified using this approach in PMA-stimulated EL4 cells
is related to mouse mammary tumor virus (MMTV). This is worth noting
because of recent reports that retrovirus envelope polypeptide sequences may, under appropriate circumstances, suppress immune responses. Thus, lymphokine researchers who use molecular cloning
technology to identify interesting "inducible" genes must be alert to the
presence as well as the possible functionality of viral genes.

The next three chapters focus on the IL-2 receptor, beginning with
Warren Leonard, who first isolated the human protein and subsequently
cloned the gene. A good summary of the isolation and cloning as well as
an excellent description of the gene structure is presented. Cosman *et al.*
discuss the cloning of both human and mouse IL-2 receptor genes and
present a good summary of the approaches being taken to address, at the
genetic level, the issue of how one gene can apparently code for both a
high-affinity and a low-affinity receptor. Cosman *et al.* and Miller *et al.*
suggest that the capacity to form a high-affinity receptor for IL-2 may be
due to factors that are cell specific since fibroblasts transfected with the
IL-2 gene usually express only the low-affinity version. That this is the
case has been recently suggested by results from T. Taniguchi and
associates.

Lomedico and colleagues present a thorough view of another growth
factor, interleukin 1, in terms of the form of IL-1 found in the mouse,
human, and rabbit. It is evident that the processing of the precursor
molecule represents another example of posttranslational regulation con-

trolling the expression of the active form(s). As is the case with IL-2, it appears that there are multiple points for the expression of a functional lymphokine by a cell, and the elements that act at these points may be both intrinsic and/or extrinsic.

The next several chapters cover an area of lymphokine molecular biology that has blossomed somewhat unexpectedly, namely, the area of effector factors: the lymphotoxins, including tumor necrosis factor and interferon-γ. It may be appropriate at this point to underscore the importance of molecular biology to cellular immunology by pointing out that the availability of cloned IFN-γ to the research community has been invaluable in enhancing our understanding of the complex regulatory role that this molecule plays in the immune system. Further, the protein sequencing and cloning of the genes for lymphotoxin and tumor necrosis factor provided a real impetus to research in this area by showing that TNF and cachectin were one and the same and by establishing the homologous but nonetheless unique nature of lymphotoxin as compared to TNF. The close linkage of the human lymphotoxin gene and the TNF gene (795 base pairs apart) raises some interesting questions about gene regulation since these two genes are expressed rather exclusively by quite different cell types. Tavernier *et al.* further raise important questions about the role of TNF/cachectin in inflammation and immunity, the implication being that the role of TNF as both an effector factor and regulatory factor may make it more analogous to a molecule such as IFN-γ in its range of activities.

Another area that has developed very quickly in the last two years is represented by four chapters covering hematopoietic growth factors, including interleukin 3. Kelso and Gough provide insights into the complex area of hematopoiesis and the regulation of IL-3/Multi-CSF and GM–CSF production in T cell clones. In light of the observation by many workers (initially by Glasebrook, Fitch, and colleagues) that individual T cell clones may produce multiple factors, it is noteworthy that Kelso and Gough report that, on maturation, a given T cell clone takes on a stable phenotype with respect to the lymphokines it produces. Given this observation, the nature of the mechanisms responsible for gene activation becomes a key question; the complexity of the problem is well presented by Kelso and Gough and should be viewed in tandem with the chapters by Kaempfer *et al.* and Paetkau *et al.* Campbell *et al.* continue the theme, presenting their studies on the cloning and analysis of IL-3 (Multi-CSF). Of particular interest are the retrovirus expression studies designed to test whether in some cases (e.g., WEHI-3) constitutive production of a growth factor by cells possessing the receptor for that growth factor may be associated with the development of a tumorigenic state.

Related to this are their studies on the IL-3 gene in WEHI-3B cells that contain an intracisternal A particle, IAP (head-to-head orientation); transfection studies clearly suggest that the IAP contributes to the constitutive production of IL-3 by these cells. Otsuka *et al.* and Culpepper and Lee present a detailed molecular map of the IL-3 and GM–CSF genes and indicate how glucocorticoids may play a role in regulating lymphokine production, particularly IL-3/Multi-CSF and GM–CSF.

Last, Bleackley and colleagues (Lobe *et al.*) present a look at where we may be headed in the future by using differential screening of cDNA libraries to probe the distinct gene set active in one subclass of cells, cytolytic T cells. Their successful recovery of at least one gene responsible for defining the cytolytic capacity of these cells points to the power of the methodology for attacking problems that heretofore have largely been the province of cellular immunology.

As everyone is aware, the pace of work in this area continues to increase. Notably absent from this volume at the time of its inception were chapters covering B cell growth factors and suppressor factors. Recent journal publications as well as past experience clearly suggest that another volume on the cloning of lymphokines dealing exclusively with those not covered here will be possible in a very short time. The editors wish to thank all of the authors for a job well done, and we particularly acknowledge the support and encouragement provided by Drs. E. Pick and M. Landy in bringing this volume to fruition.

DAVID R. WEBB
DAVID V. GOEDDEL

Strategies for Cloning Mouse and Human Lymphokine Genes Using a Mammalian cDNA Expression Vector

TAKASHI YOKOTA,[1] FRANK LEE,[1] NAOKO ARAI,[1] DONNA RENNICK,[2] ALBERT ZLOTNIK,[2] TIM MOSMANN,[2] ATSUSHI MIYAJIMA,[1] YUTAKA TAKEBE,[1] ROBERT KASTELEIN,[1] GERARD ZURAWSKI,[1] AND KEN-ICHI ARAI[1]

[1]Department of Molecular Biology and [2]Department of Immunology, DNAX Research Institute of Molecular and Cellular Biology, Palo Alto, California 94304

I. Molecular Biology of T Cell-Derived Lymphokines

T lymphocytes regulate the growth and differentiation of certain lymphopoietic and hematopoietic cells through the action of secreted protein factors known as lymphokines. Helper or inducer T cells produce these factors upon activation by either antigen or lectin, such as concanavalin A (Con A). Activation of helper T cells may involve two different stages. The first is recognition of antigen by a T cell receptor which generates intracellular signals for inducing a variety of lymphokines. The second is a T cell-effector function mediated by lymphokines that regulates the growth and differentiation of target cells. Lymphokines produced by helper T cells may be classified into several types based on their targets of action (Fig. 1). IL-2 stimulates predominantly the proliferation of cells of the T cell lineage, while BCGF and BCDF stimulate proliferation and differentiation of B cells into antibody-secreting plasma cells. IL-3 and GM-CSF stimulate the proliferation and differentiation of various hematopoietic cells.

We have begun to resolve these multiple factors by cloning their respective mRNAs and expressing functional polypeptides. Our interests in T cell lymphokine systems involve (1) the organization of T cell lymphokine genes within the chromosome, (2) the regulation of expression of the lymphokine genes, (3) the biological activities of lymphokines, and (4) the interaction of lymphokines with their respective receptors and the mechanism of their action. The lymphokine–receptor interaction may produce certain intracellular signals which stimulate proliferation and/or differentiation of target cells. The elucidation of the signal transduction pathways mediated by lymphokines, along with studies of other growth factors, receptors, and *onco* genes, will provide basic knowledge on the control of growth and differentiation of mammalian cells.

1

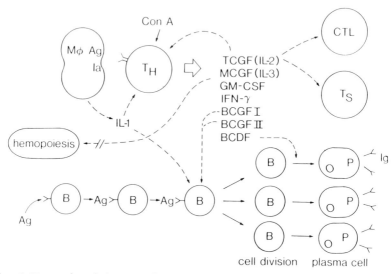

FIG. 1. Various lymphokines produced by activated helper T cells. T cell lymphokines are induced by helper T cells when antigens are presented by macrophage cells (Mϕ) in association with Ia molecules. Lectins such as concanavalin A (Con A) mimic antigen presentation by macrophage cells and induce T cells to produce various lymphokines. T$_H$, T helper cell; T$_S$, T suppressor cell; CTL, cytotoxic T lymphocyte.

II. Isolation of Lymphokine cDNA Clones Using pcD Mammalian Expression Vector

As a first step toward answering these questions, the molecular cloning of several lymphokines has been completed. There are several strategies which have been used for the isolation of cDNA clones. The first is the chemical approach which utilizes oligonucleotide probes based on protein sequence information. The second is an immunological approach using antibody probes to screen the bacterial lysates (Chang *et al.*, 1978; Villa-Komaroff *et al.*, 1978; Young and Davis, 1983). The third is a functional approach which relies on the availability of specific biological or enzymatic assays. The protein products, translated following hybrid selection of mRNA or expressed in cells by cDNA inserts, are assayed for biological activity.

Our strategy for isolating lymphokine cDNA clones mainly relies on the functional approach. Using a pcD cDNA library prepared with mRNA from Con A-activated mouse and human T cell lines, we have developed a screening procedure employing transfection of plasmid DNAs into mammalian cells followed by assaying the transfected cell supernatants for lymphokine activities of interest. Important aspects of

TABLE I

LYMPHOKINE ACTIVITIES IN MOUSE AND HUMAN T CELL SUPERNATANTS

	IL-3	GM-CSF	BCGF	IL-2	BCDF	IFN-γ
Mouse T cell lines						
D9	+	+	+	−	+	−
LB2-1	+	+	+	+	+	+
E1	+	+	ND^a	+	ND	+
C5	+	+	ND	+	ND	+
Human T cell lines						
T7		+	ND	+	ND	+
Clone 2		+	ND	+	ND	+
Clone 3		+	ND	ND	ND	±
5C10		+	+	+	+	+
2D8		+	+	+	+	+
2F1		+	+	+	+	+
Peripheral blood		+	ND	+	ND	+

^{a}ND, Not determined.

this cloning protocol include (1) the use of a reliable and sensitive bioassay for lymphokine activities, (2) the use of T cell lines as an enriched source of biologically active lymphokine mRNAs, and (3) the construction of a cDNA library in a pcD mammalian expression vector. Our results demonstrate that the identification of full-length cDNA clones for many lymphokines may be achieved entirely on the basis of detection of the functional polypeptides produced by transfected mammalian cells.

The pcD mammalian expression vector developed by Okayama and Berg (1983) is composed of pcDV1 primer and pL1 linker plasmids. This vector contains the SV40 early region promoter, the late splicing junction, and replication origin, and permits the expression of cDNA inserts in COS-7 monkey kidney cells which provide T antigen for amplification of the plasmid copy number. Table I summarizes the lymphokine activities we have detected so far in the supernatants of mouse and human T cell clones used for molecular cloning. We have constructed cDNA libraries using mRNA from antigen-specific as well as non-antigen-specific T cell clones.

Figure 2 shows an outline of our cDNA screening protocol. About 10,000 clones are picked into microtiter plates and divided into pools of plasmid DNA, each containing 48 cDNA clones. Plasmid DNA from each pool is transfected into COS-7 monkey cells using DEAE-dextran. Since lymphokines may be secreted in mammalian cells, the supernatants from the transfected cells are assayed for biological activity after a

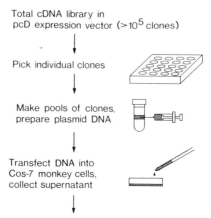

Total cDNA library in
pcD expression vector ($>10^5$ clones)

↓

Pick individual clones

↓

Make pools of clones,
prepare plasmid DNA

↓

Transfect DNA into
Cos-7 monkey cells,
collect supernatant

↓

Test supernatant for biological activity

FIG. 2. Screening of cDNA library by direct expression in mammalian cells.

3-day incubation. Positive pools are further subdivided to identify single cDNA clones which give biological activity after transfection.

In the course of screening for the IL-3 cDNA clone, an IL-3-dependent mast cell clone (MC/9) (Nabel *et al.*, 1981), was used for the proliferation assay. Mouse IL-2 was measured by a proliferation assay using the HT2 T cell line (Watson, 1979). To assay for mouse GM-CSF, either a proliferation assay using a GM-CSF-dependent myeloid leukemia cell line, NFS60, or a colony-formation assay with mouse bone marrow cells (Metcalf *et al.*, 1979) was used. For human GM-CSF, we relied on a similar colony-formation assay using either human bone marrow or cord blood cells.

A. MOUSE IL-3

An IL-3 cDNA clone (Yokota *et al.*, 1984; Fung *et al.*, 1984) was isolated from a mouse T cell cDNA library on the basis of its ability to direct the synthesis of MCGF activity, although mRNA hybrid selection followed by oocyte translation was used for initial screening. The IL-3 cDNA, selected this way, produced high levels of MCGF activity in the COS-7 cells, almost all of which was secreted into the cell's supernatant.

The cDNA insert of pcD IL-3 plasmid (Fig. 3) is about 1 kb and contains a single open-reading frame (Fig. 4). The first ATG codon is found 28 nucleotides downstream of the 5′ end and is followed by 166 codons before the termination codon TAA. The NH_2-terminal segment of the predicted IL-3 protein sequence is a hydrophobic signal peptide. The 5′ end of the shorter cDNA insert of clone B4 is at nucleotide

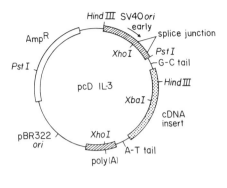

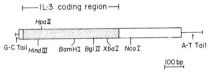

Fig. 3. (Top) Diagram of pcD IL-3, a plasmid carrying the functional mouse IL-3 cDNA insert (Yokota *et al.*, 1984). (Bottom) Restriction endonuclease cleavage map of cDNA insert. The IL-3 coding region is shaded by dots and the noncoding regions are lightly shaded.

position 41. This shorter cDNA clone B4 lacks the first methionine codon but still produces active MCGF upon introduction into COS-7 cells. The much shorter cDNA clone, B20, starts at nucleotide position 83, lacks the first and second methionine codons, and did not produce MCGF activity. These results suggest that the second methionine codon may be the translation initiation site. Initial studies suggested that the NH_2-terminal amino acid residue for IL-3 isolated from WEHI-3 cells is aspartic acid, 20 amino acids downstream of the second ATG codon (Ihle *et al.*, 1983). Recently, others have shown that the NH_2-terminus of IL-3 starts at alanine, 6 amino acids upstream of the aspartic acid (Clark-Lewis *et al.*, 1984; J. Watson, personal communication).

Mature IL-3 would consist of 134 or 140 amino acid residues with a calculated molecular weight of about 15,000. Ihle *et al.* (1982) have shown that mouse IL-3 is glycosylated and has an apparent molecular weight of 28,000. Judging from the deduced amino acid sequence of the mouse IL-3 clones, there are four potential N-glycosylation sites (Asn-X-Ser at positions 42–44, 70–72, 77–79, and 112–114). The discrepancy between the reported size of IL-3 and the calculated molecular weight of IL-3 deduced from our clones may be partly due to the glycosylation of the molecule.

```
B6
 1                                                                              B20
                     20                    B4                    60             80↓
                                           40↓                                  ↓
GGGGGGGGGG GGGAACCCCT TGGAGGACCA GAACGAGACA ATG GTT CTT GCC TCT ACC AGC ATC AGC ACC ATG CTC CTG CTG CTC TTC CAC CTG GGA
                                            MET Val Leu Ala Ser Thr Ser Thr Ile His Thr MET Leu Leu Leu Leu MET Phe His Leu Gly
                                             1                  10                      20

100            IL-3                  140             160             180           5G      200
                ↓120                                                               ↓
CTC CAA GCT TCA ATC AGT GGC CGG GAT ACC CGT TTA ACC AGA ACG TTG AAT TGC AGC TCT ATT GTC AAG GAG ATT ATA GGG AAG GTG CCA GAA CTC AAA
Leu Gln Ala Ser Ile Ser Gly Arg Asp Thr Arg Leu Thr Arg Thr Leu Asn Cys Ser Ser Ile Val Lys Glu Ile Ile Gly Lys Val Pro Glu Leu Lys
                         30                      40                      50                      60

                  220             240             260             280             300
ACT GAT GAT GAA CCC TCT CTG AGG AAT AAG AGC TTT CGG AGA GTA AAC CTG TCC AAA TTC GTG GAA GTG GAT GAA GGA GAT CCT GAG GAC AGA TAC GTT ATC
Thr Asp Asp Glu Pro Ser Leu Arg Asn Lys Ser Phe Arg Arg Val Asn Leu Ser Lys Phe Val Glu Val Asp Glu Gly Asp Pro Glu Asp Arg Tyr Val Ile
               70                      80                              90

320             340             360             380             400             420
AAG TCC AAT CTT CAG AAA CTT AAC TGC TGC CTG CCT ACA TCT GCG AAT GAC TCT GCG CTG CCA GGG GTC TTC ATT CGA GAT CTG GAT GAC TTT CGG AAG AAA CTG AGA
Lys Ser Asn Leu Gln Lys Leu Asn Cys Cys Leu Pro Thr Ser Ala Asn Asp Ser Ala Leu Pro Gly Val Phe Ile Arg Asp Leu Asp Asp Phe Arg Lys Lys Leu Arg
       100                     110                     120                     130

440             460             480             500             520
TTC TAC ATG GTC CAC CTT AAC GAT CTG GAG ACA GTG CTA GCC TCT AGA CCA CCT CAG CCC GCA TCT GGC TCC GTC CCT CCT AAC CGT GGA ACC GTG GAA TGT TAA .
Phe Tyr Met Val His Leu Asn Asp Leu Glu Thr Val Leu Ala Ser Arg Pro Pro Gln Pro Ala Ser Gly Ser Val Pro Pro Asn Arg Gly Thr Val Glu Cys
       140                     150                     160
```

Fig. 4. Nucleotide sequence and predicted amino acid sequence of the IL-3 coding region. The nucleotide sequence of clone B9 begins with position 1 at the first nucleotide following the oligo(dG) segment. The amino acid sequence begins with the first in-phase ATG codon for the single long open-reading frame. The underlined amino acids from 33–41 are those that are identical to the partial sequence reported by Ihle *et al.* (1983) for IL-3. The nucleotide sequences of incomplete clones (B4, B20, and 5G) begin with position 41, 84, and 191, respectively, at the first nucleotides following the oligo(dG) segment.

B. Mouse IL-2

Mouse IL-2 cDNA-clone identification (Yokota *et al.*, 1985; Kashima *et al.*, 1985) was based entirely on the synthesis of a functional product in mammalian cells. A sublibrary enriched for cDNA inserts 1–2 kb long from the LB2-1 library was screened for TCGF activity (Table II). Bacterial clones were pooled into groups of 48 clones, and plasmid DNA was isolated from 58 such pools as described above. Supernatants from transfected cells were assayed for TCGF activity, and positive pools were subdivided. We have identified four functionally active mouse IL-2 cDNA clones (MT-1, MT-18, MT-20, and MT-28) using this procedure.

The mouse IL-2 cDNA contains a single open-reading frame consisting of 169 codons corresponding to a protein with a calculated molecular weight of 19,000, whereas the human IL-2 cDNA contains 153 codons (Taniguchi *et al.*, 1983). Overall, there is about 70% homology between the mouse IL-2 cDNA and the human IL-2 cDNA sequence. Of the predicted 169 amino acid residues of mouse IL-2, 94 are conserved in human IL-2 (Fig. 5). However, the trinucleotide sequence CAG, which is repeated 12 times within the mouse IL-2 cDNA coding region, is not present in the human IL-2 cDNA. Downstream of the putative initiation codon in both is a region rich in hydrophobic amino acids. The mature form of the secreted mouse IL-2 begins with an alanine residue and the preceding 20 amino acids constitute the putative leader sequence that is removed by proteolytic processing.

C. Human GM-CSF

Isolation of human GM-CSF cDNA clone (Lee *et al.*, 1985; Wong *et al.*, 1985) was carried out by the procedures described above using an *in vitro* semisolid agar-colony-formation assay with human bone marrow cells. For the first screening of the human T7 library, plasmid DNAs from 40 pools of 48 clones were transfected into COS-7 cells. Four positive pools were identified. Further subdivision of active pools resulted in the isolation of four individual active clones.

The human GM-CSF cDNA insert contains a single open-reading frame with 144 codons. The amino acid sequences of human and mouse GM-CSF (Gough *et al.*, 1984; Miyatake *et al.*, 1985a) deduced from nucleotide sequences are compared in Fig. 6. Human and mouse amino acid sequences are approximately 50% homologous while nucleotide sequences are approximately 70% homologous. The NH_2-terminal segment of the predicted GM-CSF amino acid sequence is hydrophobic as would be expected for a signal peptide. Cleavage of the precursor polypeptide occurs after the Ser residue at position 17 (Gasson *et al.*, 1984; Wong *et al.*, 1985).

TABLE II

DNA Transfection Assay for TCGF Activity from Pools
of Plasmid DNA

	DNA	Units (ml)
First screening[a,b]	1–5	Each <10
	6	144
	7–32	Each <10
	33	128
	34–39	Each <10
	40	128
	41–55	Each <10
	56	140
Second screening[a]	a and b	Each <10
(group 33)	c	1669
	d–h	Each <10
Third screening[a]	1 and 2	Each <10
(group C)	3 (MT-18)	9020
	4–6	Each <10
Fourth screening[c]	MT-1	5851
(hybridization with MT-18	MT-2 –MT-5	Each <10
cDNA)	MT-7	<10
	MT-17	<10
	MT-19	<10
	MT-20	6800
	MT-21–MT-23	Each <10
	MT-26	<10
	MT-28	8200
	MT-29	<10
Mock transfected EL-4 COS-7[d]		<10
PMA-stimulated EL-4		107,126
Supernatant human COS IL-2		51,100

[a]The first, second, and third screenings were performed with pools of 48 and 6 cDNA clones and a single cDNA clone, respectively.

[b]Positive clones MT-1, MT-20, and MT-28 that express TCGF activity were isolated from groups 6, 10, and 56, respectively, in the first screening.

[c]For the fourth screening, the same 58 pools of the sublibrary were screened by colony hybridization using MT-18 cDNA probe.

[d]Mock-transfected COS-7 cells were treated identically but DNA was omitted.

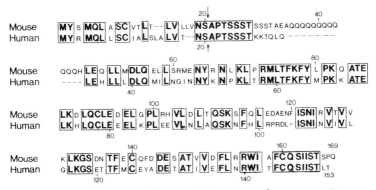

FIG. 5. Comparison of mouse and human IL-2 amino acid sequences. Two sequences deduced from nucleotide sequences of their cDNA clones were aligned to maximize the homology between the two IL-2 peptides. Identical residues are shown with boxes. The possible processing site is indicated by the arrows.

D. MOUSE AND HUMAN BSF-1 (IL-4)

A novel mouse interleukin cDNA (Lee *et al.*, 1986; Noma *et al.*, 1986) that expresses the activity to stimulate B cells, T cells, and mast cells was identified. This factor not only stimulates the proliferation of T cell and mast cell lines (Smith and Rennick, 1986) but also induces Ia expression on resting B cells and enhances IgG_1 and IgE production by B cells, two properties of BSF-1 (Roehm *et al.*, 1984; Coffman and Carty, 1986; Vitetta *et al.*, 1985). On the basis of these multiple biological activities, it has been proposed that this lymphokine be called IL-4 rather than BSF-1 (Lee *et al.*, 1986; Noma *et al.*, 1986). The single open-reading frame in the mouse IL-4 cDNA clone consists of 140 amino acid residues (Fig. 7). The mature polypeptide would be 120 amino acid residues long and begin with a histidine residue. There are three potential N-glycosylation sequences (Asn-X-Thr or Asn-X-Ser at positions 61–63, 91–93, and 117–119). Despite the biological activities of IL-4 that are similar to the activities of IL-2 and IL-3, there is no significant sequence homology between IL-4 and either IL-2 or IL-3.

A human cDNA clone which is homologous to the mouse IL-4 cDNA and expresses B cell and T cell stimulating activities was isolated. This cDNA clone encodes a protein of 153 amino acid residues (Yokota *et al.*, 1986) containing two potential N-glycosylation sequences (Asn-X-Thr or Asn-X-Ser at positions 62–64 and 129–131, respectively). Amino acid sequences of the mouse and human polypeptides share extensive homology with the exception of about 40 amino acids near the middle portion (Fig. 7). Supernatants of COS-7 monkey cells transfected with the

```
                                        10
MET Trp Leu Gln Ser Leu Leu Leu Leu Gly Thr Val Ala Cys Ser Ile Ser Ala
            Asn             Phe     Ile     Val Tyr     Leu

 20
Pro Ala Arg Ser Pro Ser Pro Ser Thr Gln Pro Trp Glu His Val Asn Ala Ile
Thr         Ile Thr Val     Arg         Lys     Glu

             40                                  50
Gln Glu Ala Arg Arg Leu Leu Asn Leu Ser Arg Asp Thr Ala Ala Glu Met Asn
Lys         Leu Asn         Asp Asp Met Pro Val     Leu Asn

            *   60     *   *           *       *   *   * 70
Glu Thr Val Glu Val Ile Ser Glu Met Phe Asp Leu Gln Glu Pro Thr Cys Leu
    Val         Phe                 Lys|Lys                           Val
        Ser|Asn

                        80
Gln Thr Arg Leu Glu Leu Try Lys Gln Gly Leu Arg Gly Ser Leu Thr Lys Leu 90
            Lys Ile Phe Glu                 Asn Phe

Lys Gly Pro Leu Thr Met Met Ala Ser His Thr Lys Gln His Cys Pro Pro Thr
        Ala     Asn     Thr     Thr     Gln Thr Tyr     100

110
Pro Glu Thr Ser Cys Ala Thr Gln Ile Ile Thr Phe Glu Ser Phe Lys Glu Asn
        Asp     Glu         Val Thr     Tyr Ala Asp     Ile Asp Ser
                                        120

        130
Leu Lys Asp Phe Leu Leu Val Ile Pro Phe Asp Cys Trp Glu Pro Val Gln Glu
        Thr     Thr Asp             Glu         Lys Lys     Ser     Lys
                                                        140
```

FIG. 6. Comparison of the deduced amino acid sequence for human GM-CSF. Upper line is the complete human sequence. The underlined amino acid residues are identical between mouse and human GM-CSF, while the residues in the mouse sequence that are different are shown below the human sequence. Adjustments were made to maximize the homology between the two sequences; there are two positions (57–58 and 65) of the human sequence that have no amino acids corresponding to those present in mouse GM-CSF, shown below, and indicated with a vertical line. There are also several amino acids(*) present only in the human sequence.

human cDNA clone stimulated proliferation of human helper T cell clones and anti-IgM-activated human B cells, two of the properties of BSF-1 in the mouse assay system. These results indicate that this human cDNA clone encodes a protein structurally and functionally homologous to mouse BSF-1.

E. OTHER LYMPHOKINE AND RECEPTOR cDNA CLONES ISOLATED FROM T CELL pcD LIBRARIES

Using a similar procedure, we have isolated various lymphokine cDNA clones from both mouse and human T cell pcD libraries (Table III). These lymphokine cDNA clones generally represent about 0.05–1% of total Con A activated T cell libraries. For example, mouse and human IFN-γ (Gray et al., 1982; Gray and Goeddel, 1983), mouse GM-CSF

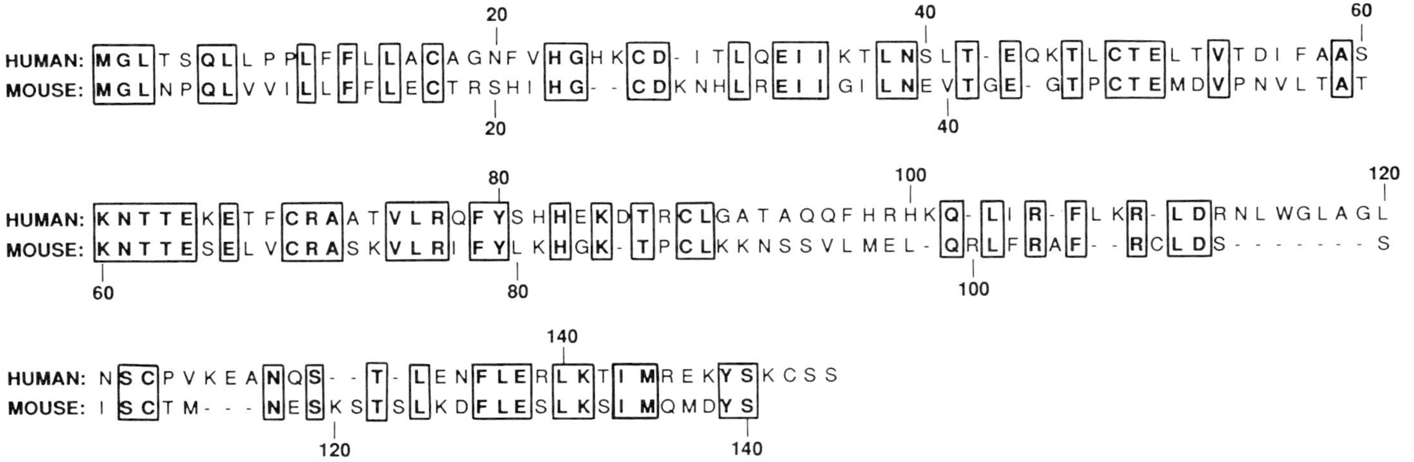

FIG. 7. Comparison of human and mouse IL-4 amino acid sequences. Two sequences deduced from the nucleotide sequences of the cDNA clones were aligned to maximize homology between the two IL-4 peptides. Identical residues are shown with boxes.

TABLE III
EXPRESSIBLE LYMPHOKINE cDNA
CLONES ISOLATED FROM HELPER
T CELL LIBRARIES

	Mouse	Human
IL-3	Yes	
GM-CSF	Yes	Yes
IL-2	Yes	Yes
BSF-1 (IL-4)	Yes	Yes
IFN-γ	Yes	Yes
IL-2 receptor	Yes	Yes
T cell receptor	Yes	

(Gough *et al.*, 1984; Miyatake *et al.*, 1985a), human IL-2, and mouse and human IL-2 receptors (Leonard *et al.*, 1984; Nikaido *et al.*, 1984; Shimizu *et al.*, 1985) isolated from several pcD libraries could transiently express active products in COS-7 cells. A set of cDNA clones encoding either the α or β chain of the antigen-specific T cell receptor (Patten *et al.*, 1984; Becker *et al.*, 1985), Thy 1 (Hiraki *et al.*, 1986), and P53 (N. Arai *et al.*, unpublished) was also isolated from antigen-specific mouse T cell pcD libraries. These results also suggest that cDNA clones encoding some cell surface receptors may be identified by detection of the polypeptide on mammalian cells. Availability of these T cell-derived lymphokine and receptor cDNA clones expressible in mammalian cells should aid molecular studies of T cell activation and lymphokine action.

III. Expression of Lymphokine cDNA Clones in Various Host–Vector Systems

Recombinant lymphokines expressed in COS-7 cells provide convenient sources for evaluating their biological activities in the absence of other T cell-specific products. However, COS-7 cells allow replication of the pcD plasmid only transiently, so this system is not as useful as stable mammalian cell lines which produce lymphokines continuously, or *Escherichia coli* or yeast expression systems. To obtain larger amounts of lymphokines for biochemical and biological characterization. we have therefore transferred lymphokine cDNA inserts into other appropriate expression vector systems.

A. EXPRESSION IN MAMMALIAN CELLS

Expression in mammalian cells has distinct advantages in producing the native forms of lymphokine polypeptides. Unlike expression in *E.*

coli or yeast, cloned lymphokine cDNA can be expressed and secreted in mammalian cells without specific modifications such as the removal of signal sequences. Mouse L cells cotransfected with pcD IL-3 and pSV2neo plasmids yielded cell lines carrying multiple copies of IL-3 cDNA integrated into the chromosome. These cell lines produce and secrete IL-3 constitutively with the expression level being 10–400% of transfected COS-7 cells (Miyatake *et al.*, 1985b). Mouse IL-3 genomic DNA or cDNA placed downstream of the SV40 early region promoter has been cloned into a bovine papilloma virus (BPV) vector, pdBPV-MMTneo (342-12) (Law *et al.*, 1983) (Fig. 8). Transfected mouse fibroblast cells secreted high levels of IL-3 into the medium. In Fig. 7, mouse

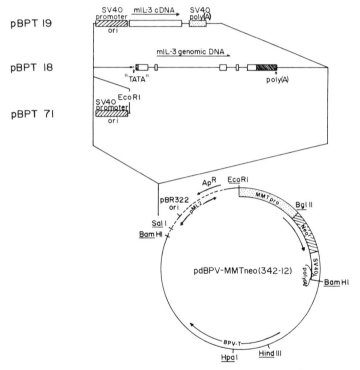

FIG. 8. BPV-mouse IL-3 recombinant plasmids and the activities of mouse IL-3 in the supernatant of the transfected mouse fibroblast C127 cells. The orientation of the mouse IL-3 transcription unit in each plasmid is the same as that of the β-lactamase gene (Ap^R). Mouse C127 cells were transfected with the recombinant plasmid and stable transformants were isolated. Mouse IL-3 activity in the supernatant of each stable transformant was measured by the proliferation of MC/9 mast cells and is expressed as a relative value compared to the supernatant activity in B9/COS-7 cells acutely transfected with the pcD mIL-3 plasmid: pBPT 19, $\frac{1}{8} \sim \frac{1}{2}$; pBPT 18, $\frac{1}{16} \sim \frac{1}{8}$; pBPT 71, $\frac{1}{2} \sim 1$.

IL-3 activities are expressed as relative values compared to COS-7 cells transfected transiently with the original pcD IL-3 plasmid. Retrovirus- or Epstein–Barr virus (EBV)-based vectors may have advantages for the introduction and expression of lymphokine genes in lymphocytes.

B. Expression in Saccharomyces cerevisiae

The yeast mating pheromone α-factor is initially synthesized as a pre- pro α-factor carrying signal and leader sequence. This precursor is cleav- ed at several specific sites. By using the first processing site in the leader, we have constructed a general expression vector, pMFα8, which con- tains the promoter of the mating pheromone (α-factor), its downstream leader sequence, and the TRP5 terminator (Miyajima et al., 1985). This vector allows the synthesis and secretion of processed gene products in S. cerevisiae. The cDNA segments encoding mature mouse IL-2 and IL-3, and mouse and human GM-CSFs were fused immediately down- stream of the α-factor leader sequence. The resulting recombinant plas- mids directed the synthesis of lymphokines in S. cerevisiae, with most of the activity secreted into the culture fluid and extracellular space. Figure 9 shows the fusion of the α-factor leader with mature mouse and human

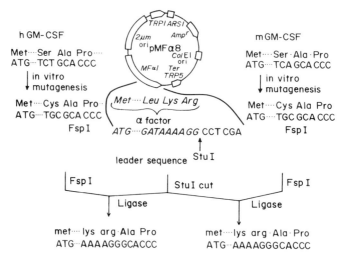

Fig. 9. Construction of α-factor–GM-CSF fusion genes. Both human and mouse GM- CSF cDNA were mutagenized in vitro by using oligonucleotides to create a unique FspI restriction site at the junction between the putative signal sequence and the mature protein. The DNA fragment coding for the mature protein was inserted at the StuI site of the secretion vector pMFα8 which is located right after the first processing point of the prepro-α-factor. Since pMFα8 contains all the necessary elements for plasmid mainte- nance in yeast, the recombinant plasmids were directly introduced into S. cerevisiae.

GM-CSF coding sequences. Yeast cells carrying the fusion plasmid secrete biologically active GM-CSF into the medium with much higher activity than COS-7 supernatants.

C. EXPRESSION IN *Escherichia coli*

Various vector systems have been used to direct the expression of mouse and human lymphokines either in the cytoplasm or in the periplasm of *E. coli*. The latter approach seems feasible since all lymphokines are naturally secreted proteins in mammalian cells. Expression of a lymphokine in the *E. coli* periplasmic space has the advantage of easy recovery (via osmotic shock) of the product in a soluble form while synthesis in the cytoplasm may result in insoluble protein forms. Fortunately, lymphokines are relatively stable proteins, so both approaches have proven useful. Besides the appropriate transcriptional and translational elements, a bacterial signal sequence preceeding the mature lymphokine is necessary to express and direct the product to the periplasmic space. For this purpose the signal sequence of the outer membrane protein (*OmpA*) is used. After tailoring the lymphokine cDNA to an appropriate size, it is fused to the *OmpA* signal sequence in such a way that correct processing would result in secretion of the exact mature lymphokine. This approach has been successful for the expression and secretion of lymphokines including both mouse and human IL-2 and mouse GM-CSF. Interestingly, the percentage of product that is correctly processed and secreted varies even for homologous lymphokines such as mouse and human IL-2. In both cases expression is high, but while mouse IL-2 is almost entirely secreted, human IL-2 is found mainly as a precursor in the cytoplasm (Kastelein *et al.*, unpublished). This latter result shows that sequences within the protein to be expressed are critical in determining the extent of processing and secretion through the *E. coli* membrane.

IV. Biological Characterization of Recombinant Lymphokines

In vivo, antigen-stimulated helper T cells may affect hematopoiesis by producing GM-CSF and IL-3. The term IL-3 was introduced to describe a factor responsible for the expression of 20α-steroid dehydrogenase (20α-SDH) in splenic lymphocytes (Ihle *et al.*, 1981). Recent studies suggest that more than 10 additional biological activities are associated with IL-3, which had been called different names by different investigators. By using IL-3 expressed in COS-7 cells and yeast, we have confirmed that recombinant IL-3 induces both 20α-SDH and Thy 1 expression and supports the growth of IL-3-dependent cell lines. Fur-

TABLE IV
SUMMARY OF BIOLOGICAL ACTIVITIES OF IL-3 (MCGF)

Activity/factor	Purified IL-3	COS IL-3	Yeast IL-3
Induction of 20α-SDH	Yes	Yes	Not done
Thy 1-inducing activity (TIF)	Yes	Yes	Not done
P cell stimulating factor, mast cell growth factor (MCGF)	Yes	Yes	Yes
Growth factor of hematopoietic cell lines	Yes	Yes	Yes
Burst-promoting activity (BPA)	Yes	Yes	Yes
Maintains CFU-S in culture	Yes	Yes	Not done
Multilineage CSF	Yes	Yes	Yes

thermore, it has burst-promoting activity and maintains CFU-S in culture. We have also confirmed that recombinant IL-3 is in fact a multi-CSF (Table IV; Rennick et al., 1985). Table V shows the cellular composition of colonies stimulated by yeast IL-3 and COS IL-3. Most of the colonies were composed of granulocytes, macrophages, or granulocyte/macrophage mixtures, while a few were mixed colonies including erythrocytes. COS IL-3 and yeast IL-3 stimulate the growth and differentiation of committed progenitor cells of all lineages. These results suggest that recombinant IL-3 also stimulates multipotential progenitor cells.

By contrast, COS GM-CSF or yeast GM-CSF stimulates primarily the formation of granulocyte and macrophage colonies (Lee et al., 1985). Both human and mouse recombinant GM-CSFs produced by COS-7 cells are species-specific (Table VI). Mouse GM-CSF does not stimulate colony formation using human cord blood cells. Human GM-CSF does

TABLE V
CELLULAR COMPOSITION OF COLONIES STIMULATED BY YEAST
MCGF AND COS MCGF

Colony	COS MCGF (%)	Yeast MCGF (%)
Macrophage	29	28
Granulocyte	14	20
Macrophage/granulocyte	46	39
Mast cells	2	1
Erythrocytes	1	2
Mixed composition	8	10

TABLE VI

SPECIES SPECIFICITY OF MOUSE AND HUMAN GM-CSF CLONES

cDNA clone transfected	Human		Mouse
	Bone marrow	Cord blood	Bone marrow
	Colonies Per 10^5 Cells		
Mock transfection	<5	<5	<5
Mouse GM-CSF clone			
E1-11	ND	0	230
Human GM-CSF clone			
7-1a	56	186	0
14-1e	65	85	0
204	41	120	0

[a]ND, Not determined.

not stimulate in the mouse system, although it induces colony formation of granulocytes, macrophages, and eosinophils in semisolid human bone marrow cultures. These features suggest that our human GM-CSF clone is similar to what has been described for CSF-α previously (Nicola *et al.*, 1979; Das *et al.*, 1981; Lusis *et al.*, 1981). From these results we conclude that in both mouse and human there is only one class of GM-CSF, and our human GM-CSF is a homologue of mouse GM-CSF. Human CSF-β, which is active in the mouse system, may be encoded by a human gene other than GM-CSF.

REFERENCES

Becker, D. M., Patten, P., Chien, Y., Yokota, T., Eshhar, Z., Giedlin, M., Gasgoigne, N. R. J., Goodnow, C., Wolf, R., Arai, K., and Davis, M. M. (1985). *Nature (London)* **317**, 430–434.

Chang, A. C. Y., Nunberg, J. H., Kaufman, R. J., Erlich, H. A., Schimke, R. T., and Cohen, S. N. (1978). *Nature (London)* **275**, 617–624.

Clark-Lewis, I., Kent, S. B. H., and Schrader, J. W. (1984). *J. Biol. Chem.* **259**, 7488–7494.

Coffman, R. L., and Carty, J. (1986). *J. Immunol.* **136**, 949–954.

Das, S. K., Stanley, E. R., Guilbert, L. J., and Forman, L. W. (1981). *Blood* **58**, 630–641.

Fung, M. C., Hapel, A. J., Ymer, S., Cohen, D. R., Johnson, R. A., Campbell, H. D., and Young, I. G. (1984). *Nature (London)* **307**, 233–237.

Gasson, J. C., Weisbert, R. H., Kaufman, S. E., Clark, S. C., Hewick, R. M., Wong, G. G., and Golde, D. W. (1984). *Science* **226**, 1339–1342.

Gough, N. M., Gough, J., Metcalf, D., Kelso, A., Grail, D., Nicola, N. A., Burgess, A. W., and Dunn, A. R. (1984). *Nature (London)* **309**, 763–767.

Gough, N. M., Metcalf, D., Gough, J., Grail, D., and Dunn, A. R. (1985). *EMBO J.* **4**, 645–653.

Gray, P. W., and Goeddel, D. V. (1983). *Proc. Natl. Acad. Sci. U.S.A.* **80**, 5842–5846.

Gray, P. W., Leung, D. W., Pennica, D., Yelverton, E., Najarian, R., Simonsen, C. D.,

Derynck, R., Sherwood, P. J., Wallace, D. M., Berger, S. L., Levinson, A. D., and Goeddel, D. V. (1982). *Nature (London)* **295**, 503–508.

Hiraki, D. D., Nomura, D., Yokota, T., Arai, K., and Coffman, R. L. (1985). *J. Immunol.* **136**, 4291–4926.

Ihle, J. N., Pepersack, L., and Rebar, L. (1981). *J. Immunol.* **126**, 2184–2189.

Ihle, J. N., Keller, J., Henderson, L., Frederick, K., and Palaszynski, E. (1982). *J. Immunol.* **129**, 2431–2436.

Ihle, J. N., Keller, J., Oroszlan, S., Henderson, L. E., Copeland, T. D., Fitch, F., Prystowsky, M. D., Goldwasser, E., Schrader, J. W., Palaszynski, E., Dy, M., and Lebel, B. (1983). *J. Immunol.* **131**, 282–287.

Kashima, N., Nishi-Takaoka, C., Fujita, T., Taki, S., Yamada, G., Hamuro, J., and Taniguchi, T. (1985). *Nature (London)* **313**, 402–404.

Kasteline, R. (1985). In preparation.

Law, M., Byrne, J. C., and Howley, P. M. (1983). *Mol. Cell. Biol.* **3**, 2110–2115.

Lee, F., Yokota, T., Otsuka, T., Gemmell, L., Larson, N., Luh, J., Arai, K., and Rennick, D. (1985). *Proc. Natl. Acad. Sci. U.S.A.* **82**, 4360–4364.

Lee, F., Yokota, T., Otsuka, T., Meyerson, P., Villaret, D., Coffman, R., Mosmann, T., Rennick, D., Roehm, N., Smith, C., Zlotnik, A., and Arai, K. (1986). *Proc. Natl. Acad. Sci. U.S.A.* **83**, 2061–2065.

Leonard, W. J., Depper, J. M., Crabtree, G. R., Rudikoff, S., Pumphrey, J., Robb, R. J., Kronke, M., Svetlik, P. B., Peffer, N. J., Waldmann, T. A., and Greene, W. C. (1984). *Nature (London)* **311**, 626–631.

Lusis, A. J., Quan, D. H., and Golde, D. W. (1981). *Blood* **57**, 13–21.

Metcalf, D., Johnson, G. R., and Mandel, T. E. (1979). *J. Cell. Physiol.* **98**, 401–420.

Miyajima, A., Bond, M. W., Otsu, K., Arai, K., and Arai, N. (1985). *Gene* **37**, 155–161.

Miyatake, S., Otsuka, T., Yokota, T., Lee, F., and Arai, K. (1985a). *EMBO J.* **4**, 2561–2568.

Miyatake, S., Yokota, T., Lee, F., and Arai, K. (1985b). *Proc. Natl. Acad. Sci. U.S.A.* **82**, 316–320.

Nabel, G., Galli, S. J., Dvorak, A. M., Dvorak, H. F., and Cantor, H. (1981). *Nature (London)* **291**, 332–334.

Nicola, N. A., Metcalf, D., Johnson, G. R., and Burgess, A. W. (1979). *Blood* **54**, 614–627.

Nikaido, T., Shimizu, A., Ishida, N., Sabe, H., Teshigawara, K., Maeda, M., Uchiyama, T., Yodoi, J., and Honjo, T. (1984). *Nature (London)* **311**, 631–635.

Noma, Y., Sideras, P., Naito, T., Bergstedt-Lindquist, S., Azuma, C., Severinson, E., Tanabe, T., Kinashi, T., Matsuda, F., Yaoita, Y., and Honjo, T. (1986). *Nature (London)* **319**, 640–646.

Okayama, H., and Berg, P. (1983). *Mol. Cell. Biol.* **3**, 280–289.

Patten, P., Yokota, T., Rothbard, J., Chien, Y., Arai, K., and Davis, M. M. (1984). *Nature (London)* **312**, 40–46.

Rennick, R. M., Lee, F. D., Yokota, T., Arai, K., Cantor, H., and Nabel, G. J. (1985). *J. Immunol.* **134**, 910–914.

Roehm, N. W., Leibson, H. J., Zlotnik, A., Kappler, J. W., Marrack, P., and Cambier, J. C. (1984). *J. Exp. Med.* **160**, 679–694.

Shimizu, A., Kondo, S., Takeda, S., Yodoi, J., Ishida, N., Sabe, H., Osawa, H., Diamantstein, T., Nicaido, T., and Honjo, T. (1985). *Nucleic Acids Res.* **13**, 1505–1516.

Smith, C. A., and Rennick, D. M. (1986). *Proc. Natl. Acad. Sci. U.S.A.* **83**, 1857–1861.

Taniguchi, T., Matsui, H., Fujita, T., Takaoka, C., Kashima, N., Yoshimoto, R., and Hamuro, J. (1983). *Nature (London)* **302**, 305–310.

Villa-Komaroff, L., Efstratiadis, A., Broome, S., Lomedico, P., Tizard, R., Naber, S. P., Chich, W. L., and Gilbert, W. (1978). *Proc. Natl. Acad. Sci. U.S.A.* **75**, 3727–3731.
Vitetta, E. S., Ohara, J., Meyers, C., Layton, J., Krammer, P. H., and Paul, W. E. (1985). *J. Exp. Med.* **162**, 1726–1731.
Watson, J. (1979). *J. Exp. Med.* **150**, 1520–1519.
Wong, G. G., Witek, J. S., Temple, P. A., Wilkens, K. M., Leary, A. G., Luxenberg, D. P., Jones, S. S., Brown, E. L., Kay, R. M., Orr, E. C., Shoemaker, C., Golde, D. W., Kaufmann, R. J., Hewick, R. M., Wang, E. A., and Clark, S. C. (1985). *Science* **228**, 810–815.
Yokota, T., Lee, F., Rennick, D., Hall, C., Arai, N., Mosmann, T., Nabel, G., Cantor, H., and Arai, K. (1984). *Proc. Natl. Acad. Sci. U.S.A.* **81**, 1070–1074.
Yokota, T., Arai, N., Lee, F., Rennick, D., Mosmann, T., and Arai, K. (1985). *Proc. Natl. Acad. Sci. U.S.A.* **82**, 68–72.
Yokota, T., Otsuka, T., Mosmann, T., Banchereau, J., DeFrance, T., Blanchard, D., De Vries, J., Lee, F., and Arai, K. (1986). *Proc. Natl. Acad. Sci. U.S.A.* **83**, 5894–5898.
Young, R. A., and Davis, R. W. (1983). *Proc. Natl. Acad. Sci. U.S.A.* **80**, 1194–1198.

Identification and Expression of cDNA Plasmids Corresponding to Human Interferon-Gamma (IFN-γ) and Interleukin 2 (IL-2)

RENE DEVOS,* HILDE CHEROUTRE,†,1
GEERT PLAETINCK,†,2
AND WALTER FIERS†

*Biogent, 9000 Ghent, Belgium, and †Laboratory of Molecular Biology,
State University of Ghent, 9000 Ghent, Belgium

I. Introduction

Studies in cellular immunology have led to the insight that the immune system is regulated by products secreted by activated lymphoid cells. Beside small molecules such as prostaglandins and leukotrienes, many proteins have been identified which mediate various regulating functions such as growth, cytotoxicity, chemotaxis, differentiation, and other alterations of cell behavior. These lymphokines act at very low concentrations and could only be assayed and quantified by making use of their biological properties. Better insights into the existence of multiple-protein entities responsible for the various activities not only came from recent advances made in purification procedures but also from the application of recombinant DNA technology. In view of the interest to produce large amounts of pure, recombinant lymphokines, the cDNA corresponding to the mRNA coding for some of these proteins was isolated from appropriate libraries of colonies of recombinant *Escherichia coli* or plaques of recombinant phage λ. Once a library is constructed, the success of identifying a recombinant cDNA molecule is primarily dependent on the screening methodology used. From a partial amino acid sequence deduced from a purified protein, one can derive a chemically synthesized oligonucleotide to use as a probe to isolate an exon sequence from a genomic DNA library or to directly identify a cDNA plasmid. However, if the corresponding mRNA is relatively small and easily detectable by *in vitro* translation using a biological assay, a correct clone can be identified on the basis of specific hybridization.

Lymphokines such as IFN-γ and lL-2 can be assayed with very high sensitivity, and their corresponding mRNAs are easily detected by injec-

---

[1]Present address: Division of Biology, California Institute of Technology, Pasadena, California 91125.

[2]Present address: Isrec, Epalinges, 1066 Lausanne, Switzerland.

21

tion into *Xenopus laevis* oocytes and assaying the products secreted by these cells. We have used the latter screening methodology to successfully isolate human IFN-γ and human IL-2 cDNA plasmids from libraries derived from appropriately stimulated human spleen cells. While this work was in progress, Gray and associates (1982) and Taniguchi and associates (1983) published the structure of the human IFN-γ gene and the human IL-2 gene, respectively. None of their sequence information has been used in our laboratory to isolate the cDNA plasmids. In this article we summarize our work on the cloning and expression of both these human lymphokines (Devos *et al.*, 1982a, 1983) and some of the observed biological activities of the recombinant products.

II. Bioassay for Human IFN-γ and IL-2

Interferon-γ titers were determined by measuring the inhibition of the cytopathogenic effect of *Encephalomyocarditis* virus using human FS4 cells as described in Devos *et al.* (1982b). Originally, units were referred to the WHO First Int. Prep 69/19 IFN-α standard and the NIH IFN-α standard, while later the assay was calibrated against NIH IFN-γ reference standard Gg23-901-530. Interleukin 2 was assayed by measuring the short-term proliferation ([^{3}H]thymidine incorporation) of human peripheral blood-derived PHA blasts (cultured in IL-2-containing medium for 2 weeks and stored in liquid nitrogen) essentially as described by Gillis *et al.* (1978). Later on, stable, IL-2-dependent mouse T cell lines were used for routine testing.

III. Preparation of Human Spleen Cell Cultures and Induction of IFN-γ and IL-2

Since fresh human spleens were readily obtainable from Belgian hospitals (approximately 40 spleens were worked up per year), we chose to use these organs as a source of human lymphoid cells rather than peripheral blood or a long-term human leukemic T cell line for the production of IFN-γ and IL-2. Splenocytes were isolated as described in Devos *et al.* (1982b) and 5-liter cultures ($2-10 \times 10^6$ cells/ml) were set up in RPMI 1640 medium plus 10% FCS in spinner flasks. Each fresh spleen yielded approximately 2×10^{10} living cells. It has been shown by Langford *et al.* (1979) that *Staphylococcus* enterotoxin A (SEA) is a very efficient inducer for synthesis of IFN-γ. *Staphylococcus* enterotoxin A was purified from the supernatant (Schantz *et al.*, 1972) of *Staphylococcus aureus* strain 13N2909 (Friedman and Howard, 1971) cultures and used at a final concentration of 0.3 μg/ml. After 2–3 days at 37°C, when the cultures became slightly acidic, the IFN titer in the splenocyte

culture supernatant reached 10^4 units/ml. Since many other lymphokines beside IFN-γ are certainly induced in SEA-activated human
spleen cell cultures, it should be possible to use this material as a source
of both IFN-γ and IL-2 mRNA. However, since it was shown that the
supernatant of human peripheral blood lymphocytes (PBL) stimulated
with PHA and a phorbol ester (TPA) yielded high titers of IL-2 (Farrar *et
al.*, 1980), the latter activation conditions were chosen. Hence, cultures
of human spleen cells were prepared and stimulated with 10 μg/ml
PHA–10 ng/ml TPA for 40 hr at 37°C.

IV. Detection of mRNA Corresponding to Human IFN-γ and IL-2

A. Preparation of Poly(A)$^+$ RNA

After 72 and 40 hr for IFN-γ and IL-2, respectively, the induced
spleen cells were collected and lysed immediately with a solution of
guanidinium thiocyanate (Chirgwin *et al.*, 1979). Total RNA was isolated
by sedimentation of the homogenized cell lysate through a CsCl cushion
and further purified by precipitation out of a guanidinium hydrochloride
solution. Poly(A)$^+$ RNA was isolated by oligo(dT)-cellulose chromatography and fractionated on a neutral sucrose gradient prepared by freezing
and thawing a 15% sucrose solution. An average of 20 mg total RNA was
obtained per spleen, yielding approximately 0.5 mg poly(A)$^+$ RNA after
one single oligo(dT)-cellulose chromatographic step. More than 60% of
this RNA is still ribosomal RNA.

B. Injection in *Xenopus Laevis* Oocytes

Of each sucrose gradient fraction, 50 nl was microinjected into each of
15–20 *X. laevis* oocytes, and after 3 days at 23°C the oocyte bathing
medium (modified Barth medium containing 0.1% polyethylene glycol
6000, 0.5 mg/ml BSA, 0.4% aprotinin, 2 mM 6-aminocaproic acid, 10
μg/ml soybean trypsin inhibitor) was used for measuring the antirival
activity and the [^{3}H]thymidine incorporation in PHA-stimulated IL-2-
dependent human PBLs. As shown in Table I a reproducible signal of
IFN-γ and IL-2 could be detected in these supernatants. The IFN-γ
activity corresponded to a mRNA sedimenting around 13 S and was 30–
100 times lower than the antirival activity obtained in the splenocyte
medium. The IL-2 activity was observed at a position corresponding to
mRNA which sedimented at 10 S and was 15 times lower than the IL-2
activity of the spleen cells' conditioned medium. We estimate that the
sucrose gradient fractionation of the poly(A)$^+$ RNA resulted in at least a
10-fold enrichment for the lymphokine-specific mRNA species.

TABLE I

COMPARISON OF IFN-γ AND IL-2 ACTIVITY[a]

	Supernatant	
Activity	Spleen	Oocyte
IFN-γ ($\log_{10}$ IFN/ml)		
Experiment 1	3.0	1.5
Experiment 2	4.0	2.0
Experiment 3	3.5	2.5
IL-2 (units/ml)		
Experiment 1	64	5
Experiment 2	100	16

[a]Comparisons were obtained after microinjection of oocytes with splenocyte poly(A)+ RNA fractionated on sucrose gradients with the corresponding activity found in the splenocyte culture supernatant.

C. SEDIMENTATION HETEROGENEITY OF mRNA

Occasionally we found evidence for some heterogeneity of the IFN-γ-specific mRNA as a shoulder or even a small amount of faster moving mRNA in the nondenaturing sucrose gradients, while in the presence of formamide we observed two peaks of IFN-γ mRNA activity (12 S and 15 S) in sucrose gradients (Devos *et al.*, 1982b). Possibly this sedimentation heterogeneity is linked to different steps in denaturation and/or aggregation. For the IL-2 mRNA activity we observed no sedimentation heterogeneity in sucrose gradients, although after injection of poly(A)+ RNA derived from PHA/TPA-stimulated human tonsil cells, Efrat *et al.* (1984) reported that IL-2-specific mRNA sedimented as two peaks.

V. Identification of cDNA Plasmids Corresponding to Human IFN-γ and IL-2

A. PREPARATION OF cDNA LIBRARIES

It was shown by Gheysen and Fiers (1982) that, after transfection of cultured AP8 monkey cells with a pSV529 plasmid (a eukaryotic expression vector) (Fig. 1) containing the human IFN-β cDNA under the control of SV40 late transcription, one could detect the IFN-β synthesized and secreted by these cells. Very low amounts (0.03 μg) of plasmid DNA could be detected by measuring the antiviral activity of the cell medium. These experiments led us to use this pSV529 plasmid as a

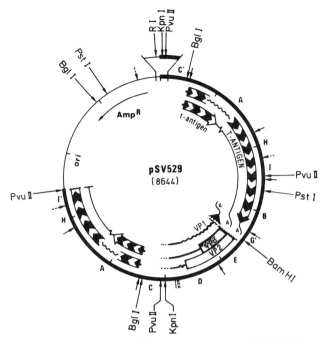

FIG. 1. Physical and genetic map of the expression vector pSV529. The thin segment part of the circle represents the pBR322 DNA sequence. SV40 sequences are shown as a heavy line and contain a partially duplicated DNA replication and early region of the SV40 genome. The coding regions for the early and late proteins are shown as dark arrows. The dotted 5′ ends and wavy poly(A) 3′ ends indicate the span of the mRNAs [for more details on the construction of pSV529, refer to Gheysen and Fiers (1982)]. A gene inserted into the unique *Bam*HI site of pSV529 is under transcriptional control of the late SV40 promotor. This figure is reproduced with permission from Gheysen and Fiers (1982), "Expression and excretion of human IFN-β in monkey cells after transfection with a recombinant SV40 plasmid vector," *J. Mol. Appl. Genet.* **1**, 385.

cloning vector since they suggested that—providing the cDNA copy is (1) full length and (2) inserted in the correct orientation relative to the SV40 late promotor—a sensitive screening method could be derived based on direct expression.

Double stranded cDNA was synthesized using sucrose gradient-fractionated, human spleen-derived IL-2-specific and IFN-γ-specific mRNA from a single donor essentially as described in Devos *et al.* (1979), fractionated by polyacrylamide gel electrophoresis. Appropriate size classes (ranging between 800 and 1000, 1000 and 1250, and 1250 and 1400 bp for IFN-γ, and ranging between 600 and 750, and 750 and 1000 bp for IL-2) were inserted into the unique *Bam*HI site of pSV529 DNA (Fig. 1) via

G/C homopolymer tailing and used to transform *E. coli* (strain DH1 for IFN-γ, and strain HB101 for IL-2). Between 5000 and 10,000 colonies were obtained for each size group. Plasmid DNA was prepared from mixtures of 50 individual clones from the IFN-γ cDNA library and used to transfect AP8 monkey cells (Gheysen and Fiers, 1982). After testing 8000 clones (160 groups of 50 colonies), not one group of 50 clones led to a significant IFN activity in the supernatant of the transfected cells. We concluded that either no full length IFN-γ cDNA copy, inserted in the correct orientation, was present in our library or IFN-γ was expressed below the detection limit of our assay.

Later (Devos *et al.*, 1982a), we showed that our cDNA library indeed contained a IFN-γ cDNA clone which resulted in the appearance of IFN-γ activity after transfection of AP8 cells, but that the level of expression was about 100 times lower than the IFN activity of IFN-β produced after transfection of AP8 cells under similar conditions with a homologous IFN-β cDNA containing plasmid. Our inability to identify an IFN-γ cDNA clone using this direct-screening method led us to use cDNA–mRNA hybridization followed by translation in oocytes to screen our IFN-γ and IL-2 cDNA libraries. Human spleens proved to be a reliable source of both IFN-γ and IL-2 mRNA necessary for the successful identification of both IFN-γ- and IL-2-cDNA clones.

B. PREPARATION OF cDNA INSERTS

For the identification of specific cDNA clones by mRNA selection, groups of individual recombinant plasmids are immobilized on nitrocellulose filters, hybridized with mRNA and bound mRNA, eluted, and translated *in vitro* (Derynck *et al.*, 1980; Parnes *et al.*, 1981). To increase the hybridization efficiency, and thus the potential signal after translation, we decided to immobilize only insert DNA onto the filters instead of binding total plasmid DNA. On the other hand, since the insert DNA comprises 10% of the total plasmid DNA, binding only insert DNA allows the screening of a greater number of different colonies per filter. Insert DNA from mixtures of 50 individual clones was prepared by *Bam*HI digestion (the *Bam*HI site of the vector pSV529 was restored by filling in the 5′ protruding ends before the dC homopolymer tailing), purified by sucrose gradient centrifugation (Fig. 2), and bound on nitrocellulose filters (Kafatos *et al.*, 1979). We estimated that at least 10 inserts were present per group of 50 colonies and that approximately 5 μg insert DNA per group or 0.5 μg of each insert was immobilized on each filter. Assuming that 10 ng of each mRNA species can hybridize to each individual insert [10% of total poly(A)⁺ RNA, see below] and that

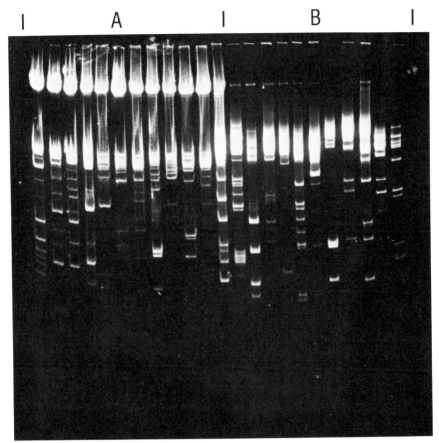

FIG. 2. Purification of BamHI-excised insert DNA derived from mixtures of 50 individual cDNA plasmids. Plasmid DNA was prepared from mixtures of 50 bacterial colonies, digested with Bam HI, and the excised insert DNA purified by sucrose gradient centrifugation. Aliquots were analyzed on 4% polyacrylamide gels before (A) and after (B) centrifugation.

3 ng of this material can be recovered, taking up the eluted mRNA in 2 μl of H_2O will yield around 0.1 ng (50 nl) of each mRNA species for injection into one oocyte. Since for the detection of IL-2 or IFN-γ mRNA approximately 50 ng of sucrose gradient-enriched poly(A)$^+$ RNA per oocyte will lead to a positive signal, if we estimate that the frequency of these lymphokine mRNA is 0.1%, then approximately 0.05 ng of lL-2 or IFN-γ mRNA per oocyte is easily detectable. We therefore conclude that if at least 100 μg poly(A)$^+$ RNA is used for the hybridization, the

presence of an IFN-γ or IL-2-specific insert cDNA on the filters should
be identified.

C. HYBRID SELECTION

1. Interferon-Gamma

Using sucrose gradient-enriched poly(A)+ RNA derived from SEA-
induced human splenocytes, 20 filters each containing insert cDNA corresponding to 50 cDNA plasmids constructed with dscDNA ranging in
size between 1000 and 1250 bp were utilized for hybrid selection of
IFN-γ-specific mRNA. Three groups were found to be reproducibly
(three times) positive. Hybrid selection using insert cDNA from subdivi-
sions of one of these groups finally resulted in the identification of a
plasmid, pHIIF-SVγ0, which specifically retained IFN-γ mRNA. Colony
hybridization (Hanahan and Meselson, 1980) on 3000 colonies of this
cDNA library with a radioactively labeled restriction fragment (*Dde*I
fragment), derived from pHIIF-SVγ0, resulted in the identification of 8
more IFN-γ cDNA-containing plasmids (pHIIF-SVγ1–8) (Table II). All
these plasmids contained an insert between 1000 and 1250 bp in length,
and all except one were excisable with *Bam*HI. From the results obtained by restriction analysis it was apparent that these plasmids contained an almost full-length IFN-γ cDNA insert and that the cDNA in
pHIIF-SVγ1 was inserted in the correct orientation relative to the SV40
late promotor. Therefore, pHIIF-SVγ1 was the only clone which led to
expression of IFN-γ (100 units/ml) after transfection of AP8 monkey

TABLE II

IDENTIFICATION OF IFN-γ AND IL-2 cDNA-CONTAINING PLASMIDS

IFN-γ ("insert DNA" 1000–1250 bp)	IL-2 ("insert DNA" 600–750 bp)
20 Filters (50 clones each) ↓ 3 Positive filters	18 Filters (50 clones each) ↓ 2 Positive filters
Subgroups of 50 clones ↓ pHIIF-SVγ0	Subgroups of 50 clones ↓ pSV-HIL2-0
Colony hybridization (3000 clones) ↓ pHIIF-SVγ1–8	Colony hybridization (1300 clones) ↓ pSV-HIL2-1

cells, proving that the clones we had isolated did actually code for human IFN-γ.

2. *Interleukin 2*

Hybridization of 18 filters each containing cDNA derived from 50 plasmids with poly(A)⁺ RNA, derived from PHA–TPA-induced splenocytes and subsequent elution, microinjection into oocytes, and assay of the oocyte medium for IL-2 activity yielded 2 filters which gave a clear positive signal. Further hybridization of subgroups led to the identification of an IL-2 cDNA-containing plasmid pSV-HIL2-0 containing an insert of approximately 750 bp in length. Colony hybridization of 1300 colonies with an internal *Hin*f fragment derived from pSV-HIL2-0 resulted in the identification of one additional clone, pSV-HIL2-1 (Table II), containing an insert of only 250 bp in length and corresponding to an internal sequence within insert DNA derived from pSV-HIL2-0. This second clone was derived from a group of 50 plasmids which corresponded to one of the two original filters which scored positive in the hybrid-selection assay, proving that our screening method is indeed sensitive.

D. STRUCTURE OF HUMAN IFN-γ AND IL-2 AS DEDUCED FROM THE NUCLEOTIDE SEQUENCE

A physical map of human IFN-γ and IL-2 mRNA as determined from the nucleotide sequence of the cDNA inserts of the pHIIF-SV plasmids and from pSV-HIL2-0 is shown in Fig. 3. For IFN-γ an open-reading

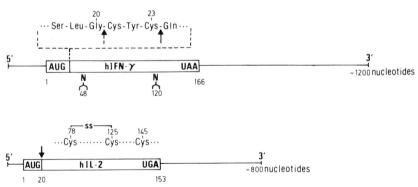

FIG. 3. Structure of human IFN-γ and IL-2. The boxed area represents the region coding for a signal sequence and the mature polypeptide. Above the coding region the positions of the cysteine residues are shown. The amino acid residues are numbered starting from the initiation methionine. The assigned signal sequence cleavage position is indicated by a vertical arrow, N represents potential N-glycosylation sites.

frame coding for a polypeptide of 166 amino acids was identified. The 20 amino terminal residues have been assigned as a signal sequence. Rinderknecht *et al.* (1984) showed that the natural mature human IFN-γ does not contain cysteine residues and started at amino acid position 24, so that the protein would then have a length of 143 amino acids. There are two potential N-glycosylation sites which are responsible for the heterogeneity after SDS–polyacrylamide gel electrophoresis of natural IFN-γ or recombinant IFN-γ expressed by eukaryotic cells (Devos *et al.*, 1984a; Rinderknecht *et al.*, 1984; Scahill *et al.*, 1983).

Since part of the 5′ coding region (signal sequence) was missing from the IL-2 cDNA, the nucleotide sequence for IL-2 was completed with sequence information from a genomic IL-2 clone (Degrave *et al.*, 1983). A unique reading frame was identified coding for a polypeptide of 153 amino acids and containing a putative signal sequence of 20 amino acids, resulting in a mature protein of 133 amino acids. Three cysteine residues are present of which two are involved in an intramolecular disulfide bridge (Wang *et al.*, 1984). Since no potential N-glycosylation sites are present, heterogeneity of molecular weight of the natural IL-2 can be explained by other posttranslational modification, such as O-glycosylation (Robb and Smith, 1981).

VI. Expression of Human IFN-γ and IL-2

A. EXPRESSION OF HUMAN IFN-γ AND IL-2 IN *Escherichia coli*

1. Interferon-Gamma

Several hybrid plasmids have been constructed in which the phage λ P_L promotor, and a ribosome binding site derived from the phage MS2-replicase gene or the *E. coli* tryptophan attenuator was fused to the mature human IFN-γ sequence. Using a temperature-sensitive phage λ C_I repressor on a compatible plasmid or on the bacterial chromosome (Remaut *et al.*, 1981), these plasmids directed the high-level synthesis of IFN-γ after induction of the promotor at 42°C (Simons *et al.*, 1984). Almost all the IFN-γ produced in *E. coli* is in an insoluble form and has to be renatured to reach the same specific biological activity as the glycosylated IFN-γ produced in mammalian cells.

2. Interleukin 2

Mature human IL-2 was expressed in *E. coli* under control of the *E. coli* tryptophan promotor or using a combination of the phage λ P_L promotor and a ribosome binding site derived from phage Mu (Devos *et*

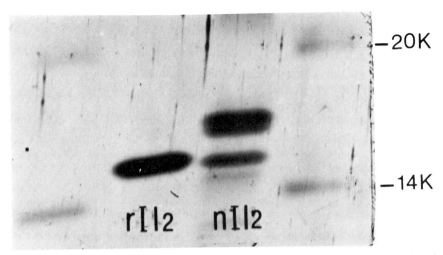

Fig. 4. SDS–polyacrylamide gel electrophoresis of human recombinant IL-2 (rIL2) expressed in *E. coli* and spleen-derived human natural IL-2 (nIL2) purified by affinity chromatography on a rabbit–antihuman rIL-2–Sepharose column.

al., 1983). The IL-2 present in bacterial extracts remained insoluble and has a molecular weight of 15,000 in SDS–polyacrylamide gels (Fig. 4). After renaturation and purification, recombinant human IL-2 of high specific activity can be obtained which has the same affinity for the IL-2 receptor as the IL-2 produced by human T cells (M. Nabholz, personal communication).

B. EXPRESSION OF HUMAN IFN-γ IN CHINESE HAMSTER OVARY CELLS

High levels of human IFN-γ (5 mg/liter) are secreted by cultures of Chinese hamster ovary cells transformed with a combination of a plasmid-encoding mouse dihydrofolate reductase (Kaufman and Sharp, 1982) and a plasmid-encoding human IFN-γ (Scahill *et al.*, 1983). Since the IFN-γ cDNA gene used is under the transcriptional control of the SV40 early promotor, the IFN-γ production was constitutive. The recombinant IFN-γ was purified as in Devos *et al.* (1984a) and its molecular weight, as determined by gel filtration, is about 50,000, corresponding to a dimer structure. The purified product migrated in SDS–polyacrylamide gel as two bands having molecular weights of 25,000 and 20,000, consistent with the doubly and singly glycosylated forms of human IFN-γ produced in mitogen-stimulated lymphocyte cultures (Yip *et al.*, 1982).

VII. Biological Studies Using Recombinant IFN-γ and IL-2

Using the recombinant human IFN-γ and IL-2, a more precise functional analysis of their biological activities has been initiated. Of special interest is the induction of class II-HLA antigen by IFN-γ on human monocyte cell lines (Virelizier *et al.*, 1984; Kelley *et al.*, 1984), on human thymic epithelial cells (Berrih *et al.*, 1985), and on human endothelial cells and dermal fibroblasts (Pober *et al.*, 1983a,b). This finding underscores the importance of IFN-γ as a modulator of the immune response. Moreover it was demonstrated that IFN-γ can act as a very potent macrophage-activating factor for tumor cytotoxicity (Schultz and Kleinschmidt, 1983) and for enhancing the killing of intracellular parasites (Nathan *et al.*, 1983). More recently it was shown that IFN-γ acts synergistically with tumor necrosis factor (TNF) for *in vitro* lysis of tumor cell lines (Fransen *et al.*, 1985). These studies clearly demonstrate the potential clinical usefulness of recombinant IFN-γ, and it is anticipated that they will lead to a better understanding of the mechanisms of the immune-defense system. Purified recombinant human IL-2 very efficiently induces the generation of cytolytic cells in both human PBL and mouse spleen cell cultures (Devos *et al.*, 1984b). This phenomenon is related to the nonspecific, secondary cytotoxic T lymphocyte activation. and these cells may be identical to the lymphokine-activated killer (LAK) cells, described by Grimm *et al.* (1982). The high cytolytic activity toward tumor cells obtained with recombinant IL-2 is being explored with regard to its possible role in cancer immunotherapy (Mule *et al.*, 1985).

It is now well established that human B cells activated *in vitro* can express the IL-2 receptor (Muraguchi *et al.*, 1985; Waldmann *et al.*, 1984) and that these cells can respond to recombinant IL-2 by proliferation, suggesting that IL-2 is one of the lymphokines directly involved in the activation of B lymphocytes. Using purified human B cells activated with *S. aureus* strain Cowan I (SAC) particles, we have shown (Devos *et al.*, 1985) that human rIL-2 also promotes the differentiation of these cells toward immunoglobulin secretion and thus that IL-2 could also act as a B cell differentiation factor. In conclusion, the use of homogeneous recombinant IFN-γ and recombinant IL-2 has clearly demonstrated that various cells are susceptible to signals provided by these lymphokines and has proved that these reagents are uniquely useful for examining new hypotheses concerning lymphokine functions.

ACKNOWLEDGMENTS

We thank Mrs. M. C. Vermeire and Mr. W. Drijvers for their help in preparing this manuscript. This work was supported by BIOGEN, N.V.

REFERENCES

Berrih, S., Arenzana-Seisdedos, F., Cohen, S., Devos, R., Charron, D., and Virelizier, J. L. (1985). *J. Immunol.* **135**, 1165.

Chergwin, J. M., Przybyla, A. E., MacDonald, R. J., and Rutter, W. J. (1979). *Biochemistry* **18**, 5294.

Degrave, W., Tavernier, J., Duerinck, F., Plaetinck, G., Devos, R., and Fiers, W. (1983). *EMBO J.* **2**, 2349.

Derynck, R., Content, J., De Clercq, E., Volckaert, G., Tavernier, J., Devos, R., and Fiers, W. (1980). *Nature (London)* **285**, 542.

Devos, R., Van Emmelo, J., Contreras, R., and Fiers, W. (1979). *J. Mol. Biol.* **128**, 595.

Devos, R., Cheroutre, H., Taya, Y., Degrave, W., Van Heuverswyn, H., and Fiers, W. (1982a). *Nucleic Acids Res.* **10**, 2487.

Devos, R., Cheroutre, H., Taya, Y., and Fiers, W. (1982b). *J. Interferon Res.* **2**, 409.

Devos, R., Plaetinck, G., Cheroutre, H., Simons, G., Degrave, W., Tavernier, J., Remaut, R., and Fiers, W. (1983). *Nucleic Acids Res.* **11**, 4307.

Devos, R., Opsomer, C., Scahill, S. J., Van Der Heyden, J., and Fiers, W. (1984a). *J. Interferon Res.* **4**, 461.

Devos, R., Plaetinck, G., and Fiers, W. (1984b). *Eur. J. Immunol.* **14**, 1057.

Devos, R., Jayaram, B., Vandenabeele, P., and Fiers, W. (1985). *Immunol. Lett.* **11**, 101.

Efrat, S., and Kaempfer, R. (1984). *Proc. Natl. Acad. Sci. U.S.A.* **81**, 2601.

Farrar, J. J., Mizel, S. B., Fuller-Farrar, J., Farrar, W. L., and Hilfiker, M. L. (1980). *J. Immunol.* **125**, 793.

Fransen, L., Van Der Heyden, J., Ruysschaert, R., and Fiers, W. (1986). *Eur. J. Cancer Clin. Oncol.* **22**, 419.

Friedman, M. E., and Howard, M. B. (1971). *J. Bacteriol.* **106**, 289.

Gheysen, D., and Fiers, W. (1982). *J. Mol. Appl. Genet.* **1**, 385.

Gillis, S., Ferm, M. M., Ou, W., and Smith, K. A. (1978). *J. Immunol.* **120**, 2027.

Gray, P. W., Leung, D. W., Pennica, D., Yelverton, E., Najarian, R., Simonsen, C. C., Derynck, R., Sherwood, P. J., Wallace, D. M., Berger, S. L., Levinson, A. D., and Goeddel, D. V. (1982). *Nature (London)* **295**, 503.

Grimm, E. A., Mazumder, A., Zhang, H. Z., and Rosenberg, S. A. (1982). *J. Exp. Med.* **155**, 1823.

Hanahan, D., and Meselson, M. (1980). *Gene* **10**, 63.

Kafatos, F. C., Jones, C. W., and Efstratiadis, A. (1979). *Nucleic Acids Res.* **7**, 1541.

Kaufman, R. J., and Sharp, P. A. (1982). *Mol. Cell Biol.* **2**, 1304.

Kelley, V. E., Fiers, W., and Strom, T. B. (1984). *J. Immunol.* **132**, 240.

Langford, M. P., Georgiades, J. A., Stenton, G. J., Dianzani, F., and Johnson, H. M. (1979). *Infect. Immun.* **26**, 36.

Mingari, M. C., Gerosa, F., Moretta, A., Zubler, R. H., and Moretta, L. (1985). *Eur. J. Immunol.* **15**, 193.

Mule, J. J., Shu, S., and Rosenberg, S. A. (1985). *J. Immunol.* **135**, 646.

Muraguchi, A., Kehrl, J. H., Longo, D. L., Volkman, D. J., Smith, K. A., and Fauci, A. S. (1985). *J. Exp. Med.* **161**, 181.

Nathan, C. F., Murray, H. W., Wiebe, M. E., and Rubin, B. Y. (1983). *J. Exp. Med.* **158**, 670.

Parnes, J. R., Velan, B., Felsenfeld, A., Ramanathan, L., Ferrini, U., Appella, E., and Seidman, J. G. (1981). *Proc. Natl. Acad. Sci. U.S.A.* **78**, 2253.

Pober, J. S., Collins, T., Gimbrone, M. A., Cotran, R. S., Gitlin, J. D., Fiers, W., Clayberger, C., Krensky, A. M., Burakoff, S. J., and Reiss, C. S. (1983a). *Nature (London)* **305**, 726.

Pober, J. S., Gimbrone, M. A., Cotran, R. S., Reiss, C. S., Burakoff, S. J., Fiers, W., and Sult, K. A. (1983b). *J. Exp. Med.* **157**, 1339.

Remaut, E., Stanssens, P., and Fiers, W. (1981). *Gene* **15**, 81.

Rinderknecht, E., O'Connor, B. H., and Rodriguez, H. (1984). *J. Biol. Chem.* **259**, 6790.

Robb, R. J., and Smith, K. A. (1981). *Mol. Immunol.* **18**, 1087.

Scahill, S. J., Devos, R., Van Der Heyden, J., and Fiers, W. (1983). *Proc. Natl. Acad. Sci. U.S.A.* **80**, 4654.

Schantz, E. J., Roessler, W. G., Woodburn, M. J., Lynch, J. M., Jacoby, H. M., Silverman, S. J., Gorman, J. C., and Spero, L. (1972). *Biochemistry* **11**, 360.

Schultz, R. M., and Kleinschmidt, W. J. (1983). *Nature (London)* **305**, 239.

Simons, G., Remaut, E., Allet, B., Devos, R., and Fiers, W. (1984). *Gene* **28**, 55.

Taniguchi, T., Matsui, H., Fujita, T., Takaoka, C., Kashima, N., Yoshimoto, R., and Hamuro, J. (1983). *Nature (London)* **302**, 305.

Virelizier, J. L., Perez, N., Arenzana-Seisdedos, F., and Devos, R. (1984). *Eur. J. Immunol.* **14**, 106.

Waldmann, T. A., Goldman, C. K., Robb, R. J., Depper, J. M., Leonard, W. J., Sharrow, S. O., Bongiovanni, K. F., Korsmeyer, S. J., and Greene, W. C. (1984). *J. Exp. Med.* **160**, 1450.

Wang, A., Lu, S.-D., and Mark, D. F. (1984). *Science* **224**, 1431.

Yip, Y. K., Barrowclough, B. S., Urban, C., and Vilcek, J. (1982). *Science* **215**, 411.

T Cell Growth Factor (Interleukin 2) Gene: Organization and Expression in Human T Lymphotropic Virus-Infected Cells in Leukemia and AIDS

SURESH K. ARYA AND ROBERT C. GALLO

*Laboratory of Tumor Cell Biology, National Center Institute,
National Institutes of Health,
Bethesda, Maryland 20892*

I. Introduction

T cells play a central role in immune regulation, affecting the development of immmune response in many diverse ways. Apart from the direct action of cytotoxic T cells, many of the immune modulatory effects of T cells are brought about by the release of soluble factors collectively called lymphokines. One of the more important T cell lymphokines is the T cell growth factor (TCGF), alternatively termed interleukin 2 (IL-2). This factor is required for the growth and proliferation of activated T lymphocytes. The demonstration that a distinct molecular entity (TCGF) stimulates the proliferation of activated T cells had a major impact on immunological research. It stimulated the search for other lymphokines involved in cellular and humoral immunity and shifted the focus from phenomenology to the development of well-defined systems to dissect interacting components of the immune system in health and disease.

Human TCGF was first identified in preparations of conditioned mediums of mitogen-stimulated human T lymphocyte cultures (Morgan *et al.*, 1976). Though mitogens stimulate short-term proliferation of activated T cells, TCGF is required for long-term growth (Ruscetti *et al.*, 1977; Smith, 1980; Ruscetti and Gallo, 1981). Ability to grow T cells in culture has made it possible to develop T cell clones of defined phenotypic specificity (Gillis and Smith, 1977; Lotze *et al.*, 1980; Schrier *et al.*, 1980; von Boehmer and Haas, 1981), thus allowing functional studies of different subsets of T cells and developing adaptive immunotherapeutic measures in human cancers and other disorders (Rosenberg *et al.*, 1982). In addition to or concomitant with its effects on T cell proliferation, TCGF is implicated in the production and function of other lymphokines. For example, TCGF reportedly modulates the production of B cell growth factor (BCGF) (Howard *et al.*, 1983) and/or B cell differentiation factor (Miedema *et al.*, 1985) and IFN-γ (Farrar *et al.*, 1982; Kasahara *et al.*, 1983). Whether this is a direct effect or a result of the expansion of a

35

BCGF- or IFN-γ-producing cell population is not yet clear. Recently, receptors for TCGF have been detected on some human B cells, raising the possibility that TCGF directly stimulates the proliferation and differentiation of B cells and thus has a direct effect on humoral immunity (Tsudo *et al.*, 1984; Jung *et al.*, 1984; Waldmann *et al.*, 1984; Ralph *et al.*, 1984; Nakagawa *et al.*, 1985).

Availability of preparations of TCGF and the consequent ability to maintain human neoplastic T cells in culture allowed the isolation of the first genuine human retrovirus—a finding of considerable practical as well as heuristic importance. Retrovirus particles were first isolated from TCGF-maintained lymphocyte cultures of patients with cutaneous T cell lymphoma (Poiesz *et al.*, 1980) and with Sezary T cell leukemia (Poiesz *et al.*, 1981). Subsequently, many other virus isolates were obtained by coculturing lymphocytes from adult T cell leukemia (ATL) patients with human T cell-enriched populations (Miyoshi *et al.*, 1981; Yoshida *et al.*, 1982; Gallo *et al.*, 1982; Popovic *et al.*, 1983a,b). These isolates have been collectively termed human T lymphotropic virus Type I (HTLV-I) (Gallo *et al.*, 1984a). A distinct but related retrovirus was isolated from lymphocytes of a patient with a benign form of hairy cell leukemia (Kalyanaraman *et al.*, 1982) which has been termed HTLV-II. The experience with maintaining T cells in culture and the isolation of retroviruses played a crucial role in our more recent isolation and full characterization of retrovirus associated with human acquired immune deficiency syndrome (AIDS) (Popovic *et al.*, 1984; Schupbach *et al.*, 1984; Sarngadharan *et al.*, 1984; Gallo *et al.*, 1984b). Since this virus has some structural and functional similarities to HTLV-I and HTLV-II (Arya *et al.*, 1984a; Ratner *et al.*, 1985; Starcich *et al.*, 1985a), we termed it HTLV-III. A similar virus, termed LAV, has been isolated from patients with lymphoadenopathy syndrome (Barre-Sinoussi *et al.*, 1983). By now more than 100 isolates of HTLV-III/LAV have been reported from our laboratory (Salahuddin *et al.*, 1985); many of these have been propagated in human T lymphocytes and some have been molecularly cloned and sequenced (Hahn *et al.*, 1984; Shaw *et al.*, 1984; Arya *et al.*, 1985). Most of these isolates show substantial genomic diversity whereas some are more closely related to our prototype HTLV-III(B) or to other isolates (Starcich *et al.*, 1986).

II. TCGF Synthesis in Normal and HTLV-Infected Human Cells

T cell growth factor is produced by mature T lymphocytes upon appropriate stimulation. The major producer cell type appears to be the OKT4⁺ T lymphocyte, particularly with helper/inducer phenotype

(Schrier and Iscove, 1980; Ruscetti and Gallo, 1981; Palacois, 1982), although it has not been ruled out that T cells with other phenotypes are incapable of producing TCGF (Moretta, 1985). Elaboration of TCGF from normal human lymphocytes apparently requires at least two signals (Larsson et al., 1980; Palacois, 1982). One of these is provided by interleukin 1 (IL-1) produced by accessory macrophages, and the second signal can be either specific antigen or mitogen. For practical purposes, human TCGF is generally obtained by stimulation of T cell-enriched peripheral blood lymphocytes with mitogen and phytohemagglutinin (PHA). A cloned human leukemic T cell line, Jurkat, can be induced with PHA and tumor promoter 12-O-tetradecanoylphorbol-13-acetate (TPA) to produce TCGF (Gillis and Watson, 1980), as if TPA in this case mimics what IL-1 does for normal lymphocytes.

T cell growth factor secreted by normal human T cells is a single polypeptide with a molecular weight of 14,000–16,000, though it migrates as a 20,000–24,000 Da protein on gel permeation, presumably due to aggregation related to the hydrophobic nature of the polypeptide (Mier and Gallo, 1980; Robb et al., 1983; Gallo et al., 1984c). Minor apparent molecular weight heterogeneities have been observed for TCGF secreted by normal lymphocytes and leukemic Jurkat cells (Robb et al., 1983; Gallo et al., 1984c). Furthermore, TCGFs produced by these two cell sources differ in such physicochemical properties as isoelectric focusing and hydrophobicity (Gallo et al., 1984c). In contrast to these cells which require induction, a human leukemic T cell line harboring HTLV-I (HuT 102) produces measurable quantities of TCGF constitutively (Gootenberg et al., 1981, 1982). Similarly, an HTLV-II-infected human leukemic T cell line (Mo) also produces some TCGF (S. C. Clark et al., personal communication). We have recently found that some other human neoplastic T cells, specifically those infected with HTLV-III, also produce TCGF constitutively (Arya and Gallo, 1985a; and unpublished observations).

III. TCGF Gene Expression and Regulation in Normal and HTLV-Infected Human Cells

Though TCGF initially played a critical role in successful isolation of HTLVs, many of the HTLV-infected T cell lines grow in culture independent of exogenously added TCGF. Many of these cell lines possess OKT4 + phenotype and are mature or nearly mature T cells. Given the backdrop of the requirement of TCGF for normal T cell growth, we initially hypothesized that HTLV-infected T cells produce and respond to their own TCGF (Gootenberg et al., 1981; Arya et al., 1984b). We surmised that these cells either employ an autostimulation mechanism for growth control, where every cell in the population produces and responds to TCGF, or employ a parastimulation mechanism where some cells in the population produce sufficient TCGF to sustain the growth of the population (Arya *et al.*, 1984c). These notions were buttressed by the fact that many HTLV-infected cells display abundant membrane receptors for TCGF (Popovic *et al.*, 1983b; Mann *et al.*, 1983) and some, though few, HTLV-infected cell lines produce TCGF (Gootenberg *et al.*, 1981). The fact that many of the HTLV-I-infected cell lines did not elaborate detectable TCGF could be explained by a rapid utilization of TCGF by these cells coupled with the lack of sensitivity of assays used to measure the release of TCGF.

To evaluate these issues and to investigate the regulation of TCGF gene expression in normal and aberrant cells, we cloned human TCGF cDNA from PHA-stimulated peripheral blood lymphocytes (Clark *et al.*, 1984). DNA sequence analysis of the clone shows that the functional part of the TCGF gene contains a coding sequence of 459 base pairs (bp), and additional 5' and 3' untranslated sequences of about 50 and 250 bp, respectively. Since we had determined the N-terminal and carboxy-terminal amino acid sequence of the purified TCGF, a comparison of the predicted amino acid sequence with the actually determined sequence allowed us to conclude that the first 60 bp of the coding sequence of the TCGF gene corresponds to signal peptides of 20 amino acid residues (Clark *et al.*, 1984)—a possibility also suggested by Taniguchi *et al.* (1983). Furthermore, this comparison also allowed us to conclude that there was no proteolytic cleavage at the carboxy-terminus to generate mature protein. Thus, mature TCGF is composed of 133 amino acid residues corresponding to 399 bp of the gene.

Taniguchi *et al.* (1983) had previously published the DNA sequence of a TCGF cDNA clone derived from human leukemic Jurkat cells. This allowed us to inquire into the basis of physicochemical differences between normal (PBL) and leukemic (Jurkat) TCGFs. These differences could result from posttranslational modifications of the protein or from polymorphism of the gene itself. It was possible that TCGF was derived from a gene family with multiple members, only one of which was expressed in a given cell type. However, comparison of the DNA sequence of our PBL cDNA clone with that of the Jurkat cDNA clone showed them to be identical except for one nucleotide difference which did not change the amino acid sequence of the protein (Clark *et al.*, 1984). This inference is supported by the sequence of a cDNA clone from normal human splenocytes (Devos *et al.*, 1983). We therefore concluded that the differences in physicochemical properties of the two proteins were due

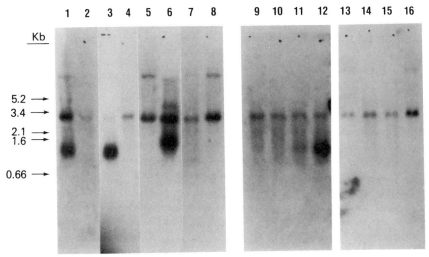

FIG. 1. Expression of TCGF gene in human cells. Lanes 1–16 are as follows: 1, PHA-stimulated lymphocytes; 2, unstimulated lymphocytes; 3, pHA + TPA-stimulated Jurkat cells; 4, unstimulated Jurkat cells; 5, 6G1 cells; 6, MLA 144 cells; 7, MOLT-4 cells; 8, HL-60 cells; 9, unstimulated Jurkat cells; 10, TPA-stimulated Jurkat cells; 11, PHA-stimulated Jurkat cells; 12, PHA + TPA-stimulated cells; 13, Daudi cells; 14, Raji cells; 15, trophoblast 3A cells; and 16, SD cells. TCGF-specific RNA appears as a 900-nucleotide band (100 nucleotides for MLA 144 cells). The 2300-nucleotide band is for an abundant mRNA species constitutively expressed in many cell types. Adopted from Clark *et al.* (1984).

to posttranslational modifications (Clark *et al.*, 1984; Gallo *et al.*, 1984c). This has now been confirmed by detection of O'-linked glycosylation of threonine at position 3 of the TCGF amino acid sequence (Robb *et al.*, 1983, 1984).

We also demonstrated unequivocally that the production of TCGF is regulated at the level of TCGF mRNA synthesis (Clark *et al.*, 1984). The induction of TCGF is primarily the induction of TCGF gene transcription (Clark *et al.*, 1984; Arya and Gallo, 1984). Using Northern blot analysis, we showed that the TCGF mRNA could be detected only in those human cells which were known to produce TCGF (Fig. 1; Table I). To understand further the induction of TCGF mRNA synthesis, and hence TCGF production, we inquired whether the regulation occurred at the level of initiation of gene transcription or whether other post-transcriptional events, such as mRNA stability, were also contributory factors. Our nuclear transcription or "run off" experiments showed that the primary induction event is the initiation of TCGF gene transcription (Fig. 2), and the degree of transcriptional activation of the TCGF gene in

TABLE I

EXPRESSION OF TCGF, IFN-γ, AND *JD15* GENES IN HUMAN CELLS

Cells	Inducer	Relative mRNA abundance[a]		
		TCGF	IFN-γ	JD15
T cells				
PBL	—	—	±	±
	PHA	+++	+++	+
	TPA	NT[b]	NT	++
	PHA + TPA	+++	+++	+++
Jurkat	—	—	—	±
	PHA	+	—	++
	TPA	±	—	++
	PHA + TPA	+++	—	+++
H4	—	+	—	+
	PHA + TPA	++	—	+++
H9	—	+	—	+
	PHA + TPA	+++	—	+++
HuT 78	—	±	—	+
CEM	—	—	—	±
	PHA + TPA	—	—	+
MOLT-4	—	—	—	±
	PHA + TPA	—	—	+
HSB-20	—	—	—	±
	PHA + TPA	—	—	+
B cells				
Daudi	—	—	—	±
	PHA + TPA	—	—	±
Raji	—	—	—	±
HTLV-I-infected T cells				
HuT 102	—	+	—	++
MI	—	—	+	++
	PHA + TPA	—	++	+++
MJ	—	—	+	++
MT2	—	—	+	++
C2/MJ	—	—	++	++
	PHA + TPA	—	+++	+++
C5/MJ	—	—	+	++
1C/UK	—	—	+	++
	PHA + TPA	—	++	+++

TABLE I (Continued)

		Relative mRNA abundance[a]		
Cells	Inducer	TCGF	IFN-γ	JD15
HTLV-II-infected T cells				
Mo	−	+	NT	+ +
HTLV-III-infected T cells				
H4/HIII	−	+	−	+ ±
	PHA	+ +	−	+ +
	TPA	+ +	−	+ +
	PHA + TPA	+ + +	−	+ + +
H9/HIII	−	+	−	+ +
	PHA + TAP	+ + +	−	+ + +
Other cells				
3A (trophoblasts)	−	−	NT	−
SD (trophoblasts)	−	−	NT	−
HL60 (myeloid)	−	−	NT	−

[a]The number of symbols (+ or −) is meant to provide an approximate description of mRNA abundance.

[b]NT, Not tested.

Jurkat cells correlates with the abundance of mRNA in cells induced with PHA, TPA, and PHA plus TPA (Arya and Gallo, 1984). PHA alone induces some gene transcription which is markedly enhanced by the inclusion of TPA along with PHA, suggesting synergy in the effect of these two inducers. The results of experiments using RNA synthesis inhibitors to block further transcription of the TCGF gene in induced cells suggest that TPA may additionally affect the half-life of TCGF mRNAs, possibly by increasing the specific degradation of TCGF mRNA or, alternatively, by increasing the rate of its translation into the protein (Arya and Gallo, 1984). We have previously noted similar posttranscriptional effects of TPA on the synthesis of mouse mammary tumor virus (Arya, 1980; see also Kaempfer et al., this volume).

Since the two inductive signals for PBL are provided by PHA and IL-1, and those for Jurkat cells by PHA and TPA, we inquired if TPA acted in Jurkat cells in a manner analogous to the action of IL-1 in PBL. If this is the case, we would expect that Jurkat cells maximally induced with TPA will not display any further induction with IL-1. However, we found that IL-1 was able to further enhance the abundance of TCGF mRNA in Jurkat cells maximally induced with TPA and PHA (Fig. 3),

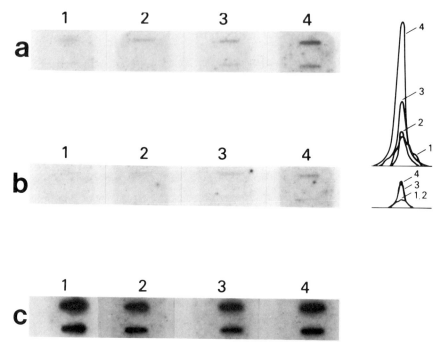

Fig. 2. Analysis of nuclear transcripts of TCGF gene from induced and uninduced Jurkat cells. (a) pTC6F; (b) pBR; (c) pJB1. Lane 1, control cells; lane 2, cells treated with TPA; lane 3, cells treated with PHA; lane 4, cells treated with PHA plus TPA. Negative and positive controls are pBR and pJBI, respectively. Curves on the right are the respective densitometer tracings of two of the bands shown on the left (top, pTCGF; bottom, pBR). Adopted from Arya and Gallo (1984). Reprinted with permission of *Biochemistry*, Copyright 1984, American Chemical Society.

and thus IL-1 was synergistic with TPA (Arya and Gallo, 1984). This implies that TPA and IL-1 act by different mechanisms in enhancing the transcriptional activity of the TCGF gene. It is likely that both of these inducers act by binding to specific membrane receptors and generate secondary mediators. The maximal inducing concentration of a given inducer may pertain to its capacity to bind the specific membrane receptors and not necessarily to the capacity of the TCGF gene to be induced by secondary mediators activated by that inducer. Thus, TPA and IL-1 could individually generate different or the same secondary mediators, which could affect TCGF gene transcription by acting in concert on the same basic process such as the rate of gene transcription.

In our original publication (Clark *et al.*, 1984), we also reported the kinetics of induction of TCGF mRNA synthesis in Jurkat cells. The TCGF-specific mRNA in these cells is readily detected at 2 hr postinduc-

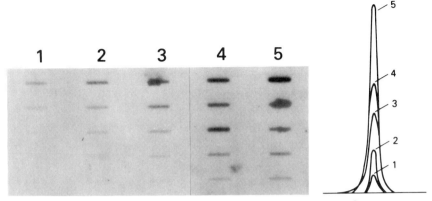

Fig. 3. Induction of TCGF mRNA in Jurkat cells by PHA, TPA, and IL-1. Lane 1, control cells; lane 2, cells treated with PHA; lane 3, cells treated with PHA plus IL-1; lane 4, cells treated with PHA plus TPA; lane 5, cells treated with PHA plus TPA plus IL-1. Curves on the right are the respective densitometer tracings of the top bands shown on the left. Adopted from Arya and Gallo (1984). Reprinted with permission of *Biochemistry*, Copyright 1984, American Chemical Society.

tion, rises to maximal levels at 4–6 hr, is maintained at these levels for 8–10 hr, and is followed by steady decline for the next 24 hr or more. These kinetics suggest a tight control of TCGF gene expression. The rather rapid decline suggests either a cessation of TCGF gene transcription or an increasing rate of disappearance of TCGF mRNA by its utilization for translation and/or degradation. These kinetic parameters for Jurkat cells are different than those reported by Efrat and co-workers for human tonsillar lymphocytes (Efrat and Kaempfer, 1984; Efrat and Kaempfer, 1984; Kaempfer *et al.*, this volume) who used oocyte translation system for evaluating functional TCGF mRNA levels. The kinetics of induction and of decay of TCGF mRNA in tonsillar lymphocytes induced with PHA is considerably delayed in comparison to Jurkat cells. Efrat *et al.* (1982) were able to demonstrate superinduction of TCGF mRNA in tonsillar lymphocytes by using protein synthesis inhibitors soon after induction. They suggest that the decline in the accumulation of TCGF mRNA was due to a shutoff of TCGF mRNA synthesis triggered by the production of a transcriptional repressor. Interestingly, although TCGF mRNA in tonsillar lymphocytes does not reach its maximal levels until 20 hr postinduction, induction with PHA for only 1 hr was apparently sufficient to generate maximal response. If confirmed, these results suggest the rapidity of initiation and continual maintenance of the intracellular events in signal transduction.

A study of the agents that down-regulate TCGF synthesis (Larsson,

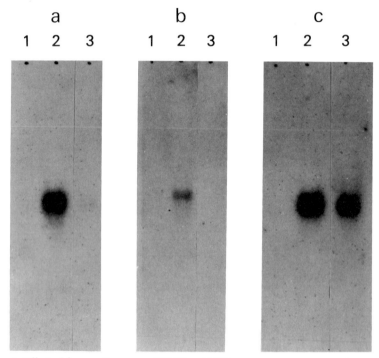

FIG. 4. Effect of dexamethasone on TCGF and IFN-γ gene transcription in human PBL and Jurkat cells. (a) TCGF mRNA in induced PBL; (b) IFN-γ mRNA in induced PBL; (c) TCGF mRNA in induced Jurkat cells. Lanes 1–3 are for uninduced cells, induced cells, and induced cells treated with dexamethasone, respectively. Adopted from Arya *et al.* (1984c). Reprinted with permission of *Biochemistry*, Copyright 1984, American Chemical Society.

1980) forms a useful adjunct in understanding gene regulation. We have investigated the effect of anti-inflammatory glucocorticoids and immunosuppressive cyclosporins on the TCGF gene expression. Both of these drugs inhibit TCGF gene transcription in PBL (Arya *et al.*, 1984c; Kronke *et al.*, 1984). Significantly, a glucocorticoid, dexamethasone, also inhibits the expression of the IFN-γ gene (Fig. 4). This dual effect of glucocorticoids on TCGF and IFN-γ gene expression may underlie or contribute to its anti-inflammatory and immunosuppressive effects *in vivo*. Surprisingly, dexamethasone did not inhibit TCGF gene expression in Jurkat cells which was not related to the presence or absence of the receptors for this hormone (Arya *et al.*, 1984c). Though other explanations are possible, these results may reflect subtle differences in the organization and/or inducibility of the TCGF gene in normal and leukemic cells.

FIG. 5. Expression of TCGF gene in HTLV-I-infected cells. Lanes 1–14 are as follows: 1, PHA plus TPA-stimulated Jurkat cells; 2, TCGF-independent HuT 78 cells, 3, TCGF-independent HuT 102 cells; 4, another preparation of TCGF-independent HuT 102 cells; 5, TCGF-independent C5/MJ cells; 6, TCGF-dependent C5/MJ cells; 7, TCGF-independent C10/MJ cells; 8, TCGF-dependent C5/MJ cells treated with TPA–PHA; 9, TCGF-independent B2/UK cells; 10, TCGF-independent B2/UK cells treated with TPA–PHA; 11, TCGF-independent MT-2 cells; 12, TCGF-dependent M1 cells; 13, TCGF-independent Mo cells; and 14, TCGF-independent MOLT-4 cells (immature T). Adopted from Arya *et al.* (1984b), with permission of *Science*, Volume **223**, pp. 927–930, Copyright 1984 by the AAAS.

The above studies clearly establish that TCGF gene expression is first and foremost regulated at the level of gene transcription. This allows us to quantitatively evaluate the basis for the autonomous growth of the HTLV-I-infected T cell lines. If these cells utilize autostimulation or parastimulation mechanisms of growth control, we should be able to detect TCGF mRNA in these cells with a sensitive Northern blot analysis utilizing a cloned TCGF probe. This would be true regardless of whether or not these cells release TCGF which they might synthesize into the medium. Our analysis of HTLV-I-infected cells has not provided any evidence for active TCGF gene transcription either constitutive or subsequent to induction with PHA and TPA in many of these cells (Fig. 5; Table I) (Arya *et al.*, 1984b). The only exceptions thus far have been the HTLV-I-infected HuT 102 cells which synthesize, at times, barely detectable TCGF mRNA, and HTLV-II-infected Mo cell line which we have not investigated in detail. We conclude that most of the HTLV-I-infected cell lines are truly independent of TCGF for growth. Curiously, HTLV-I-infected cells invariably display abundant membrane receptors for TCGF (Popovic *et al.*, 1983b; Mann *et al.*, 1983). But since these cells do not produce the ligand, TCGF, they bypass the TCGF pathway of growth control. Viewed from a different perspective, the TCGF-independent growth of these cells may precisely be among the reasons underlying their immortalization.

In contrast to the TCGF gene, the transcripts of the IFN-γ gene are readily detected in many of the HTLV-I infected cells, and abundance of

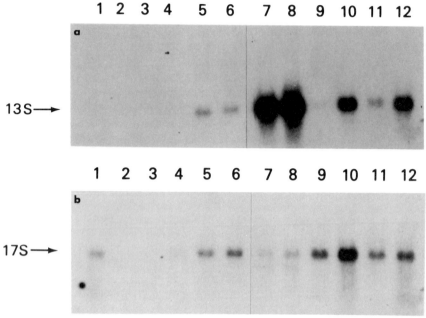

FIG. 6. Expression of IFN-γ gene (a) and *JD15* gene (b) in HTLV-infected cells. Lanes 1–12 contain the same RNAs as lanes 1–12 in Fig. 5. Adopted from Arya *et al.* (1984b), with permission of *Science*, Volume **223**, pp. 927–930, Copyright 1984 by the AAAS.

these transcripts is increased by inducing the cells with PHA and TPA (Fig. 6a) (Arya *et al.*, 1984b). Thus, while the TCGF gene is inactive, the IFN-γ gene is transcriptionally active and inducible in these cells. The case for another human T cell-specific and inducible gene (termed *JD15*), which is also transcriptionally active and inducible (Fig. 6b) (Arya *et al.*, 1984d), is similar. The lack of expression and inducibility of TCGF in these cells is thus specific to TCGF and not a result of a more widespread transcriptional repression related to HTLV-I infection (Table I).

The more recent isolation of the AIDS virus (HTLV-III/LAV) (Popovic *et al.*, 1984; Salahuddin *et al.*, 1985; Barre-Sinoussi *et al.*, 1983) has allowed us to extend our studies on the impact of retrovirus infection on lymphokine gene expression in human T cells. HTLV-III, like HTLV-I and II, is clearly T lymphotropic and shares some structural and biological similarities with HTLV–BLV group of retroviruses (Arya *et al.*, 1984a; Hahn *et al.*, 1984; Ratner *et al.*, 1985; Muesing *et al.* 1985; Wain-Hobson *et al.*, 1985; Sanchez-Pescador *et al.*, 1985; Sodroski *et al.*, 1985; Starcich *et al.*, 1985b). However, HTLV-III also differs from other HTLVs in possesssing two novel genes, *sor* (short open-reading frame) and 3'-orf (3'-open-reading frame), which may impart different biological attributes to HTLV-III than HTLV-I (Arya et al., 1985; Arya and Gallo, 1986). In fact, HTLV-III and HTLV-I have different effects on human T cells. Whereas HTLV-I is generally transforming, HTLV-III is usually cytopathic. It is this cytopathology of HTLV-III which largely underlies immune deficiency in AIDS. We thought that T cell depletion in AIDS may be due to the diminished production of TCGF by infected cells resulting in the starvation of T cells for their growth factor. The analysis of cultured HTLV-III infected cells has, however, shown that TCGF gene expression and TCGF production are not impaired in these cells (Fig. 7) (Arya and Gallo, 1985). The induction of TCGF gene expression by PHA and TPA in these cells is again a consequence of the transcriptional activation of the TCGF gene as demonstrated by nuclear transcrip-

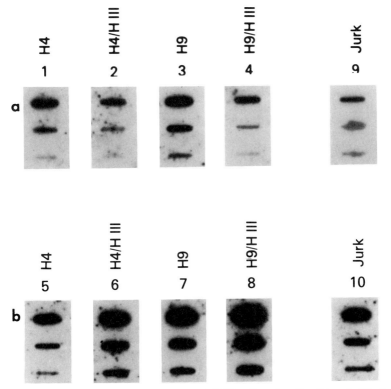

FIG. 7. Expression of TCGF gene in HTLV-III infected cells. H4 and H9 denote uninfected cells and H4/HIII and H9/HIII are the corresponding infected cells. a, Uninduced; b, induced; Jurk, Jurkat cells. Adopted from Arya and Gallo (1985a).

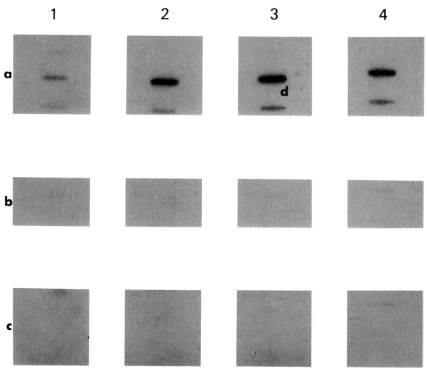

FIG. 8. Analysis of nuclear transcripts of TCGF gene from uninduced and induced HTLV-III-infected H4 cells. (a) pTCGF; (b) pIFN-γ; (c) pBR. Lane 1, uninduced cells; lane 2, cells induced with PHA; lane 3, cells induced with TPA; lane 4, cells induced with PHA plus TPA. Adopted from Arya and Gallo (1985a).

tion experiments (Fig. 8). Perhaps significantly, the induced levels of TCGF mRNA in HTLV-III-infected T cells were measurably higher than in uninfected cells, while the reverse may be the case for uninduced mRNA levels. This aspect requires further close scrutiny as it may indicate subtle differences in the regulation of TCGF gene expression in HTLV-III-infected cells. For the present, it appears that HTLV-III infection per se does not abrogate TCGF gene expression and induction. Similar observations have been made for HTLV-III-positive T cells cultured directly from the lymphocytes of AIDS patients (D. Zagury *et al.*, personal communication). It is thus likely that T cell depletion in AIDS is due to factors other than the unavailability of TCGF. On the other hand, unregulated production of TCGF by HTLV-III-infected cells may directly or indirectly affect T cell proliferation and functions.

In contrast to the TCGF gene, the IFN-γ gene in HTLV-III-infected cells is transcriptionally inactive and uninducible as is the case for the counterpart uninfected cells (Arya and Gallo, 1985). This is specific for the IFN-γ gene as, like the TCGF gene, the human T cell-specific *JD15* gene is transcriptionally active and inducible (Table I). It is notable that the TCGF gene is active in HTLV-III-infected cells but not in HTLV-I-infected cells, and the IFN-γ gene is active in HTLV-I-infected cells but not in HTLV-III-infected cells. The hypothesis has been advanced that TCGF stimulates the synthesis of IFN-γ in T cells as a part of a cascading network of lymphokine synthesis and function (Farrar *et al.*, 1982; Kasahara *et al.*, 1983; Reem and Yeh, 1984). Of the several human T cell lines we have examined, we have yet to encounter a cell line where both the TCGF and IFN-γ genes are transcriptionally active or inducible. Our consistent finding is that if the TCGF gene is transcribed, the IFN-γ gene is not, and vice versa. Clearly, the expression of these two genes is not necessarily linked or coupled. The only exception is the cultures of human PBL, but these cultures contain mixed populations of cells and we cannot rule out that subpopulations of cells are not independently induced to produce TCGF and IFN-γ. A recent report shows that some cultures of Jurkat and HuT 78 cells can be induced to synthesize both TCGF and IFN-γ mRNAs, suggesting coordinate regulation of the two genes (Wiskocil *et al.*, 1985). These results are obviously at variance with our findings (Table I). These observations again stress the importance of analyzing defined populations of cells. Many variant populations of Jurkat and HuT 78 cells exist, and we suspect that the phenotypic behavior of both Jurkat and HuT 78 cells can change during prolonged cultivation, presumably due to generational aging of the cells. If both TCGF and IFN-γ genes are active in some cultures, convincing evidence of the uniformity of the population may be needed. Even the data in this report do not support the notion that TCGF stimulates the synthesis of IFN-γ, as the authors point out (Wiskocil *et al.*, 1985).

IV. Organization and Control of the TCGF Gene

The lack of expression and inducibility of the TCGF gene in HTLV-I-infected cells poses the question, "How is this gene turned off in these cells?" This is not due to some general consequence of the retrovirus infection of T cells as this gene is expressed and inducible in HTLV-III-infected cells. It is also unlikely to be due to a direct and *in cis* down-regulation of the TCGF gene by HTLV-I genome, since HTLV-I integrates into the cell genome randomly at multiple and different sites in different infected cells. As a guide to further exploration, we postulate two broad possible mechanisms: (1) the TCGF gene is structured and chromasomally organized differently in HTLV-I-infected cells than in normal and other inducible cells; and (2) the transduced intracellular events that control the inducibility of TCGF gene are impaired in HTLV-I-infected cells. Viewed from a different perspective, we can postulate that lymphokine expression in T cells is a differentiation state-specific and/or cell cycle-specific phenomenon. We can further postulate that HTLV fixes the state of genetic expression of a cell at the time of the establishment of infection. We now need only to postulate that HTLV-I infection occurs when the TCGF gene is not expressed but the IFN-γ gene is expressed; conversely, HTLV-III infection occurs when the TCGF gene is in the expression mode and the IFN-γ gene is not.

We have shown that the TCGF gene exists as a single copy gene in normal, HTLV-I-, and HTLV-III-infected, or uninfected cells (Clark *et al.*, 1984; S. K. Arya, unpublished results). Others have made similar observations for other cell types (Holbrook *et al.*, 1984a). This is consistent with a single location of the TCGF gene on human chromosome 4q (Siegel *et al.*, 1984). We have not detected, at the level of restriction enzyme site mapping, any difference in the organization of the TCGF gene in HTLV-I-infected cells or from a variety of other cells, including HTLV-III-infected cells (Fig. 9). Thus, no rearrangement or polymorphism of the TCGF gene is detectable in producer and nonproducer cells at this level. This does not rule out subtle differences in the struc-

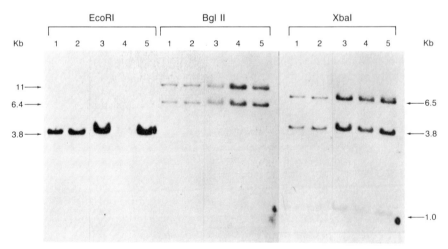

FIG. 9. Organization of TCGF gene in human cells. Lanes 1–5 are for DNA from normal PBL, leukemic Jurkat cells, HTLV-I-infected HuT 102 cells, HTLV-II-infected Mo cells, and HTLV-III-infected H9 cells, respectively.

ture and organization of the gene in HTLV-I-infected and normal cells. We need to undertake comparison at the DNA sequence level.

Genomic TCGF clones from normal human cells (PBL) have been obtained and their DNA sequence reported (Fujita *et al.*, 1983; Holbrook *et al.*, 1984a). The gene consists of four exons and three introns of varying lengths (Fig. 10). The first exon contains the 5′ untranslated region (47 bp) and codes for the first 49 amino acids (147 bp) of the protein, including 20 amino acids of signal peptide. The second and third exons encode the next 20 and 48 amino acids (60 and 144 bp), respectively. The fourth exon codes for the last 36 amino acids (108 bp) of the carboxy-terminus and also contains 216 bp of the 3′ untranslated sequence. The first, second, and third introns are, respectively, 91, 2292, and 1364 bp long. Thus, the gene encoding the 133-amino acid (399-bp) mature TCGF protein is distributed over about 5 kb of DNA length. The computer searches of the gene data banks for sequence homologies have revealed regions of TCGF gene with some homology to the core sequence of viral enhancer elements and the IFN-γ gene (Fujita *et al.*, 1983), to HTLV-I LTR (Holbrook *et al.*, 1984b), and to HTLV-III LTR (Starcich *et al.*, 1985a) (Fig. 11). The biological significance of these homologies in gene expression and cell-type specificity remains unknown.

We have now obtained TCGF genomic clones from HTLV-I-positive leukemic cells. We have not yet determined the nucleotide sequences of these clones and compared them with those of normal clones. The overall structural organization and restriction site maps of the leukemic clones are, however, identical to the normal clones, but the final word must await complete DNA sequence determination.

Alternative to structural difference is the difference in the intracellular events that control the expression and induction of the TCGF gene in HTLV-I-infected cells. We are now investigating this possiblity. A simple version of the model guiding our thinking is presented in Fig. 12. We suppose that the TCGF gene contains both positive regulatory sequence (enhancer–promoter) and negative regulatory sequence (repressor–abrogator) elements. The interaction of certain effectors with positive regulatory sequence enhances gene transcription, and interaction with negative regulatory sequence results in the abrogation of transcription. The balance between these interactions governs the transcription of the gene. We assume that inducing agents operate by transducing signals through intracellular effector molecules. While in normal cells, the positive regulatory interactions are functional,, but these interactions may not be functional, or may be dominated by negative regulatory interactions, in HTLV-I-infected cells. These notions are experimentally

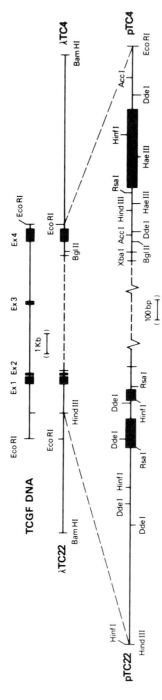

FIG. 10. Physical map of TCGF DNA and genomic clones from leukemic cells. See text for discussion.

```
TCGF      -1221  CACAAGTCTGTAAGACTTATATT--AGACTAAG  -1191
                 ||  |||||||| ||     |  |    |||||||||
HTLV-I     -281  CAGAAGTCTGAAAAGGTCAGGGCCCAGACTAAG  -249


TCGF        -24  TATAAATTGCATCTCTTGTTCAAGAG  +2
                 ||||||  |||||||||  ||||  | |
HTLV-I      -29  TATAAA--GCATCTCTCCTTCACGCG  -4


TCGF       +853  AC-CTAC-TCTGTTTGTGATTCAGTTT  +877
                 ||  |||| |||    |||   |||  ||||
HTLV-I      +71  ACTCTACGTCT--TTGT--TTC-GTTT  +93


TCGF       -292  AAAGAAAGGAG GAAAAACTGTTTCATACA  -264
                 ||   |||||||| |||  |  | |||     ||||
HTLV-III   -275  AAT-AAAGGAGAGAACACCAGCTTGTTACA  -246


TCGF      +1225  AGTTGTGCCAGTTAAGAGAGAATGAA  +1250
                 |||||| |||||  ||||  ||||   |||
HTLV-III   -302  AGTTGAGCCAGAGAAGATAGAA GAA  -259
```

FIG. 11. TCGF genomic regions homologous to HTLV-I and HTLV-III LTRs.

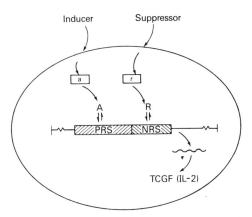

FIG. 12. A simple version of the model for TCGF gene regulation. PRS, Positive regulatory sequence; NRS, negative regulatory sequence.

testable in an *in vitro* transcriptional system using cloned TCGF DNAs with their regulatory sequences and introducing specific soluble factors from normal and HTLV-I-infected or other noninducible cells. Of course, the situation may be, and is likely to be, more complex than depicted, but elements of complexity can readily be added to this model.

In summary, the TCGF gene is an inducible lymphokine gene which exists as a single copy gene in all cell types examined. Its expression is primarily regulated at the level of gene transcription. Though other factors may play a role, they are secondary to the induced transcriptional activation of the gene. The molecular basis of the lack of expression and induction of the TCGF gene in HTLV-I-infected T cells remains to be explained, especially in light of the fact that this gene is transcriptionally active and inducible in HTLV-III-infected T cells. It is paradoxical that the TCGF gene in HTLV-I-infected cells which are immortal is inactive, while the TCGF gene in HTLV-III-infected cells which are prone to cell death is active. The case for the IFN-γ is equally intriguing. It is transcriptionally active in HTLV-I-infected cells but not in HTLV-III-infected cells. A convincing case for the coupled expression of these two lymphokine genes remains to be made. The molecular events in the transduction of extracellular events into intracellular signals influencing lymphokine gene expression are yet a mystery. The fundamentals of regulatory circuits involving these lymphokines in immune regulation are far from understood.

REFERENCES

Arya, S. K. (1980). *Nature (London)* **284**, 71–72.
Arya, S. K., and Gallo, R. C. (1984). *Biochemistry* **23**, 6690–6696.
Arya, S. K., and Gallo, R. C. (1985a). *Proc. Natl. Acad. Sci. U.S.A.*, **82**, 8691–8695.
Arya, S. K., and Gallo, R. C. (1985b). *Proc. Natl. Acad. Sci. U.S.A.* **83**, 2209–2213.
Arya, S. K., Gallo, R. C., Hahn, B. H., Shaw, G. M., Popovic, M., Salahuddin, S. Z., and Wong-Staal, F. (1984a). *Science* **225**, 927–930.
Arya, S. K., Wong-Staal, F., and Gallo, R. C. (1984b). *Science* **223**, 1086–1087.
Arya, S. K., Wong-Staal, F., and Gallo, R. C. (1984c). *J. Immunol.* **133**, 273–276.
Arya, S. K., Wong-Staal, F., and Gallo, R. C. (1984d). *Mol. Cell. Biol.* **4**, 2540–2542.
Arya, S. K., Chan, G., Josephs, S. F., and Wong-Staal, F. (1985). *Science* **229**, 69–73.
Barre-Sinoussi, F., Chermann, J. C., Rey, F., Nugeyre, M. T., Chamaret, S., Gruest, J., Dauguet, C., Axler-Blin, C., Vezinet-Brun, F., Rouzioux, C., Rosenbaum, W., and Montagnier, L. (1983). *Science* **220**, 868–870.
Clark, S. C., Arya, S. K., Wong-Staal, F., Matsumoto-Kobayashi, M., Kay, R. M., Kaufman, R. J., Brown, E. L., Shoemaker, C., Copeland, T., Oroszlan, S., Smith, K., Sarngadharan, M. G., Lindner, S. G., and Gallo, R. C. (1984). *Proc. Natl. Acad. Sci. U.S.A.* **81**, 2543–2547.
Devos, R., Plaetinck, G., Cheroutre, H., Simons, G., Degrave, W., Tavernier, J., Remaut, E., and Fiers, W. (1983). *Nucleic Acids Res.* **11**, 4307–4322.
Efrat, S., and Kaempfer, R. (1984). *Proc. Natl. Acad. Sci. U.S.A.* **81**, 2601–2605.

Efrat, S., Pilo, S., and Kaempfer, R. (1982). *Nature (London)* **297**, 236–239.

Farrar, J. J., Benjamin, W. R., Hilfiker, M. L., Howard, M., Farrar, W. L., and Fuller-Farrar, J. (1982). *Immunol. Rev.* **63**, 129–166.

Fujita, T., Takaoka, C., Matsui, H., and Taniguchi, T. (1983). *Proc. Natl. Acad. Sci. U.S.A.* **80**, 7437–7441.

Gallo, R. C., Mann, D., Broder, S., Ruscetti, F. W., Maeda, M., Kalyanavaman, V. S., Robert-Guroff, M., and Reitz, M. S., Jr. (1982). *Proc. Natl. Acad. Sci. U.S.A.* **79**, 5680–5683.

Gallo, R. C., Essex, M., and Gross, L., eds. (1984a). *In* "Human T-Cell Leukemia/Lymphoma Virus." Cold Spring Harbor Laboratory, Cold Spring Harbor, New York.

Gallo, R. C., Salahuddin, S. Z., Popovic, M., Shearer, G. M., Kaplan, M., Haynes, B. F., Palker, T. J., Redfield, R., Okeske, J., Safai, B., White, C., Foster, P., and Markham, P. D. (1984b). *Science* **224**, 500–503.

Gallo, R. C., Arya, S. K., Lindner, S. G., Wong-Staal, F., and Sarngadharan, M. G. (1984c). *In* "Thymic Hormones and Lymphokines" (A. L. Goldstein, ed.), pp. 1–17. Plenum, New York.

Gillis, S., and Smith, K. A. (1977). *Nature (London)* **268**, 154–155.

Gillis, S., and Watson, J. (1980). *J. Exp. Med.* **152**, 1709–1719.

Grimm, E. A., Robb, R. J., and Roth, J. A., Neckers, L. M., Lachman, L. B., Wilson, D. J., and Rosenberg, S. A. (1983). *J. Exp. Med.* **158**, 1356–1361.

Gootenberg, J. E., Ruscetti, F. W., Mier, J. W., Gazdar, A., and Gallo, R. C. (1981). *J. Exp. Med.* **154**, 1403–1418.

Gootenberg, J. E., Ruscetti, F. W., and Gallo, R. C. (1982). *J. Immunol.* **129**, 1499–1502.

Hahn, B., Shaw, G. M., Arya, S. K., Popovic, M., Gallo, R. C., and Wong-Staal, F. (1984). *Nature (London)* **312**, 166–169.

Holbrook, N., Smith, K. A., Fornace, A. J., Comean, C., Wiskocil, R. L., and Crabtree, G. R. (1984a). *Proc. Natl. Acad. Sci. U.S.A.* **81**, 1634–1638.

Holbrook, N. J., Lieber, M., and Crabtree, G. R. (1984b). *Nucleic Acids Res.* **12**, 5005–5013.

Howard, M., Mates, L., Malek, T. R., Shevach, E., Kell, W., Cohn, P., Nakanishi, K., and Paul, W. E., (1983). *J. Exp. Med.* **158**, 2024–2039.

Jung, L., Hara, T., and Fu, S. M. (1984). *J. Exp. Med.* **160**, 1597–1602.

Kalyanaraman, V. S., Sarngadharan, M. G., Robert-Guroff, M., Miyoshi, I., Blayncy, D., Golde, D., and Gallo, R. C. (1982). *Science* **218**, 571–573.

Kasahara, T., Hooks, J. J., Dougherty, S. F., and Oppenheim, J. J. (1983). *J. Immunol.* **130**, 1784–1787.

Kronke, M., Leonard, W. J., Depper, J. M., Arya, S. K., Wong-Staal, F., Gallo, R. C., Waldmann, T. A., and Greene, W. C. (1984). *Proc. Natl. Acad. Sci. U.S.A.* **81**, 5214–5218.

Larsson, E. L. (1980). *J. Immunol.* **124**, 2828–2835.

Larsson, E. L., Iscove, N. N., and Coutinho, A. (1980). *Nature (London)* **283**, 664–666.

Lotze, M. T., Strausser, J. L., and Rosenberg, S. A. (1980). *J. Immunol.* **124**, 2972–2978.

Mann, D. L., Popovic, M., Murray, C., Neuland, C., Strong, D. M., Sarin, P., Gallo, R. C., and Blattner, W. A. (1983). *J. Immunol.* **131**, 2021–2024.

Miedema, F., van Oostreen, J. W., Saurwein, R. W., Terpestra, F. G., Aarden, L. A., and Melief, C. J. (1965). *Eur. J. Immunol.* **15**, 107–112.

Mier, J. W., and Gallo, R. C. (1980). *Proc. Natl. Acad. Sci. U.S.A.* **77**, 6134–6138.

Miyoshi, I., Kubonishi, I., Yoshimoto, S., Akagi, T., Ohtsuki, Y., Shiraishi, Y., Nagato, K., and Hinuma, Y. (1981). *Nature (London)* **294**, 770–771.

Moretta, A. (1985). *Eur. J. Immunol.* **15**, 148–155.

Morgan, D. A., Ruscetti, F. W., and Gallo, R. C. (1976). *Science* **193**, 1007–1008.

Muesing, M. A., Smith, D. H., Cabradilla, C. D., Benton, C. V., Lasky, L. A., and Capon, D. J. (1985). *Nature (London)* **313**, 450–458.

Nakagawa, T., Hirano, T., Nakagawa, N., Yoshizaki, K., and Kishmoto, T. (1985). *J. Immunol.* **134**, 959–965.

Palacios, R. (1982). *Immunol. Rev.* **63**, 73–110.

Poiesz, B. J., Ruscetti, F. W., Gazdar, A. F., Bunn, P. A., Minna, J. D., and Gallo, R. C. (1980). *Proc. Natl. Acad. Sci. U.S.A.* **77**, 7415–7419.

Poiesz, B. J., Ruscetti, F. W., Reitz, M. S., Kalyanaraman, V. S., and Gallo, R. C. (1981). *Nature (London)* **294**, 268–271.

Popovic, M., Sarin, P. S., Robert-Guroff, M., Kalayanayaman, V. S., Mann, D., Minnowada, J., and Gallo, R. C. (1983a). *Science* **219**, 850–859.

Popovic, M., Lange-Wantzin, G., Sarin, P. S., Mann, D., and Gallo, R. C. (1983b). *Proc. Natl. Acad. Sci. U.S.A.* **80**, 5402–5406.

Popovic, M., Sarngadharan, M. G., Read, E., and Gallo, R. C. (1984). *Science* **224**, 497–500.

Ralph, P., Jeong, G., Welte, K., Mertelsmann, R., Rabin, H., Henderson, L. E., Souza, L. M., Boon, T. C., and Robb, R. J. (1984). *J. Immunol.* **133**, 2442–2245.

Ratner, L., Haseltine, W., Patarca, R., Livak, K. J., Starcich, B., Josephs, S. F., Doran, E. R., Rafalski, J. A., Whitehorn, E. A., Baumeister, K., Ivanoff, L., Petteway, S. R., Pearson, M. L., Lautenberger, J. A., Papas, T. S., Ghrayeb, J., Chang, N. T., Gallo, R. C., and Wong-Staal, F. (1985). *Nature (London)* **313**, 227–284.

Reem, G., and Yeh, N. H. (1984). *Science* **225**, 429–430.

Robb, R. J., Kutny, R. M., and Chowdhry, V. (1983). *Proc. Natl. Acad. Sci. U.S.A.* **80**, 5990–5994.

Robb, R. J., Kutny, R. M., Panico, M., Morris, H. R., and Chowdhry, V. (1984). *Proc. Natl. Acad. Sci. U.S.A.* **81**, 6486–6490.

Rosenberg, S. A., Grimm, E. A., Lotze, M. T., and Muzunder, A. (1982). *Lymphokines* **1**, 213–248.

Ruscetti, F. W., and Gallo, R. C. (1981). *Blood* **57**, 379–394.

Ruscetti, F. W., Morgan, D. A., and Gallo, R. C. (1977). *J. Immunol.* **119**, 131–138.

Salahuddin, S. Z., Markham, M., Popovic, M., Sarngadharan, M. G., Orndorff, S., Flandagar, A., Patel, A., Gold, J., and Gallo, R. C. (1985). *Proc. Natl. Acad. Sci. U.S.A.* **82**, 5530–5534.

Sanchez-Pescador, R., Power, M. D., Barr, P. J., Steimer, K. S., Stempien, M. M., Brown-Shimer, S. L., Gee, W. W., Renard, A., Randolph, A., Levy, J. A., Dina, D., and Luciw, P. A. (1985). *Science* **227**, 484–492.

Sarngadharan, M. G., Popovic, M., Bruch, L., Schupbach, J., and Gallo, R. C. (1984). *Science* **224**, 506–508.

Schrier, M. H., and Iscove, N. N. (1980). *Nature (London)* **287**, 229–232.

Schrier, M. H., Iscove, N. N., Tees, R., Aardon, L., and von Boehmer, H. (1980). *Immunol. Rev.* **51**, 314–336.

Schupbach, J., Popovic, M., Gilden, R. V., Gonda, M. A., Sarngadharan, M. G., and Gallo, R. C. (1984). *Science* **224**, 503–504.

Shaw, G. M., Hahn, B. H., Arya, S. K., Groopman, J. E., Gallo, R. C., and Wong-Staal, F. (1984). *Science* **226**, 1165–1171.

Siegel, L. J., Harper, M. E., Wong-Staal, F., Gallo, R. C., Nash, W. G., and O'Brien, S. J. (1984). *Science* **223**, 175–178.

Smith, K. A. (1980). *Immunol. Rev.* **51**, 337–356.

Sodroski, J., Rosen, C., Wong-Staal, F., Popovic, M., Arya, S. K., Gallo, R. C., and Haseltine, W. A. (1985). *Science* **227**, 171–173.

Starcich, B., Hahn, B. H., Shaw, G. M., McNeely, P. D., Modrow, S., Wolf, H., Parks, E. S., Parks, W. P., Josephs, S. F., Gallo, R. C., and Wong-Staal, F. (1986). *Cell* **45**, 637–648.

Starcich, B., Ratner, L., Josephs, S. F., Okamoto, T., Gallo, R. C., and Wong-Staal, F. (1985). *Science* **227**, 538–540.

Taniguchi, T., Matsui, H., Fujita, T., Takaoka, C., Kashima, N., Yoshimoto, R., and Hamuro, J. (1983). *Nature (London)* **301**, 306–310.

Tsudo, M., Uchiyama, T., and Uchino, H. (1984). *J. Exp. Med.* **160**, 612–617.

von Boehmer, H., and Haas, W. (1981). *Immunol. Rev.* **54**, 27–56.

Wain-Hobson, S., Sonigo, P., Danos, O., Cole, S., and Alizon, M. (1985). *Cell* **40**, 9–17.

Waldmann, T. A., Goldman, C. K., Robb, R. J., Depper, J. M., Leonard, W. J., Sharrow, S. O., Bongiovanni, K. F., Korsmeyer, S. J., and Greene, W. C. (1984). *J. Exp. Med.* **160**, 1450–1466.

Wiskocil, R., Weiss, A., Imboden, J., Kamin-Lewis, R., and Stobo, J. (1985). *J. Immunol.* **134**, 1599–1603.

Yoshida, M., Miyoshi, I., and Hinuma, Y. (1982). *Proc. Natl. Acad. Sci. U.S.A.* **79**, 2031–2134.

Regulation of Human Interleukin 2 Gene Expression

RAYMOND KAEMPFER, SHIMON EFRAT, AND SUSAN MARSH

Department of Molecular Virology, The Hebrew University-Hadassah Medical School, 91010
Jerusalem, Israel

I. Introduction

Interleukin 2 (IL-2), or T cell growth factor, is an inducible lympho-kine produced by T cells upon antigenic or mitogenic stimulation (Morgan *et al.*, 1976; Gillis and Smith, 1977; Gillis *et al.*, 1978a). This key immunoregulatory protein is absolutely required for the proliferation of activated T cells of various types (Gillis *et al.*, 1978b; Zarling and Bach, 1979; Tees and Schreier, 1980; Henney *et al.*, 1981). It is thought that the strength of the immune response is determined to a large extent by the amount of IL-2 made available for T cell growth in response to a stimulus (Gillis and Smith, 1977; Andersson *et al.*, 1979; Smith, 1981). Study of the control of IL-2 gene expression is, therefore, of direct relevance to understanding the molecular basis for the regulation of the strength of the immune response.

We show here that induction of the human gene encoding interleukin 2 (IL-2) leads to the appearance of a brief wave of IL-2 mRNA. *De novo* synthesis of IL-2 mRNA molecules is followed promptly by cessation of transcription and decay of mRNA sequences (half-life, about 15 hr). IL-2 mRNA activity, quantitated by microinjection analysis, appears coordinately with IL-2 mRNA sequences, quantitated by Northern blotting, and IL-2 synthesis by the lymphocytes; thus, translational control does not determine the observed wave of IL-2 mRNA. Formation of IL-2 mRNA is tightly controlled by the early appearance of a labile protein repressor whose neutralization by any one of a series of translation inhibitors causes extensive (up to 60-fold) superinduction of both IL-2 mRNA in tonsil cells and IL-2 in the culture medium. Superinduction of the human IL-2 gene is not accompanied by any increase in primary transcription or in the stability of IL-2 mRNA. Instead, superinduction conditions cause a greatly increased flow of large IL-2 RNA precursors into mature IL-2 mRNA molecules. Our data support the concept that IL-2 gene expression in human T cells is controlled at transcription and, in addition, by a labile repressor that acts posttranscriptionally to reduce, by up to 98%, the processing of IL-2 mRNA precursors. This labile repressor mechanism determines the magnitude of the IL-2 mRNA wave over an approximately 50-fold range and, thereby, the strength of the

59

eventual IL-2 signal in the immune response. Normally, the human IL-2 gene is, therefore, expressed to only about 2% of its potential. This mode of regulation by a labile repressor allows for dramatic up-regulation of the gene within a short time span.

II. Results and Discussion

A. INDUCTION AND SHUTOFF OF BIOLOGICALLY ACTIVE IL-2 mRNA FORMATION

Figure 1A depicts the kinetics of accumulation of mRNA encoding IL-2 in human tonsil lymphocytes cultured in the presence of the mitogen, phytohemagglutinin (PHA). In this experiment, total mRNA was isolated from the cells at the time intervals and microinjected at a constant concentration into oocytes of *Xenopus laevis* (Efrat *et al.*, 1982; Efrat and Kaempfer, 1984a,b). It is evident that the appearance of IL-2 mRNA during induction is followed by a prompt shutoff, giving rise to a wave of IL-2 mRNA activity in the induced lymphocytes.

When DRB (5,6-dichloro-1-β-D-ribofuranosylbenzimidazole), a reversible inhibitor of primary transcription, was present from 4 hr of induction, little, if any, IL-2 mRNA activity appeared up to 22 hr of induction (Fig. 1A). Induction of IL-2 mRNA activity thus involves synthesis of new mRNA molecules. DRB. when added at 20 hr, did not significantly affect the rate of decline of IL-2 mRNA activity (Fig. 1A), showing that little, if any, synthesis of additional active IL-2 mRNA takes place during the decline period. Therefore, this decline is the result of an inactivation or breakdown process only. The functional half-life of human IL-2 mRNA may be estimated from the upper curve of Fig. 1A at about 15–20 hr.

In Fig. 1B, the expected accumulation of IL-2 activity during induction, predicted from the amount of active IL-2 mRNA present in the cell during successive time intervals in Fig. 1A, is compared with the accumulation of IL-2 activity actually observed in the medium. The extremely close correspondence between predicted and observed values shows that the mRNA levels quantitated by the method used in Fig. 1A accurately reflect intracellular concentrations of active IL-2 mRNA. Since IL-2 synthesis by lymphocytes is precisely that predicted from active mRNA levels, translational control does not determine the observed wave of IL-2 mRNA.

B. SUPERINDUCTION OF IL-2 AND IL-2 mRNA

To examine the nature of the mechanisms that regulate the level of IL-2 mRNA activity, induction was studied in the presence of reversible

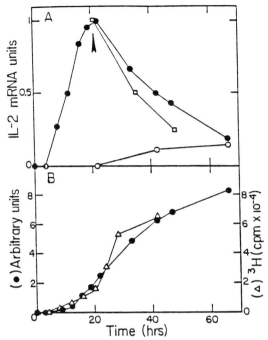

FIG. 1. Kinetics of accumulation of IL-2 mRNA during induction of human tonsil lymphocytes (oocyte micoinjection analysis). (A) Induction. (●) Normal induction, (○) induction with DRB (40 μM) added at 4 hr, (□) induction with DRB added at 21 hr (arrow). (B) Comparison between expected accumulation curve of IL-2 activity, calculated from the mRNA values in A (●), and actual IL-2 activity in conditioned medium (△). From Efrat and Kaempfer (1984a).

inhibitors of macromolecule synthesis. Accumulation of IL-2 activity was followed in cell cultures that had been preincubated for 20 hr in the presence of PHA and then transferred to fresh medium lacking PHA. Cycloheximide (CHX) and/or DRB were included during part of the preincubation period, and their effect on the accumulation of IL-2-encoding capacity was assessed upon their removal at the end of the preincubation period when expression of this capacity was allowed in fresh medium.

Figure 2 depicts the kinetics of accumulation of IL-2 activity under various conditions of induction. The presence of CHX during the 4- to 20-hr time interval led to extensive superinduction of IL-2 relative to the control incubated only with PHA. Superinduction by CHX was manifested both by a far earlier appearance of IL-2 and by greatly increased levels; by 48 hr the extent of superinduction was about 15-fold. In spite of this great increase in IL-2 synthesis, the rate of accumulation of IL-2 in

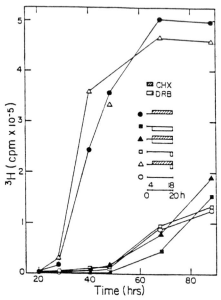

FIG. 2. Superinduction of IL-2. Cycloheximide (20 μg/ml) or DRB was added to lymphocyte cultures at 4 or 18 hr after induction as indicated. At 20 hr, all cultures were washed and the cells were resuspended in fresh PHA-free medium. At the indicated times, IL-2 activity in the medium was assayed. From Efrat and Kaempfer (1984a).

the CHX-treated culture began to decline with roughly the same kinetics as during normal induction (Fig. 1B).

When DRB was present during the 4- to 20-hr time interval, the subsequent appearance of IL-2 was delayed relative to the control. This delay might be expected because IL-2 mRNA synthesis is inhibited in the presence of DRB (Fig. 1A). Even at later times, however, there was no indication of superinduction subsequent to the removal of DRB. Indeed, the presence of DRB from 4 to 20 hr prevented almost totally the CHX-mediated superinduction, implying that superinduction depends on *de novo* transcription. When DRB was added after 18 hr of induction, it no longer affected the subsequent formation of IL-2 in normal or superinduced cell cultures.

The results of Fig. 3 show that the superinduction of IL-2 seen in the presence of CHX involves changes in the level of active IL-2 mRNA. In the presence of CHX, the amount of biologically active IL-2 mRNA increased dramatically, reaching 7.5-fold higher levels by 20 hr and 30-fold higher levels by 48 hr of induction. Note that by 8 hr, only 4 hr after addition of CHX, superinduction of IL-2 mRNA is already at least 6-fold.

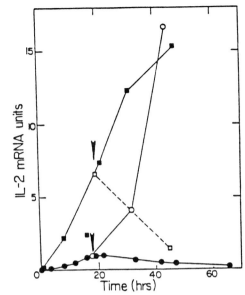

FIG. 3. Superinduction of active IL-2 mRNA. IL-2 mRNA activity was assayed by microinjection as for Fig. 1. CHX was added at 4 hr (■), at 18 hr (○) (arrow), or at 4 hr and removed at 19 hr (□) (arrow). For comparison, mRNA values for normal induction (from Fig. 1A) are plotted on the same scale (●). Note the scale change between Figs. 1A and 3. From Efrat and Kaempfer (1984a).

This implies that the CHX-sensitive mechanism starts to act early during induction.

In view of the relatively long half-life of IL-2 mRNA observed in both the presence or absence of DRB (Fig. 1A), about 15 hr, stabilization of mRNA by CHX cannot account for the observed superinduction. Even if CHX were to stabilize IL-2 mRNA completely, this would yield at most a 2-fold superinduction at late times.

In Fig. 3, the IL-2-encoding capacity of equal amounts of microinjected mRNA is measured. Clearly, CHX does not act merely by inhibiting the accumulation of non-IL-2 mRNA, for its presence led to an absolute increase in IL-2 produced in culture (Fig. 2).

When CHX was added at 18 hr, a time when shutoff of active IL-2 mRNA formation normally follows (Fig. 1A), there was an immediate and dramatic rise in IL-2 mRNA activity and neither shutoff nor decrease in mRNA level was observed (Fig. 3). Furthermore, removal of CHX at 20 hr resulted in immediate cessation of active IL-2 mRNA accumulation and a decline in mRNA level at a practically normal rate (Fig. 3).

The superinduction of active IL-2 mRNA formation in the presence of

CHX represents a true increase in active mRNA encoding IL-2, as judged by the sensitivity to anti-Tac antibody of IL-2 activity elicited by this mRNA in microinjected oocytes (Efrat and Kaempfer, 1984a).

C. SUPERINDUCTION OF IL-2 mRNA SEQUENCES: DEMONSTRATION OF TWO DISTINCT REPRESSION MECHANISMS

Apparently, IL-2 gene expression is tightly controlled by a labile protein repressor. In Fig. 4, a cloned IL-2 cDNA probe (Taniguchi *et al.*, 1983) was used to quantitate IL-2 mRNA sequences in total RNA prepared at time intervals after induction. This probe detects an RNA species migrating at about 1000 nucleotides, the expected size of IL-2 mRNA (Taniguchi *et al.*, 1983; Devos *et al.*, 1983). As seen in Fig. 4A, the presence of CHX results in an equally striking superinduction of IL-2 mRNA sequences by a factor of at least 25- to 35-fold. The extensive increase in mature IL-2 mRNA cannot be due to a pool effect since IL-2

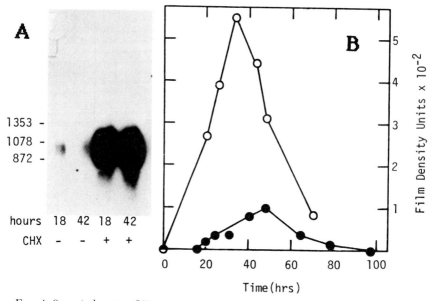

FIG. 4. Superinduction of IL-2 mRNA sequences. Human lymphocytes were induced with PHA. Where indicated CHX (20 μg/ml) was included from 4 hr onwards. At the indicated times, total RNA was extracted, subjected to formaldehyde/agarose gel electrophoresis, and blot hybridized with nick-translated, ^{32}P-labeled p3-16 DNA (specific activity 6 × 10[8] cpm/μg) carrying an insert of human IL-2 cDNA (Taniguchi *et al.*, 1983). A, Autoradiograph. B, Microdensitometric quantitation of similar RNA blots sampled at the indicated times from cultures incubated with (○) or without (●) CHX. Size markers denote nucleotide length of single-stranded φX174 RF DNA (*Hae*III digest).

mRNA sequences (Fig. 4A) and IL-2 mRNA activity (Fig. 3) rise commensurately with IL-2 production by the lymphocytes in culture (Fig. 2).

The most likely interpretation of this finding is that IL-2 gene expression is controlled over a wide range by a labile protein repressor that disappears rapidly when protein synthesis is blocked by cycloheximide. Superinduction of IL-2 mRNA activity is already evident at very early stages of induction, indicating that this repressor mechanism begins to act soon after the onset of IL-2 gene expression (Fig. 3). However, even at later stages of induction, the addition of cycloheximide results in an immediate and extensive stimulation of IL-2 mRNA formation, while its removal causes a rapid reestablishment of repression (Fig. 3). These results strongly suggest that human IL-2 gene expression is tightly controlled by the early appearance of a labile repressor whose neutralization causes extensive superinduction.

This conclusion is based on the assumption that cycloheximide exerts its action exclusively at the level of protein synthesis. Conceivably, this inhibitor could influence IL-2 mRNA formation via other processes. However, the following experiment argues against that possibility. As seen in Fig. 5, T-2 toxin, pactamycin, and sparsomycin, inhibitors that affect different stages of translation, all cause a superinduction of IL-2 mRNA sequences similar to that seen with cycloheximide (Efrat *et al.*, 1984).

Both T-2 toxin and sparsomycin inhibit peptide bond formation by affecting the acceptor site of the peptidyltransferase center in the large ribosomal unit. While sparsomycin inhibits both eukaryotic and prokaryotic ribosomes, T-2 toxin is active only on eukaryotic ones. Cycloheximide, on the other hand, blocks elongation factor 2-dependent translocation of the growing polypeptide chain in the 60 S subunit. Pactamycin, by contrast, acts at low concentrations on the small subunit of both prokaryotic and eukaryotic ribosomes to prevent positioning of Met-tRNA$_f$ into the donor site during initiation of protein synthesis (see Efrat *et al.*, 1984). In this experiment, cycloheximide yielded an 8-fold superinduction of IL-2 mRNA. The extent of superinduction of IL-2 mRNA by the other inhibitors of translation was in the same range.

The finding that four different inhibitors, each acting with distinct characteristics to inhibit translation, all result in a comparable extent of superinduction of IL-2 mRNA argues convincingly in favor of the interpretation that superinduction of the human IL-2 gene is caused by the neutralization of a labile protein that controls the formation of IL-2 mRNA.

Figure 4B depicts a kinetic analysis of IL-2 mRNA sequences present in a culture that was normally induced as compared to a culture that also

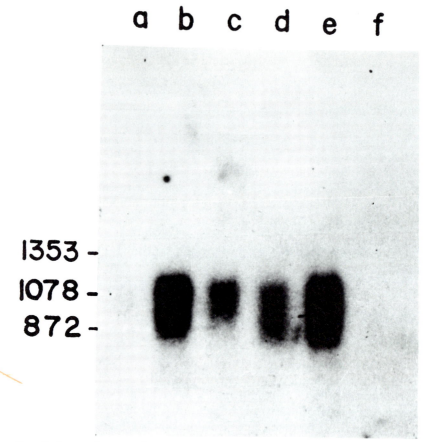

FIG. 5. Superinduction of IL-2 mRNA sequences by translation inhibitors. Human tonsillar lymphocytes were induced with PHA in culture. At 4 hr, individual cultures received no inhibitor (lane a), 20 ng/ml of T-2 toxin (lane b), 0.1 μg/ml of pactamycin (lane (c), 10 μg/ml of sparsomycin (lane d), 20 μg/ml of cycloheximide (lanes e and f), and 40 μM of DRB (lane f). The concentrations used in b–e inhibited protein synthesis to an extent of 70–85%. At 20 hr, total RNA was extracted. Of the total RNA from each culture, 50 μg was subjected to agarose gel electrophoresis, blotted onto nitrocellulose paper, and hybridized with nick-translated ^{32}P-labeled p3-16 DNA. The autoradiogram of the gel is depicted. Size markers are on left. From Efrat *et al.* (1984).

received CHX. In spite of the fact that the presence of CHX results in a pronounced superinduction of IL-2 mRNA sequences at every time tested, it is clear that the shutoff and decline observed during normal induction (Figs. 1 and 4B) also occur during superinduction (Fig. 4B).

While the general features of IL-2 gene expression are preserved in individual lymphocyte cultures, the actual timing of shutoff and the extent of superinduction are somewhat variable. The displacement in time between the peaks in Fig. 4B is due to this variability rather than to CHX treatment. Timing variation can also explain why the shutoff of IL-2 mRNA formation was not seen in the superinduced culture of Fig. 3 yet is clearly observed in the experiment of Fig. 4B.

Whether IL-2 gene expression is induced normally or is superinduced, shutoff is followed by decay of mRNA. Although cell viability does decrease after long incubations with CHX, the rate is too slow to account for the observed decay of IL-2 mRNA (Efrat and Kaempfer, 1984a); in addition, equal amounts of RNA were compared in Fig. 4. The half-life of IL-2 mRNA in this experiment is 12–15 hr, again showing that CHX does not stabilize IL-2 mRNA.

These results demonstrate the existence of two distinct repression mechanisms that regulate the accumulation of IL-2 mRNA sequences. One is sensitive to CHX, and its neutralization causes extensive superinduction. The other, apparently insensitive to CHX, is responsible for the shutoff observed both during normal induction and during superinduction. Since induction of IL-2 mRNA depends on *de novo* transcription, as shown by the inhibitory effect of DRB (Fig. 1), and since decay of translatable IL-2 mRNA after shutoff is not noticeably affected by DRB (Fig. 1), transcription apparently ceases upon shutoff. Hence, the most plausible interpretation of our findings is that the CHX-insensitive repressor mechanism acts to shut off transcription.

D. The Labile Repressor Acts Posttranscriptionally

In Fig. 4A, the striking superinduction of IL-2 mRNA sequences in the presence of CHX is not accompanied by a detectable rise in RNA sequences migrating as larger IL-2 mRNA precursors, as might have been expected if transcription were increased. Figure 6 presents direct evidence that primary transcription of the IL-2 gene in superinduced cells does not exceed that observed in normally induced cells. In this experiment, nuclear run-on transcription is quantitated in nuclei from cells induced in the presence or absence of CHX. It is seen that the extent of hybridization of IL-2 RNA molecules, labeled in nuclei from normally induced cells, to the IL-2 cDNA probe increases linearly with input radioactivity. IL-2 RNA sequences labeled in nuclei from superinduced cells hybridize within this linear range. It is clear from Fig. 6 that their amount is not increased over that observed for nuclei from normally induced cells and, indeed, is actually somewhat less. In repeats of this experiment, we never observed a greater response in nuclei from superinduced cells.

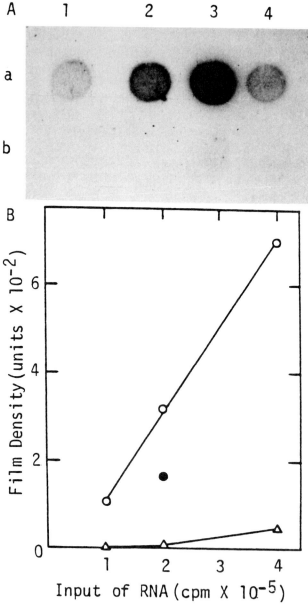

FIG. 6. Quantitation of nascent IL-2 transcripts during normal induction and superinduction. RNA labeled with [α-^{32}P]UTP in nuclei (Schibler *et al.*, 1983) from normally induced (1–3) (○) or superinduced cells (4) (●) was hybridized with IL-2 cDNA (a) or pBR322 DNA (b) (△). (A) Dot blots. (B) Microdensitometric analysis of hybridized IL-2 RNA plotted vs total input RNA.

E. The Labile Repressor Affects RNA Processing

To further analyze the mode of action of CHX-sensitive repressor, we studied IL-2 gene induction in the presence of cordycepin (3'-deoxy-yadenosine). This agent inhibits the polyadenylation of nuclear mRNA precursors and, hence, their subsequent processing, but is thought not to affect primary transcription (Penman et al., 1970; Abelson and Penman, 1972). Lymphocyte cultures were induced by PHA in the absence or presence of CHX and given cordycepin 2 hr before RNA was extracted. The RNA was analyzed by electrophoresis and blot hybridization with the IL-2 cDNA probe. As seen in Fig. 7a and b, cordycepin treatment results in the visualization of sequences migrating as larger than Il-2 mRNA, even in the absence of CHX. In its presence, the amount of such sequences does increase, but not nearly as extensively as mature IL-2 mRNA sequences (Fig. 7c and d). These larger sequences are likely to be precursors of IL-2 mRNA. Even if cordycepin was to induce the formation of abnormal intermediates, such RNA molecules must have arisen in a processing pathway and their amount thus is a measure of processing activity. Two peaks may be discerned in the putative precursor profile. We designate these as small and larger precursors, with a mean size of approximately 1800 and 3200 nucleotides, respectively. The size of the large precursors is well within the genomic length of the human IL-2 gene, about 5000 nucleotides (Fujita et al., 1983; Devos et al., 1983), indicating that they are smaller than the primary transcription product and, hence, most probably already partially processed.

Table I summarizes the effect of CHX on the distribution of IL-2 RNA sequences into precursors and mature mRNA analyzed by integration of the microdensitometer scans depicted in Fig. 7. In the presence of CHX, IL-2 RNA sequences migrating as large precursors increase about 3-fold. By contrast, small precursors increase by a factor of 24, and mature IL-2 mRNA increases by a factor of 58. A marked difference in distribution of sequences between precursors and mature mRNA is observed. Without CHX large precursors are in 4-fold excess over mature mRNA (78 vs 19%); in the presence of CHX this ratio is reversed (18 vs 77%). The proportion of small precursors, on the other hand, does not change appreciably. Superinduction thus causes a greater increase in IL-2 RNA sequences as they approach the size of mature IL-2 mRNA. We assume that, as for mature mRNA, the changes in precursor levels are not the result of a change in RNA pool size. Superinduction of the human IL-2 gene by CHX, as expressed by a very pronounced increase in IL-2 mRNA sequences and IL-2 mRNA activity, thus appears to be correlated with a strongly increased flow of precursor RNA molecules into mature IL-2 mRNA.

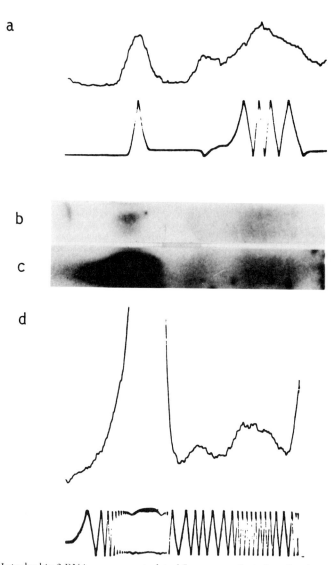

FIG. 7. Interleukin 2 RNA sequences isolated from normally induced and superinduced cells after treatment with cordycepin. Lymphocyte cultures, induced with PHA in the absence (a, b) or presence (c, d) of CHX (from 4 hr onward), received cordycepin (50 μg/ml) at 19 hr. Two hours later, total RNA was prepared and analyzed as for Fig. 4. In (a) the microdensitometer tracing of the film in (b) is shown (top), together with the peak integration (bottom). In (d) corresponding traces of (c) are depicted.

TABLE I

EFFECT OF CYCLOHEXIMIDE ON THE DISTRIBUTION OF IL-2 RNA
SEQUENCES INTO PRECURSORS AND MATURE mRNA

RNA species	Film density (%)[a]		Ratio +CHX/−CHX
	−CHX	+CHX	
Large precursors	39.5 (78)[b]	126 (18)	3.2
Small precursors	1.5 (3)	36 (5)	24
Mature mRNA	9.5 (19)	549 (77)	58

[a]Film density, expressed in arbitrary units, was obtained by integration of the scans shown in Fig. 7.

[b]Numbers in parentheses represent proportion of each RNA species within one scan, expressed as a percentage.

F. IMPLICATIONS OF THE LABILE REPRESSOR SYSTEM FOR IMMUNOREGULATION

The concept that the strength of the immune response is determined to a large extent by the amount of IL-2 available for T cell growth emphasizes the biological importance of the regulation of IL-2 production. These experiments demonstrate that two repression mechanisms act to control expression of the human IL-2 gene. One mechanism apparently shuts off the transcription of this gene. This transcriptional control is independent of continued protein synthesis. The second repression mechanism apparently acts posttranscriptionally and causes 95% or more of the nuclear IL-2 mRNA precursors to be degraded; only a few of these sequences are processes to mature, translationally active IL-2 mRNA in the cell. This posttranscriptional repression mechanism is sensitive to CHX and therefore represents the labile repressor first revealed by mRNA microinjection analysis (Efrat and Kaempfer, 1984a). This repressor may act to inhibit processing of precursor RNA, to destabilize such precursors, or both. Due to this labile, posttranscriptional repressor, the human IL-2 gene is normally expressed to only 1–5% of its potential.

While the mechanisms that generate the wave of IL-2 gene expression following induction do not depend on continued translation, the magnitude of this wave is controlled over a 30- to 60-fold range by an unstable posttranscriptional repressor. Since the magnitude of the IL-2 mRNA wave determines the strength of the eventual IL-2 signal, it appears from our results that the labile repressor mechanism has major importance for regulation of the strength of the immune response.

The fact that the labile posttranscriptional repressor mechanism prevents up to 99% of the maturation of IL-2 mRNA during normal induction has an interesting consequence. Any decrease, even a very small one, in the strength of this repression mechanism will result in greatly increased IL-2 production. For example, a decrease of 10% in repression will reduce it from 99 to 90%, increasing thereby the IL-2 mRNA signal 10-fold. In terms of the actual IL-2 signal produced, this means a 100-fold amplification of the change.

Therefore, any mechanism that acts to perturb the posttranscriptional repressor system that we have described here even slightly is expected to have a profound effect on the strength of the immune response.

ACKNOWLEDGMENTS

We thank Dr. T. Taniguchi for the IL-2 cDNA probe and Avivah Yeheskel for excellent assistance. Supported by grants from the National Council for Research and Development (Israel) and from the Cancer Research Institute (New York).

REFERENCES

Abelson, H. T., and Penman, S. (1972). *Biochim. Biophys. Acta* **277**, 129–133.

Andersson, J., Gronvik, K. O., Larsson, E. L., and Coutinho, A. (1979). *Eur. J. Immunol.* **9**, 581–587.

Devos, R., Plaetinck, G., Cheroutre, H., Simons, G., Degrave, W., Tavernier, J., Remaut, E., and Fiers, W. (1983). *Nucleic Acids Res.* **11**, 4307–4323.

Efrat, S., and Kaempfer, R. (1984a). *Proc. Natl. Acad. Sci. U.S.A.* **81**, 2601–2605.

Efrat, S., and Kaempfer, R. (1984b). *Cell. Immunol.* **88**, 207–212.

Efrat, S., Pilo, S., and Kaempfer, R. (1982). *Nature (London)* **297**, 236–239.

Efrat, S., Zelig, S., Yagen, B., and Kaempfer, R. (1984). *Biochem. Biophys. Res. Commun.* **123**, 842–848.

Fujita, T., Takaoka, C., Matsui, H., and Taniguchi, T. (1983). *Proc. Natl. Acad. Sci. U.S.A.* **80**, 7437–7441.

Gillis, S., and Smith, K. A. (1977). *Nature (London)* **268**, 154–156.

Gillis, S., Ferm, M. M., Ou, W., and Smith, K. A. (1978a). *J. Immunol.* **120**, 2027–2032.

Gillis, S., Baker, P. E., Ruscetti, F. W., and Smith, K. A. (1978b). *J. Exp. Med.* **148**, 1093–1098.

Henney, C. S., Kuribayashi, K., Kern, D. E., and Gillis, S. (1981). Nature (London) **291**, 335–338.

Morgan, D. A., Ruscetti, F. W., and Gallo, R. (1976). *Science* **193**, 1007–1008.

Penman, S., Rosbash, M., and Penman, M. (1970). *Proc. Natl. Acad. Sci. U.S.A.* **67**, 1878–1885.

Schibler, U., Hagenbüchle, O., Wellauer, P. K., and Pittet, A. C. (1983). *Cell* **33**, 501–508.

Smith, K. A. (1981). *In* "Lymphokines" (E. Pick, ed.), Vol. 2, pp. 21–30. Academic Press, New York.

Taniguchi, T., Matsui, H., Fujita, T., Takaoka, C., Kashima, N., Yoshimoto, R., and Hamuro, J. (1983). *Nature (London)* **302**, 305–310.

Tees, R., and Schreier, M. H. (1980). *Nature (London)* **283**, 780–81.

Zarling, J. M., and Bach, F. H. (1979). *Nature (London)* **280**, 685–688.

Expression Patterns of Lymphokines and Related Genes

VERNER PAETKAU, JENNIFER SHAW, JOHN F. ELLIOTT, CALLIOPI HAVELE,
BILL POHAJDAK, AND R. CHRIS BLEACKLEY

Department of Biochemistry, University of Alberta, Edmonton, Alberta, Canada T6G 2H7

I. Introduction

In the past three years our understanding of what lymphokines are and how they act has undergone a significant enhancement, brought about by molecular approaches to what was until recently a field defined by phenomenology alone. Conventional, "precloning," biochemistry has been useful and important, and a number of cytokines and lymphokines have been defined by it. The power of molecular cloning in providing detailed molecular information is amply demonstrated by the rapid accumulation of DNA and implied protein sequence information on lymphokines which were difficult to purify and study as proteins. Expression of recombinant lymphokine genes now provides essentially unlimited quantities of individual lymphokines uncontaminated by others.

The availability of cloned lymphokine and cytokine genes is useful in assigning biological effects to particular molecular structures. This is in keeping with the classical approach to chemical biology, in which a new substance is identified by its phenomonology, purified on the basis of a bioassay, and then synthesized to confirm its identity. The understanding of the biological function of lymphokines will presumably be further widened and substantiated by using recombinant DNA products. However, an equally exciting prospect is that the expression of the relevant genes can be studied using molecular probes.

In this article we will describe a distinctive phenotypic change which is induced in cytotoxic T lymphocytes (CTL) by exposure to high levels of purified or recombinant IL-2.[1] The role of IL-2 receptor (IL-2-R) transcription in the activation of specific CTL will be examined. In the second major part, we delineate patterns of lymphokine mRNA expression in T lymphocytes responding to inducers and suppressors. It will be shown that lymphokines form a subset of genes whose induction

---

[1]Abbreviations: CsA, cyclosporin A (cyclosporine); CTL, cytotoxic T lymphocytes; ED_{50}, an amount of activity which, in 1 ml, produces 50% of the maximal response; GM-CSF, colony stimulating factor for granulocytes and macrophages; IFN-α, -β, -γ, various interferons; IL-2, interleukin 2; IL-2-R, IL-2 receptor; MMTV, mouse mammary tumor virus; PBL, peripheral blood leukocytes; PMA, phorbol 12-myristate 13-acetate (also TPA).

73

and suppression have common features not shared by the rest of the genetic repertoire of such cells. Finally, we will show how these patterns of expression provide the basis for a novel method of identifying new lymphokine genes and other genes which share the unusual expression characteristics of lymphokines.

II. Phenotypic Conversion of Cytotoxic T Lymphocytes

A. THE CONVERSION OF TYPE I CTL TO TYPE II CELLS

In addition to antigen-specific CTL, there are several other forms of cytotoxic lymphocytes, including natural killer (NK), natural cytotoxic, and lymphokine-activated killer cells (Hercend et al., 1983; Grimm et al., 1982; Dennert, 1980; Nabel et al., 1981). The relationships between these cells are understood only poorly. Patterns of altered specificity of CTL can occur under certain culture conditions, leading to different, but still relatively limited, target specificity (Reimann and Miller, 1985). On the other hand, specific, cloned CTL lines can attain the target range found in classical NK cells upon exposure to high concentrations of IL-2 for a few days (Brooks, 1983; Brooks et al., 1983). Even more effective in this regard were the interferons α and β (IFN-α, IFN-β), but not IFN-γ (Brooks et al., 1985). The conversion from specific CTL to the NK phenotype was reversible. However, in the same studies, longer exposure to the same lymphokines induced a shift toward almost complete lack of target specificity. This is sometimes referred to as "anomolous" or "promiscuous" killing.

In addition to target specificity, T lymphocyte lines vary in their growth requirements, some requiring antigen, some responding to IL-2 directly. It has been widely supposed that dependence on antigen for growth is a result of the antigen inducing a higher level of expression of IL-2-R, thus making the cells more responsive to IL-2. An increased level of IL-2-R protein on the cell membrane has been found for some cytotoxic (Kaplan et al., 1984; Andrew et al., 1985; Lowenthal et al., 1985) and helper T lymphocyte lines (Hemler et al., 1984).

Several years ago, we observed that the type of CTL produced from mixed leukocyte cultures (MLC) depended on the lymphokine preparation used to induce their outgrowth. Beginning with a crude culture supernatant generated by stimulating cells of the mouse T lymphoma line EL4.E1 with PMA, lymphokine preparations of various stages of purity and definition were produced (Riendeau et al., 1983). Crude supernatant purified by dialysis and concentration using diafiltration, and then separated from high and low molecular weight impurities by chromatography on Sephadex G-100, is referred to as Fraction 3. Fraction 3 was also purified to biochemical homogeneity by a series of further steps. MLC cultures grown out with Fraction 3 lymphokine preparations invariably yielded cells with indiscriminate cytotoxic activity, not fulfilling the criteria for either antigen-specific CTL or NK cells. However, when purified IL-2 was used to support growth, only highly specific CTL resulted.

We initially assumed that these two types of cytotoxic cells had little relationship to each other. However, after cloning the specific CTL, it was found that they could be converted in their cytotoxicity to a nonspecificity which was indistinguishable from that of the cells produced with Fraction 3 lymphokine (Havele *et al.*, 1985). The essential condition for conversion was exposure for about 3 days to Fraction 3 lymphokine in the presence of the nominal antigen. To facilitate discussion of these results, we refer to the antigen-specific CTL generated by induction in the presence of purified IL-2 as "Type I" cells. The nonspecific cells produced either by initial growth in Fraction 3 lymphokines or by conversion from Type I are called "Type II" cells.

A typical specific CTL line, MTL23.2(I) (the roman numeral indicates that it is of Type I) has the growth requirements shown in Fig. 1. It proliferates in response to IL-2 only in the presence of the appropriate antigen, as shown in Fig. 1A. Irrelevent antigen is without effect (Havele *et al.*, 1985), and recombinant human IL-2 works as well as purified mouse "natural" IL-2 (data not shown). Type I cells do not proliferate in the absence of antigen, but they do persist in a quiescent state with a half-life of 2–3 weeks if IL-2 is present. In the absence of IL-2, they die rapidly. The requirements for expressing cytotoxicity are the same as for growth, namely, exposure to the correct antigen and IL-2. Phorbol myristate acetate (PMA) can replace antigen in both the proliferation and cytotoxicity responses.

Fraction 3 lymphokine preparations contain IL-2, which was present at 5–10 ED_{50} U/ml during the conversion of Type I to II cells. We refer to this as a low IL-2 level. Beside exposure to Fraction 3, which contains lymphokines other than IL-2, two other conditions were found to cause efficient conversion. These were exposure to high levels of IL-2 (50–100 ED_{50} U/ml) in the presence of either antigen or PMA. The line MTL23.2(I) was converted to the Type II phenotype by exposure to antigen and 65 ED_{50} U/ml purified mouse IL-2 to generate a line identified as MTL23.2(II). This Type II line grew in response to IL-2 alone, and antigen had virtually no effect on its growth (Fig. 1B). Its cytotoxicity was nonspecific and did not show a restriction to either the original alloantigen or to the pattern of targets exhibited by classical NK cells.

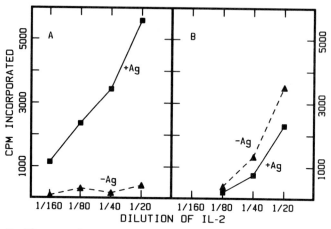

Fɪɢ. 1. Proliferation of Type I and Type II CTL. Type I CTL requires antigen to proliferate in response to IL-2, Type II cells do not. (A) The Type I CTL line MTL23.2(I) was of CBA/J origin and was specific for CBA/J × BALB/c alloantigen (H-2^k anti-H-2$^{k/d}$). It was propagated in purified natural mouse IL-2 with periodic exposure to irradiated CBA/J × BALB/c spleen cells. The cells were allowed to come to quiescence for 15 days in IL-2, and converted to the Type II phenotype by exposure to 100 ED$_{50}$ U/ml purified mouse IL-2 plus 10 ng/ml PMA. The two types of cells were assayed for growth by incorporation of [^{125}I]dIUdR into DNA. (B) The derived MTL23.2(II) line was assayed 8 weeks after conversion, and the MTL23.2(I) parental line 11 days after the last exposure to antigen.

The conversion of Type I cells has been carried out on some 20 different CTL lines with the same result. Most of the derived Type II cells retain a high level of killing of the original target superimposed on a nonspecific cytotoxic activity. In addition to their cytotoxicities and growth requirements, Types I and II also differed in morphology, with Type I cells being small and nonadherent to the plastic culture dishes and Type II cells being much larger and strongly adherent to plastic.

B. Sɪɴɢʟᴇ Tʏᴘᴇ I Cᴇʟʟs Aʀᴇ Cᴏɴᴠᴇʀᴛᴇᴅ ᴛᴏ Tʏᴘᴇ II ʙʏ IL-2 Aʟᴏɴᴇ

Single cells of Type I character can be converted to Type II phenotypes in limiting dilution experiments. In one such experiment, cells of the lineage MTL21.9(I) were seeded at an average density of 1/well in microtiter trays containing irradiated alloantigenic spleen cells and either a low (6.5 ED$_{50}$ U/ml) or high (65 ED$_{50}$ U/ml) level of recombinant human IL-2. By 12 days, 34 of 96 wells given the high IL-2 level contained colonies which were of Type II (the cells were large, adherent, capable of growth in IL-2 alone, and had a broad cytotoxic range of targets). None of the wells with a low IL-2 level contained such colonies, although 23 of 96 contained original Type I cells. At the high IL-2 level, there were also 16 wells containing exclusively Type I cells, and 10 containing mixed colonies. The overall cloning efficiency at high IL-2 levels was very near 1.0, as seen by the frequency of empty wells (predicted 36, observed 36).

Several conclusions follow from these results, which are described in detail elsewhere (Havele *et al.*, 1985, 1986). First, conversion is not a matter of selection of variant cells out of the starting population. If Type II cells arose in Type I populations, they would have a significant growth advantage and would soon become predominant; the Type I cells grow only in bursts and then stop for a period until fresh antigen is added, whereas Type II cells grow continuously. Second, IL-2 is the only exogenous lymphokine required for conversion, since recombinant human IL-2 or purified "natural" mouse IL-2,works equally well in the presence of either PMA or antigen as the complementary signal. Third, conversion appears to be a stochastic process, occurring some time after proliferation is initiated. This would account for the mixed colonies, in which some of the cells were converted at a time when the starting Type I population had expanded. It appears that the starting population, although recently cloned, is heterogeneous for conversion, with some cells not undergoing it despite the requisite signals being present.

Finally, Type II cells grow for long periods (weeks and months) in recombinant human IL-2, indicating both that once conversion is complete antigen is not required and that IL-2 alone causes their proliferation. This is in contrast to the lack of growth in IL-2 reported elsewhere for similar cells (Olabuenaga *et al.*, 1983). Conversion may have been incomplete in that case, resulting in an intermediate phenotype. Indeed, it is important to recognize that phenotypic conversion, although occurring relatively quickly in our experiments, is not an all-or-none process. From parallels with the reported work of Brooks and colleagues (Brooks, 1983; Brooks *et al.*, 1983, 1985), we expect that before conversion to Type II is complete there is an intermediate stage with the cytotoxic specificity of classical NK cells. This conversion (CTL to NK phenotype) is reversible, and the cells revert to Type I behavior on removal of the conditions promoting conversion.

Although the significance of conversion for normal CTL responses is not clear, there are several interesting features to it. First, at early stages it generates cells with a phenotype identical to that of classical, blood-derived NK cells (Brooks *et al.*, 1983). Second, the promiscuous or anomolous cytotoxicity of Type II cells may have potent antitumor activity (Grimm *et al.*, 1982). Finally, Type II cells occasionally convert to

IL-2-independent growth and, in that state, are capable of forming tumors in syngeneic mice (Giglia *et al.*, 1985). Thus, conversion may mark a progression from normal memory-like CTL, requiring both antigen and IL-2 to grow and express cytotoxicity, to autonomously growing tumorigenic cells, induced by intracellular changes as yet undefined. This progression would presumably be rare *in vivo* because conditions of chronically elevated IL-2 are uncommon, and cells with indiscriminate cytotoxicity may be deleted by regulatory mechanisms such as the presence of "veto" cells (Claesson and Miller, 1984).

C. WHAT IS THE ROLE OF IL-2-R mRNA SYNTHESIS IN THE ACTIVATION OF ANTIGEN-SPECIFIC CTL?

Exposure to antigen induces a rapid and massive increase in the level of IL-2-R expressed on the surfaces of a number of cytotoxic and helper T lymphocyte lines (Andrew *et al.*, 1985; Hemler *et al.*, 1984; Lowenthal *et al.*, 1985). To date, most of these studies have used antireceptor antibodies, which do not distinguish between high- and low-affinity receptors (Robb *et al.*, 1984). Nevertheless, it seems quite possible that the role of antigen recognition is to induce the specific expression of IL-2-R in resting T lymphocytes. It was recently found that both IL-2 and antigen could increase the expression of IL-2-R mRNA in a T helper cell line (Malek and Ashwell, 1985). Is such an enhanced expression evident at the mRNA level in Type I cells? When total cellular RNA was examined by Northern gel analysis and probed with a cloned full-length cDNA for mouse IL-2-R, there was indeed a significantly higher concentration of IL-2-R mRNA 1 day after activation with antigen as compared to 4 days later (Table I). Separate experiments showed that there was little further decline after day 5 in IL-2-R mRNA; presumably this reflects the continued, persistent expression of IL-2-R in Type I cells. This is consistent with their continued requirement for IL-2 to maintain them in the quiescent state. Although the IL-2-R mRNA levels appeared to be induced by antigen, this was no greater than the effect on actin mRNA in the same cells (Table I). The concentrations of both mRNAs fell after exposure to antigen as cells lost their state of activation. When the same results were compared on the basis of mRNA content per cell, there was a slightly greater increase in the IL-2-R mRNA upon activation (to a level of 7 times the day 5 value), but again, actin mRNA was almost as high (6.2-fold). The expression level of IL-2-R mRNA was significantly higher in the Type II line MTL2.8.2 when expressed as concentration in total RNA or on a per-cell basis (Table I).

We have not yet analyzed the expression of functional IL-2 receptor in activated Type I cells. This would best be done by binding studies with

TABLE I

INDUCTION OF mRNA IN ACTIVATED TYPE I CTL[a]

mRNA	Activated Type I cells			MTL2.8.2(II)
	Day 1	Day 3	Day 5	
Relative mRNA concentration[b]				
IL-2-R	5.7	1.6	(1.0)	12.4
Actin	5.0	2.9	(1.0)	1.6
Relative mRNA content per cell[c]				
IL-2-R	7.0	3.18	(1.0)	39.0
Actin	6.2	5.7	(1.0)	5.0

[a]Cells of the Type I CTL line MTL21.9 were allowed to come to quiescence by maintaining them for 13 days in IL-2 following their last exposure to allogeneic cells. They were washed and stimulated with 20 ED_{50} U/ml of recombinant human IL-2 plus 15 ng/ml PMA. Samples of the activated cells were harvested 1, 3, and 5 days later. Total cellular RNA was isolated and equal quantitites electrophoretically separated on a 0.8% agarose gel containing 0.67% formaldehyde. The RNA was transferred to a nitrocellulose (BA85) filter and probed with either cloned cDNA probe for mouse IL-2 receptor (IL-2-R), or human actin (provided by Dr. L. H. Kedes, Stanford University). The table expresses the levels of the two mRNAs as determined by densitometric tracing of the autoradiograms made from the blots.

[b]The relative mRNA concentration expresses the levels at days 1 and 3, relative to day 5, on the basis of micrograms RNA loaded on the gel.

[c]This expresses the relative mRNA content of actin and IL-2-R per cell. The levels of actin mRNA fell dramatically between 3 and 5 days after stimulation, more or less in parallel to the levels of IL-2-R mRNA. Note the high level of IL-2-R mRNA in the Type II line MTL2.8.2(II) (Bleackley et al., 1982), which was analyzed in parallel.

radiolabeled IL-2 to detect high affinity receptors. Nevertheless, it seems that in these cells the primary control of activation is not the selective enhancement of IL-2-R gene transcription. It is possible that actin is a member of a small subset of genes induced by antigen in Type I cells. Clearly, further analysis at the molecular level is required. However, the difference between some Type I and II cells does appear to include the massive difference in IL-2-R mRNA levels described in Table I (40-fold higher levels in the long-term Type II cell, compared to resting, IL-2-maintained Type I cells). To summarize, the enhanced level of IL-2-R mRNA expression in antigen-activated Type I cells is consistent with the observed increase in receptor protein noted in earlier work. However, the receptor gene is certainly not alone in giving a moderately enhanced (5- to 10-fold) level of transcription. Included in the number of similarly activated genes is cellular actin, at least.

Interestingly, most newly derived Type II cells have a much higher IL-2 requirement than the Type I cells from which they arise. For example, the MTL23.2(I) line showed about a 4-fold decrease in sensitivity to IL-2 after conversion to Type II growth (Fig. 1). Preliminary evidence suggests that shortly after conversion, Type II cells may have relatively modest levels of IL-2-R mRNA, at least as compared to the long-term line MTL2.8.2 which requires much lower levels of IL-2 to grow.

III. Patterns of Lymphokine Transcription

A. LYMPHOKINES SHOW A SELECTIVE PATTERN OF INDUCTION BY T CELL ACTIVATORS AND SUPPRESSION BY CsA

The expression of IL-2-R in Type I CTL may or may not represent a specific inductive effect on gene expression. Additional experiments using other probes will be required to determine whether the enhanced levels of IL-2-R and actin mRNA represent a generalized induction or whether both are members of a set of antigen-induced genes. The induction of IL-2 mRNA synthesis and mRNA for other lymphokines, however, does represent a selective effect on a small subset of all expressible genes in certain T lymphocytes. The T lymphocyte lines EL4 (mouse) and Jurkat (human), and primary human T lymphocytes, are induced to synthesize IL-2 mRNA by a combination of PMA and T lymphocyte mitogen (Con A) (Elliott et al., 1984; Kronke et al., 1984, 1985; Paetkau, 1985). Human IFN-γ (Wiskocil et al., 1985) and mouse GM-CSF (Paetkau, 1985; Kelso and Gough, this volume) are similarly induced. On the other hand, only about 4% of the proteins synthesized by EL4.E1 cells are affected in their expression levels by PMA (Paetkau, 1985; Shaw et al., 1986), indicating that the lymphokines are a highly selected set of inducible genes. The induction of lymphokine mRNA expression is blocked by the immunosuppressive drug CsA (Elliott et al., 1984; Kronke et al., 1984; Wiskocil et al., 1985), and this effect is also highly specific. Thus, we have found no direct effects of CsA on the patterns of proteins synthesized by EL4.E1 cells, and only a subset of those proteins whose expression is affected by PMA are influenced in expression by CsA (Paetkau, 1985; Shaw et al., 1986).

The induction of IL-2 mRNA accumulation in the Jurkat human T lymphocyte line following exposure to PMA and Con A is illustrated in Fig. 2. Whereas there was no detectable IL-2 mRNA before stimulation, this mRNA was rapidly induced in the presence of PMA plus Con A. However, in the presence of CsA there was no accumulation of IL-2 mRNA. The figure further shows that this accumulation apparently required protein synthesis at the outset, since cycloheximide added at this

EXPRESSION OF LYMPHOKINES AND RELATED GENES 81

TIME OF HARVEST:

4h | 6h

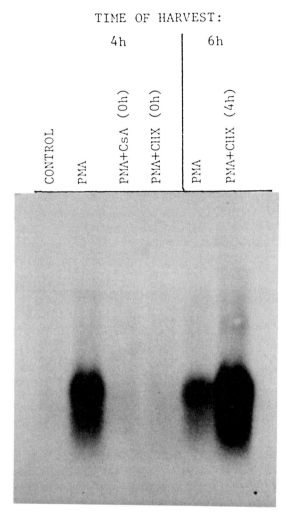

FIG. 2. Induction, suppression, and superinduction of IL-2 mRNA. IL-2 mRNA is induced by PMA, suppressed by CsA, and superinduced in the presence of cyclohexi-mide. Cells of the Jurkat human T leukemia line were stimulated with PMA (15 ng/ml) plus Con A (30 μg/ml), and total cellular RNA harvested and analyzed by gel elec-trophoresis and blotting with cloned human IL-2 cDNA as in Table I. Each track repre-sents the total RNA from 2.5 × 10⁶ cells. Cyclosporin A was present where indicated at 100 ng/ml, and cycloheximide (CHX) at 20 μg/ml. Cyclosporin A or CHX added initially completely blocked the induction by PMA (+Con A) but, added at 4 hr, CHX superin-duced IL-2 mRNA. The peak of IL-2 mRNA generally occurs between 4–6 hr and then declines.

time blocked it. Added later, however, the protein synthesis inhibitor caused a rapid increase in mRNA levels ("superinduction," see Section III,B), as has been shown for IL-2 mRNA in human tonsil leukocytes by Kaempfer and colleagues (Efrat and Kaempfer, 1984; Kaempfer et al., this volume). Since our results were obtained with a cloned, homogeneous cell line, they indicate that cycloheximide induces superinduction by a direct effect on the lymphokine-producing cell itself.

B. CsA Blocks Lymphokine mRNA Synthesis by a Mechanism Not Dependent on Protein Synthesis

In addition to blocking the induction of synthesis of lymphokine mRNA, CsA also interrupts already initiated IL-2 mRNA synthesis in EL4.E1 cells. This was seen by nuclear run-on transcription experiments, in which mRNA initiated in vivo is extended in isolated nuclei in vitro (Table II). This table also shows that unstimulated EL4.E1 nuclei

TABLE II
CsA Interrupts IL-2 mRNA Synthesis[a]

Time				Relative rate of transcription[b]
PMA	CsA	CHX	Harvest	
—	—	—	12	0.05
0	—	—	10	2.03
0	—	—	12	3.65
0	—	—	16	1.74
0	0	—	12	0.32
0	12	—	16	0.28
0	12	10	16	0.54
0	—	10	16	1.25

[a]Nuclei were harvested from EL4.E1 cells (Kronke et al., 1984) following treatment of the cells in culture as indicated. CsA was added to 100 ng/ml, cycloheximide (CHX) to 20 μg/ml, and PMA to 15 ng/ml. The nuclei were incubated under conditions for labeling nascent RNA by elongation (Kronke et al., 1984). After 15 min, reactions were stopped by the addition of 100 μg/ml of DNase I and proteinase K and incubated for 15 min at 37°C. SDS was added to a final concentration of 1%, and RNA was partially purified by extraction with phenolchloroform and precipitation with ethanol. Samples were hybridized to filters carrying either a cloned mouse IL-2 cDNA or a cloned cDNA, of unknown function, which is expressed at equal levels in stimulated and unstimulated EL4.E1 cells (probe 10) (Paetkau et al., 1985).

[b]The relative transcription rate represents the signal of IL-2 transcripts relative to probe 10 transcripts, as determined by quantitative autoradiography.

undergo very little, if any, transcription of the IL-2 gene. The rate of transcription rose to a maximum by about 12 hr and then slowly declined. Cyclosporin A initially present blocked the induction, and added at 12 hr it stopped transcription of IL-2 within the next 4 hr. The effect of adding CsA at 12 hr was only slightly reduced if cycloheximide was added at 10 hr. In other words, induction of a new protein was apparently not required for the effect of CsA. However, the action of CsA may be dependent on preexisting cellular proteins, since its ability to interrupt lymphokine mRNA transcription does appear to be less if protein synthesis is inhibited.

C. Lymphokine mRNA is Superinducible because Cycloheximide Stabilizes It

Superinduction by inhibitors of protein synthesis has been noted in a variety of responses, both *in vivo* and *in vitro*. The list of genes superinducible by cycloheximide includes IFN-β (Sehgal *et al.*, 1978) and small sets of genes induced in 3T3 cells by either PDGF (Cochran *et al.*, 1983) or mitogens (Hamilton *et al.*, 1985). The mechanism of superinduction is related to the action of the "latent" RNase (RNase L) (Slattery *et al.*, 1979), which selectively degrades inducible mRNAs, including viral RNA, giving it a relatively short half-life (cf. Newmark, 1985). RNase L activity depends on an obligatory cofactor, oligo(rA), which is itself synthesized by a rapidly turning over, and thus cycloheximide-sensitive, oligo(rA) synthetase (Slattery *et al.*, 1979; Lengyel, 1982). This mechanism predicts that superinducibility of a given mRNA is likely to reflect a short half-life.

Although IL-2 mRNA is superinducible by cycloheximide in Jurkat and EL4.E1 cells, this inhibitor blocks induction when added at the outset. This is clearly indicated by the data of Fig. 3 which show that protein synthesis is required for induction of IL-2 in Jurkat cells stimulated with PMA and Con A. In this, EL4.E1 and Jurkat cells differ from PBL, in which cycloheximide does not influence the rate of IL-2 mRNA transcription (Kronke *et al.*, 1985; our unpublished data).

Following the first hours of induction of Jurkat cells, there was a rapid shift to superinduction conditions, so that addition of cycloheximide at 6 hr led to a much higher level of IL-2 mRNA present at 10 hr (Fig. 3). The rate of increase in mRNA upon addition of cycloheximide at later times was apparently rapid, as in just 2 hr (from 8 to 10 hr) the level of mRNA rose 10-fold. If the results in EL4.E1 cells apply to the Jurkat system, it is likely that the superinduction by cycloheximide is due to stabilization of mRNA since it does not increase the rate of transcription. In fact, as seen in Table II, it reduced the rate of transcription somewhat over a 4 hr

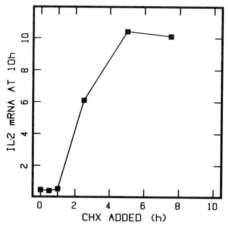

FIG. 3. IL-2 mRNA induction. Cycloheximide inhibits IL-2 mRNA induction in Jurkat cells if it is present at the onset of induction, but superinduces the mRNA if added at least 2 hr later. Jurkat cells were stimulated with PMA plus Con A, and total cellular RNA was harvested at 10 hr, as in Fig. 2. Cytodots (White and Bancroft, 1982) of total cellular RNA were analyzed by densitometry of the autoradiograms. Cycloheximide (CHX) was added at various times as indicated. The level of IL-2 mRNA at 10 hr without cycloheximide is 1.0 on the ordinate.

period (from 10 to 16 hr) when added to EL4.E1 cells. This conclusion predicts that IL-2 mRNA should have a relatively short half-life, and also suggests that it may be subject to degradation by the RNase L system.

D. INTERLEUKIN 2 mRNA HAS A SHORT HALF-LIFE IN EL4.E1 CELLS

Stabilization of mRNA is the most likely mechanism to account for the superinduction of a number of inducible mRNAs, including IL-2. For this mechanism to apply, the mRNA must have a short half-life. This is indeed the case for IL-2 in EL4.E1 cells. Relying on the fact that CsA interrupts synthesis of IL-2 (and other lymphokine) mRNA, it was possible to study the decay of this mRNA under conditions which did not perturb the general genetic expression of the cells. This is advantageous for studying the cellular half-life of mRNAs which are subject to degradation by RNase L, which is itself inhibited by RNA synthesis inhibitors such as actinomycin D.

The first order decay of IL-2 mRNA in CsA-treated cells is illustrated in Fig. 4 and supports the notion that superinducible mRNA is normally short-lived mRNA. The apparent half-life under these conditions is about 2 hr. However, this may depend on conditions such as the state of induction of the RNase L system itself. For example, in the results with Jurkat cells shown in Fig. 3, there was a 10-fold increase in the level of

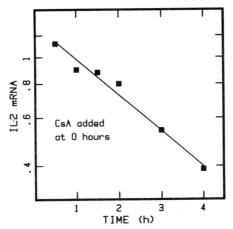

FIG. 4. Transcription blockage of IL-2 mRNA. The mRNA for IL-2 decays rapidly after its transcription is blocked with CsA. Mouse T lymphoma cells EL4.E1 were stimulated with 15 ng/ml PMA, and cellular RNA was analyzed for IL-2 mRNA by cytodot analysis as in Fig. 3. CsA was added 13 hr after induction with PMA. The levels of IL-2 mRNA were determined by densitometric analysis of the cytodot data and are expressed for CsA-treated cell samples relative to control cells harvested at the same time.

IL-2 mRNA 2 hr after the addition of cycloheximide at 8 hr, suggesting a half-life of less than 1 hr.

The summary of effects of CsA and cycloheximide on a number of lymphokines and other gene products is given in Table III. Notably, the IL-2-R gene is largely insensitive to cycloheximide or CsA, although it does undergo a modest degree of superinduction, suggesting a relatively short half-life. Actin is unaffected by CsA and cycloheximide over a moderate time span. A significant discrepancy exists between the effect of cycloheximide in blocking the induction of IL-2 in the Jurkat and EL4.E1 T cell lines and its lack of effect on the induction of human peripheral blood T lymphocytes ("CHX added early" in Table III). This lack of effect in PBL has been noted elsewhere (Kronke *et al.*, 1985). In human tonsil cells, protein synthesis inhibitors blocked induction of IL-2 mRNA expression, but this may have been due to the lack of IL-1 production of macrophages (Efrat and Kaempfer, 1984).

IV. Cloning Inducible, Suppressible Sequences

A. A Strategy for Cloning Genes Whose Expression is Induced

Numerous lymphokines have been cloned in both cDNA and genomic forms. Some lymphokines, such as those which induce the proliferation

TABLE III
PATTERNS OF INDUCTION, SUPPRESSION, AND SUPERINDUCTION[a]

		Level of expression[b]				
			PMA		CHX added	
Product	Cells	Unstimulated	(+Con A)	CsA	Early	Late
IL-2	EL4, Jurkat	−	+	−	−	+++
IL-2	PBL	−	+	−	+	+++
GM-CSF	EL4	−	+	−	−	+++
IFN-γ	PBL	−	+	−	±	++
IL-2-R	PBL, Jurkat	−	+	+	+	++
TCR-β	EL4, Jurkat	+	+	+	+	+
Actin	PBL, Jurkat	+	+	+	±	+

[a] Data for this table were compiled from Northern gel analyses of mRNA derived under the conditions of stimulation or suppression indicated. All of the observations were made more than once, and gels were stained for the presence of intact ribosomal RNA to ensure that the RNA was of good quality. In addition, actin was used to probe most blots after removing the primary probe, and found to be unchanged by PMA or CsA. Most of the clones used were full length cDNA, except IFN-γ, for which a synthetic oligonucleotide was used (provided by Dr. P. J. Barr, Chiron Corp.)

[b] The symbols (+, −, ±) indicate relative levels of expression.

of activated B lymphocytes (Farrar *et al.*, 1983) and their differentiation to antibody secretion (Nakanishi *et al.*, 1984), may be relatively difficult to clone, however, because the bioassays are more complex or because of their low abundance. The existence of additional factors required for the induction of CTL responses has been documented (Raulet and Bevan, 1982; Falk *et al.*, 1983), but these have also not yet been characterized. The conventional approaches to the molecular cloning of lymphokines include the screening of recombinant DNA for its ability either to bind the mRNA of interest or to be expressed directly into biologically or antigenically active material upon transfection into cells. Another method, successful in the cloning of human IFN-γ, is to probe a cDNA library derived from cells stimulated to produce a given lymphokine with cDNA generated either from stimulated or unstimulated cells ("plus–minus" screening) (Gray *et al.*, 1982). This approach is predicated on the assumption that only a few mRNAs are differentially expressed during stimulation and is clearly justified in some cases.

Each method of cloning has its limitations. Clearly, a definitive bioassay is essential for cloning by function, but even when such an assay exists and is relatively straightforward, this approach is still difficult. Screening with plus-minus probes may be effective only if the sequence of interest makes up at least 0.25–0.50% of the mRNA in the probe (i.e., is at least of this abundance in the "plus" sample of mRNA) (Williams, 1981). An alternative strategy for lymphokines and similar molecules can be envisaged, based on the expression patterns described above and using subtractive hybridization to overcome problems of low abundance. Lymphokine genes are inducible and many of them, including IL-2, IL-3, B cell growth factor, IFN-γ, GM-CSF, and B cell differentiation factors, are suppressed by CsA (Elliott et al., 1984; Granelli-Piperno et al., 1984; Kronke et al., 1984; Wiskocil et al., 1985; Paetkau, 1985). Several are superinduced by cycloheximide (Mizel and Mizel, 1981; Efrat and Kaempfer, 1984; Shaw et al., 1986). These differences are reflected at the level of the relevant mRNAs. Genes with these properties, expressed even at low levels after induction, can in principle be identified by subtractive cloning and screening. This method overcomes the limitations of plus-minus screening by enriching the probe sequence of interest as well as the sequences actually cloned. It was successfully applied to the cloning of T cell antigen receptors (Hedrick et al., 1984; Yanagi et al., 1984).

Upon activation, the mouse T lymphoma line EL4 synthesizes and secretes a number of lymphokines, including IL-2 (Farrar et al., 1980), IL-3 (Pearlstein et al., 1983), GM-CSF (Bleackley et al., 1983), and both growth (Howard et al., 1982) and differentiation (Pure et al., 1982) factors for B lymphocytes. Additional activities, not yet well characterized, have also been observed, including a putative "conversion factor" discussed in Section II. To apply the principle of subtractive cloning to lymphokines and similarly regulated sequences, a preparation of single-stranded cDNA from PMA-stimulated EL4.E1 cells was hybridized to mRNA from unstimulated cells (C_0t of 1680) and the hybrid molecules removed by hydroxyapatite chromatography (Hedrick et al., 1984). Unhybridized cDNA, putatively enriched for induced sequences, was converted to double-stranded form, methylated with EcoRI methylase, and adapted for cloning with EcoRI linkers along conventional lines. Following cleavage with EcoRI, cDNA products of greater than 800 bp in length were cloned in bacteriophage λgt 10.

The subtracted library was probed with a full-length cDNA probe for mouse IL-2, and found to contain 10 times as high a frequency of this sequence, known to be PMA-induced, as an unenriched library of cDNA. Of about 40,000 recombinant phages from the subtracted library, 2400 hybridized strongly to a twice-subtracted probe. Of the 2400, 80 also bound the IL-2 cDNA probe. Thus, in addition to a 10-fold enrichment of the cloned library of cDNA sequences, the use of a subtracted probe further increased the frequency of PMA-induced sequences by 17-

TABLE IV
CLONING OF PMA-INDUCED mRNA SEQUENCES[a]

Clone	Number (per 136)	Level of mRNA expression[b,c]			
		Unstimulated	PMA (+Con A)	PMA+CsA	PMA+CHX
25	1	0	+	+	+
33	3	0	+	+ +	+
14[d]	85	±	+	±	+ +
13	14	±	+	ND	ND
32	1	±	+	ND	ND
101	1	0	+	ND	ND

[a]Clones of cDNA produced from mRNA enriched for sequences induced by PMA in EL4.E1 cells were generated in λgt10 and plaque purified with subtracted probe, as described in the text. Total RNA isolated from EL4.E1 cells treated as indicated (either controls, stimulated, stimulated in the presence of CsA, or superinduced with cycloheximide) was subjected to Northern gel analysis with the individual clones.

[b]The relative expression levels under the various circumstances are indicated.

[c]0, Undetectable; ± low abundance; + and + +, increasing abundance; ND, not determined.

[d]Clone 14 and its family is MMTV related and was studied further. A map of clone 14 is given in Fig. 5.

fold as estimated from the IL-2 sequence. A second check was performed with GM-CSF, which hybridized to $\frac{1}{6}$ as many clones as did IL-2. This was about what was expected from the relative levels of IL-2 and GM-CSF mRNA produced by induced EL4.E1 cells. An initial set of 136 recombinant phages picked on the basis of their induced phenotype was analyzed by Northern gel analysis of mRNA prepared from control, PMA-induced, and PMA-induced and CsA-suppressed EL4.E1 cells with the results shown in Table IV. Most of the clones picked by this protocol were found, indeed, to represent PMA-induced genes in these cells, although of presently unknown function. One (clone 33) was apparently superinduced by CsA, a novel observation. Only one sequence, clone 14, however, was found to be suppressed by CsA in the first limited set of picked clones.

B. MOUSE MAMMARY TUMOR VIRUS EXPRESSION IS INDUCED BY PMA AND SUPPRESSED BY CsA IN EL4 CELLS

The inducible and suppressible sequence identified as clone 14 hybridized to 62% of the PMA-induced clones. DNA sequence analysis proved that these represented a closely related family of various forms of mouse mammary tumor virus (MMTV) sequences. The MMTV proviral genome is highly amplified and heterogeneous in this cell line, and its

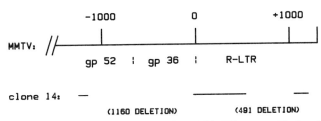

FIG. 5. A map of clone 14. Clone 14 DNA (see Table IV) was purified, subcloned into phage M13, and its sequence was determined by the dideoxy nucleoside 5'-triphosphate (NTP) incorporation method. It was found to correspond to portions of the right end of the MMTV genome, with several point mutations and two large deletions. The numbering at the top of the map is relative to the boundary of the 3' LTR of MMTV. The 491 bp deletion is precisely as described by Kwon and Weissman (1984) for their MMTV-related sequence isolated from EL4 cells, but their clone did not carry the 1160 bp upstream deletion seen here. The representation is approximately to scale. The total cDNA clone is 830 bp long. The *Hin*fI fragment used in Fig. 6 spanned the leftmost 347 nucleotides of clone 14 DNA (both *env* and LTR sequences).

induction by PMA in EL4 cells was recently described by Kwon and Weissman (1984). Furthermore, PMA induces both enhanced steady-state levels of MMTV RNA and virus production in a mammary tumor cell line (Arya, 1980). Sequence analysis of clone 14 indicated that it contained 830 nucleotides of MMTV sequence, beginning to the left of the right-hand LTR and extending through it with two large deletions (Fig. 5). The 491 bp deletion in the R-LTR region was precisely the same as in the MMTV-related sequence cloned by Kwon and Weissman (1984), but the 1160 bp deletion in clone 14 was not present in their sequence. Randomly picked clones from the 14-like family contained one or both of these deletions. It is not yet known whether any of them contain any flanking region DNA from the mouse genome.

A set of mRNAs prepared under conditions of induction, suppression, and cycloheximide treatment were probed with clone 14 with the results shown in Fig. 6. Unstimulated EL4.E1 cells expressed a low level of the 35 S RNA typically found in MMTV-producing cells (Robertson and Varmus, 1979; Sen *et al.*, 1979). Following induction with PMA, abundant MMTV sequences were found at the 24 S and 14 S positions, also typical of MMTV-expressing cells (Robertson and Varmus, 1979; Sen *et al.*, 1979). These results are similar to the data of Kwon and Weissman (1984), but differ in the predominant nature of the 14 S RNA in our experiments. The surprising result was that both the 24 S and 14 S forms were suppressed almost completely by CsA (Fig. 6), whereas the 35 S form was not significantly affected. This suggests that these forms of MMTV mRNA share regulatory features with lymphokine genes in EL4.E1 cells. The 14 S and 24 S forms, but not the 35 S form, were also

TIME OF HARVEST: 18.5h

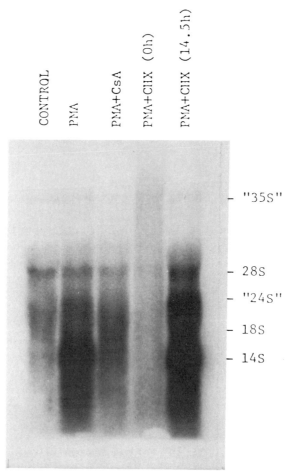

FIG. 6. Mouse mammary tumor virus (MMTV) in RNA induction and blockage. Mouse mammary tumor virus mRNA is induced by PMA in EL4 cells, and this induction is blocked by CsA. A 347 bp *Hinf*I fragment of probe 14 (Fig. 5) was used to carry out a Northern gel analysis of mRNA harvested from EL4.E1 cells treated as indicated on the figure. The 35 S, 24 S, and 14 S components correspond to MMTV species typical of mamary tumor cell lines expressing the viral sequence (Robertson and Varmus, 1979; Sen et al., 1979) and also for this T lymphoma (Kwon and Weissman, 1984). The 24 S and 14 S species, but not the intact 35 S RNA, were induced by PMA and suppressed by CsA. Their induction was also blocked by cycloheximide added at 0 hr, but they were superinduced at 14.5 hr.

superinduced by cycloheximide, added at later times, and blocked in their expression by the same drug added at the time of PMA induction (Fig. 6). The induction of MMTV RNA synthesis in EL4 cells by PMA is apparently slower (Kwon and Weissman, 1985) than that induced by glucocorticoids in mammary tumor cells (Ringold *et al.*, 1975). The blockage by cycloheximide at the time of induction in EL4.E1 also differentiates this response from the dexamethasone response, which is insensitive to cycloheximide (Ringold *et al.*, 1975). This suggests that its basis lies in the inductive and suppressive mechanisms of T lymphocytes rather than in the (virally encoded) glucocorticoid-sensitive induction of the MMTV provirus. Whether the response of the MMTV proviral DNA in EL4 cells is a property of MMTV sequences only, or depends on a flanking genetic area, is not known, but in either case this fortuitous observation may be useful in delineating the molecular basis of induction and suppression in T lymphocytes.

IV. Summary

1. Antigen-specific CTL, dependent on the presence of antigen and IL-2 for proliferation and expression of cytotoxicity (Type I cells) are converted to cells with nonspecific cytotoxicity and a growth requirement for IL-2 alone by recombinant or purified natural IL-2 at high levels. Conversion depends on costimulation with antigen or PMA.

2. Type I cells activated with antigen and IL-2 express 5- to 10-fold higher levels of IL-2-R mRNA, about the same as the enhancement of actin mRNA expression.

3. Lymphokine mRNA synthesis is selectively induced by T lymphocyte-activating molecules (mitogens and PMA) and suppressed by CsA.

4. Suppression by CsA does not require protein synthesis. CsA both blocks induction at the outset and interrupts ongoing transcription.

5. The half-life of IL-2 mRNA is relatively short (on the order of 1–2 hr), making it superinducible by the addition of inhibitors of protein synthesis.

6. The pattern of lymphokine mRNA expression can be used to isolate, by subtractive cloning, DNA sequences which are candidates for new lymphokines and similarly regulated related structures.

7. Mouse mammary tumor virus-related mRNA is induced by PMA and suppressed by CsA in EL4.E1 cells.

ACKNOWLEDGMENTS

This work was funded by the Medical Research Council of Canada, the National Cancer Institute of Canada, and the Alberta Heritage Foundation for Medical Research. We are grateful to Dr. L. H. Kedes (Stanford University) for providing the actin cDNA plasmid pHF1, and to Dr. P. J. Barr (Chiron Corp.) for the human IFN-γ oligonucleotide probe.

REFERENCES

Andrew, M. E., Churilla, A. M., Malek, T. R., Braciale, V. L., and Braciale, T. J. (1985). *J. Immunol.* **134**, 920–925.

Arya, S. K. (1980). *Nature (London)* **284**, 71–72.

Bleackley, R. C., Havele, C., and Paetkau, V. (1982). *J. Immunol.* **128**, 758–767.

Bleackley, R. C., Horak, H., McElhaney, J., Shaw, A. R. E., Turner, A. R., and Paetkau, V. (1983). *Nucleic Acids Res.* **11**, 3027–3035.

Brooks, C. G. (1983). *Nature (London)* **305**, 155–158.

Brooks, C. G., Urdal, D. L., and Henney, C. S. (1983). *Immunol. Rev.* **72**, 43–72.

Brooks, C. G., Holscher, M., and Urdal, D. (1985). *J. Immunol.* **135**, 1145–1152.

Claesson, M. H., and Miller, R. G. (1984). *J. Exp. Med.* **160**, 1702–1716.

Cochran, B. H., Reffel, A. C., and Stiles, C. D. (1983). *Cell* **33**, 939–947.

Dennert, G. (1980). *Nature (London)* **301**, 47–49.

Efrat, S., and Kaempfer, R. (1984). *Proc. Natl. Acad. Sci. U.S.A.* **81**, 2601–2605.

Elliott, J. F., Lin, Y., Mizel, S. B., Bleackley, R. C., Harnish, D. G., and Paetkau, V. (1984). *Science* **226**, 1439–1441.

Falk, W., Mannel, D. N., and Droege, W. (1983). *J. Immunol.* **130**, 2214–2218.

Farrar, J. J., Fuller-Farrar, J., Simon, P. L., Hilfiker, M. L., Stadler, B. M., and Farrar, W. L. (1980). *J. Immunol.* **125**, 2555–2558.

Farrar, J. J., Howard, M., Fuller-Farrar, J., and Paul, W. E. (1983). *J. Immunol.* **131**, 1838–1842.

Giglia, J. S., Ovak, G. M., Yoshida, M. A., Twist, C. J., Jeffery, A. R., and Pauly, J. L. (1985). *Cancer Res.* **45**, 5027–5034.

Granelli-Piperno, A., Inaba, K., and Steinman, R. M. (1984). *J. Exp. Med.* **160**, 1793–1803.

Gray, P. W., Leung, D. W., Pennica, D., Yelverton, E., Najarian, R., Simonson, C. C., Derynck, R., Sherwood, P. J., Wallace, D. M., Berger, S. L., Levinson, A. D., and Goeddel, D. V. (1982). *Nature (London)* **295**, 503–508.

Grimm, E. A., Mazumder, A., Zhang, H. Z., and Rosenberg, S. A. (1982). *J. Exp. Med.* **155**, 1823–1841.

Hamilton, R. T., Nilsen-Hamilton, M., and Adams, G. (1985). *J. Cell. Physiol.* **123**, 201–208.

Havele, C., Bleackley, R. C., and Paetkau, V. (1985). *In* "Cellular and Molecular Biology of Lymphokines" (A. Schimpl and Wecker, eds.), pp. 491–495. Academic Press, New York.

Havele, C., Bleackley, R. C., and Paetkau, V. (1986). *J. Immunol.* **137**, 1448–1454.

Hedrick, S. M., Nielsen, E. A., Kaveler, J., Cohen, D. I., and Davis, M. M. (1984). *Nature (London)* **308**, 153–158.

Hemler, E., Brenner, M. B., McLean, J. M., and Strominger, J. L. (1984). *Proc. Natl. Acad. Sci. U.S.A.* **81**, 2172–2175.

Hercend, T., Reinherz, E. L., Meuer, S., Schlossman, S. F., and Ritz, J. (1983). *Nature (London)* **301**, 158–160.

Howard, M., Farrar, J. J., Hilfiker, M., Johnson, B., Takatsu, K., Hamaoka, T., and Paul, W. E. (1982). *J. Exp. Med.* **155**, 914–923.

Kaplan, D., Braciale, V., and Braciale, T. (1984). *J. Immunol.* **133**, 1966–1969.

Kronke, M., Leonard, W. J., Depper, J. M., Arya, S. K., Wong-Stahl, F., Gallo, R. C., Waldmann, T. A., and Greene, W. C. (1984). *Proc. Natl. Acad. Sci. U.S.A.* **81**, 5214–5218.

Kronke, M., Leonard, W. J., Depper, J. M., and Greene, W. C. (1985). *J. Exp. Med.* **161**, 1593–1598.

Kwon, B. S., and Weissman, S. M. (1984). *J. Virol.* **52**, 1000–1004.

Lengyel, P. (1982). *Annu. Rev. Biochem.* **51**, 251–282.

Lowenthal, J. W., Tougne, C., MacDonald, H. R., Smith, K. A., and Nabholz, M. (1985). *J. Immunol.* **134**, 931–939.

Malek, T. R., and Ashwell, J. D. (1985). *J. Exp. Med.* **161**, 1575–1580.

Mizel, S. B., and Mizel, D. (1981). *J. Immunol.* **126**, 834–837.

Nabel, G., Bucalo, L. R., Allard, J., Wigzell, H., and Cantor, H. (1981). *J. Exp. Med.* **153**, 1582–1591.

Nakanishi, K., Cohen, D. I., Blackman, M., Nielsen, E., Ohara, J., Hamaoka, T., Koshland, M. E., and Paul, W. E. (1984). *J. Exp. Med.* **160**, 1736–1751.

Newmark, P. (1985). *Nature (London)* **317**, 380.

Olabuenaga, S. E., Brooks, C. G., Gillis, S., and Henney, C. S. (1983). *J. Immunol.* **131**, 2386–2391.

Paetkau, V. (1985). *Can. J. Biochem. Cell. Biol.* **63**, 691–699.

Paetkau, V., Bleackley, R. C., Riendeau, D., Harnish, D. G., and Holowachuk, E. W. (1985). *In* "Contemporary Topics in Molecular Immunology" (S. Gillis and F. P. Inman, eds.), Vol. 10, pp. 35–61. Plenum, New York.

Paetkau, V., Shaw, J., Ng, J., Elliott, J. F., Meerovitch, K., Barr, P. J., and Bleackley, R. C. (1986). *In* "Mediators of Immune Regulation and Immunotherapy" (K. Singhal and T. L. Delovitch, eds.), pp. 3–14. Elsevier, Amsterdam.

Pearlstein, K. T., Staiano-Coico, L., Miller, R. A., Pelus, L. M., Kirch, M. E., Stutman, O., and Palladino, M. A. (1983). *J. Natl. Cancer Inst.* **71**, 583–590.

Pure, E., Isakson, P. C., Paetkau, V., Caplan, B., Vitetta, E. S., and Krammer, P. H. (1982). *J. Immunol.* **129**, 2420–2425.

Raulet, D. H., and Bevan, M. J. (1982). *Nature (London)* **296**, 754–757.

Reimann, J., and Miller, R. G. (1985). *Cell* **40**, 571–581.

Riendeau, D., Harnish, D. G., Bleackley, R. C., and Paetkau, V. (1983). *J. Biol. Chem.* **258**, 12114–12117.

Ringold, G. M., Yamamoto, K. R., Tomkins, G. M., Bishop, J. M., and Varmus, H. E. (1975). *Cell* **6**, 299–305.

Robb, R. J., Greene, W. C., and Rusk, C. M. (1984). *J. Exp. Med.* **160**, 1126–1146.

Robertson, D. L., and Varmus, H. E. (1979). *J. Virol.* **30**, 576–589.

Sehgal, P. B., Lyles, D. S., and Tamm, I. (1978). *Virology* **89**, 186–198.

Sen, G. C., Smith, S. W., Marcus, S. L., and Sarkar, N. H. (1979). *Proc. Natl. Acad. Sci. U.S.A.* **76**, 1736–1740.

Shaw, J., Meerovitch, K., Elliott, J. F., Bleackley, R. C., and Paetkau, V. (1986). *Mol. Immunol.*, in press.

Slattery, E., Ghosh, N., Samanta, H., and Lengyel, P. (1979). *Proc. Natl. Acad. Sci. U.S.A.* **76**, 4778–4782.

White, B. A., and Bancroft, F. C. (1982). *J. Biol. Chem.* **257**, 8569–8572.

Williams, J. G. (1981). *In* "Genetic Engineering" (R. Williamson, ed.), Vol. 1, pp. 1–59. Academic Press, London.

Wiskocil, R., Weiss, A., Imboden, J., Kamin-Lewis, R., and Stobo, J. (1985). *J. Immunol.* **134**, 1599–1603.

Yanagi, Y., Yoshikai, Y., Leggett, K., Clark, S. P., Aleksander, I., and Mak, T. (1984). *Nature (London)* **308**, 145–149.

LYMPHOKINES, VOL. 13

Molecular Cloning of the Human Interleukin 2 Receptor

WARREN J. LEONARD

Cell Biology and Metabolism Branch, National Institute of Child Health and Human Development,
National Institutes of Health, Bethesda, Maryland 20892

I. Introduction

Activation of resting T lymphocytes with either antigen or mitogenic lectins stimulates the synthesis and secretion by some T cells of IL-2, formerly known as T cell growth factor (Morgan *et al.*, 1976). Another, possibly overlapping population of T cells, when activated, expresses IL-2 receptors. In the presence of IL-2, the cells with receptors proliferate, resulting in the expansion of T cells capable of mediating helper and cytotoxic functions (Watson, 1979; Coutinho *et al.*, 1979; Gillis *et al.*, 1978). IL-2 and IL-2 receptor expression are inducible events whose regulation is critically controlled. Although the antigen confers the specificity of the immune response, it is the interaction of IL-2 and IL-2 receptors that mediates the subsequent cell growth in an antigen-independent fashion that is necessary for mounting a complete T cell immune response. This model of T cell activation is depicted in Fig. 1.

Human IL-2 has been purified (Robb *et al.*, 1983), cDNAs cloned (Taniguchi *et al.*, 1983; Devos *et al.*, 1983), and a single gene (Fujita *et al.*, 1983; Holbrook *et al.*, 1984) localized to chromosome 4 (Siegel *et al.*, 1984). Interleukin 2 receptors are glycoproteins that may be sulfated and phosphorylated with apparent M_rs of approximately 55,000 on normal activated T cells (Leonard *et al.*, 1982, 1983, 1984a, 1985a; Wano *et al.*, 1984). These cells express 30,000 to 60,000 receptors per cell. Human T cell lymphotrophic virus I (HTLV-I)-infected T cells uniformly express large numbers of IL-2 receptors (several hundred thousand receptors/cell) (Depper *et al.*, 1984), and occasionally the migration of these receptors on SDS–polyacrylamide gels differs somewhat from the normal receptor (Leonard *et al.*, 1984a, 1985a; Wano *et al.*, 1984). Summarized herein is work describing the purification of IL-2 receptor protein, identification and sequencing of IL-2 receptor cDNAs (Leonard *et al.*, 1984b; Nikaido *et al.*, 1984; Cosman *et al.*, 1984), and characterization of the IL-2 receptor gene (Leonard *et al.*, 1985d). The cDNA strategy detailed here is from Leonard *et al.* (1984b).

95

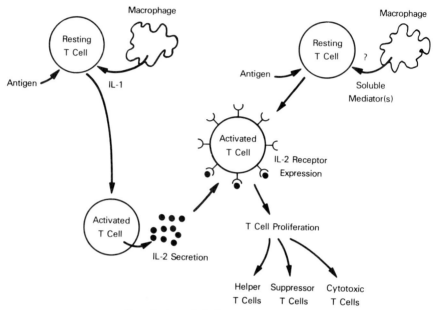

FIG. 1. A model of T cell activation.

II. Purification of IL-2 Receptor and Determination of Partial Amino Acid Sequence

Purification of the IL-2 receptor was greatly facilitated by the preparation of monoclonal anti-Tac antibody (Uchiyama *et al.*, 1981), which was originally prepared as a marker for activated T cells and subsequently demonstrated to recognize the human IL-2 receptor. The evidence in support of the specificity of anti-Tac includes the following: (1) anti-Tac blocks more than 80% of the IL-2-induced thymidine incorporation in IL-2-dependent continuous T cell lines but has no effect on IL-2-independent T cell lines (Leonard *et al.*, 1982); (2) IL-2 blocks the binding of radiolabeled anti-Tac to peripheral blood T cells activated with phytohemagglutinin (Leonard *et al.*, 1983); (3) anti-Tac, but not control antibodies, blocks the binding of radiolabeled IL-2 to HuT 102B2 cells (Leonard *et al.*, 1982); (4) both anti-Tac and IL-2 immobilized on beads bind the identical protein from extracts of receptor-positive cells (Robb and Greene, 1983); and (5) precipitations with either anti-Tac or anti-IL-2 monoclonal antibodies yield the same band on SDS–polyacrylamide gels following covalent cross-linking of IL-2 to its receptor with disuccinimidyl suberate (Leonard *et al.*, 1983).

Purification of the IL-2 receptor was also facilitated by the existence of cell lines infected with HTLV-I. As noted, these cell lines express several hundred thousand receptors per cell, approximately 5- to 20-fold more than on normal activated T cells (Depper *et al.*, 1984), and serve as a rich source of receptor protein.

The IL-2 receptor on HTLV-I-infected HuT 102B2 cells was purified to apparent homogeneity using an anti-Tac immunoaffinity column (Leonard *et al.*, 1984b). HuT-102B2 cells were extracted at 4°C in 10 m*M* Tris pH 7.4 containing 0.15 *M* NaCl, 100 μg/ml phenylmethylsulfonylfluoride, and 0.5% nonidet-P40. Nuclei and cellular debris were pelleted, and the supernatant was passed first over a control column and then over an anti-Tac Sepharose column. The column was washed extensively at varying salt concentrations, and the bound protein eluted with 2.5% acetic acid in water. The purified protein was able to bind IL-2 as evaluated by its ability to block IL-2-induced proliferation. This purified protein was used as an immunogen to produce a polyclonal antiserum against the IL-2 receptor and also to determine partial amino acid sequence data. The N-terminal amino acid sequence was determined primarily by gas-phase microsequencing. Certain positions were confirmed by sequencing receptor biosynthetically radiolabeled with select amino acids. The sequence obtained is as follows:

H$_2$N-Glu-Leu-*Cys-Asp-Asp-Asp-Pro-Pro*-Glu-Ile-Pro-His-Ala-Thr-Phe-Lys-Ala-Met-Ala-
Tyr-Lys-Glu-Gly-Thr-Met-Leu-Asn-Cys-Glu.

III. Identification of IL-2 Receptor cDNAs

A synthetic oligonucleotide probe 17 bases long with 64-fold degeneracy was prepared (by Dr. R. M. Belagaje, Lilly Research Laboratories) based on amino acids 3 through 8, italicized above, and this pool of 17-mers was used to identify cDNAs in a library prepared in λgt10 from HuT 102B2 mRNA. Details of the preparation of the cDNA library are discussed in Leonard *et al.* (1984b).

Candidate cDNA clones were identified by hybridization with the ^{32}P-end-labeled 17-mer. The inserts from three clones were subcloned into the *Eco*RI site of pBR322, and selective hybridization experiments were performed to confirm the relation of the cDNAs to the IL-2 receptor (Fig. 2). The location of the primary translation produce for IL-2 receptor mRNA is identified on the right. Clones pIL2R2, pIL2R3, and pIL2R4 (clones 2, 3, and 4) all selectively hybridized IL-2 receptor mRNA, but pBR327 and nitrocellulose without DNA did not.

The inserts of pIL2R3 and pIL2R4, the two longest clones, were sequenced by subcloning the DNA inserts or fragments of the inserts

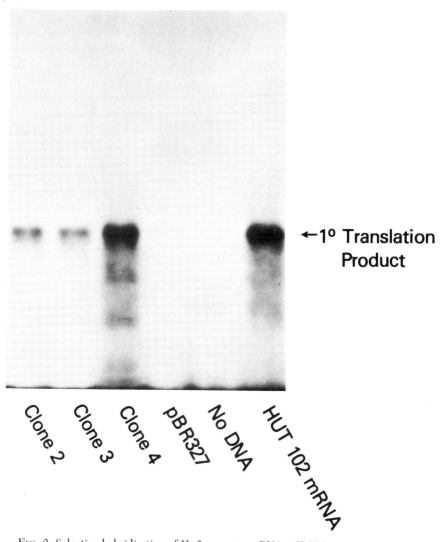

FIG. 2. Selective hybridization of IL-2 receptor mRNA. pIL2R2, pIL2R3, pIL2R4, or control pBR327 DNAs were bound to nitrocellulose as detailed in Leonard *et al.* (1984b) and hybridized to HuT 102B2 mRNA. The filters were washed and the filter bound mRNA eluted, translated in a wheat germ cell-free translation system, immunoprecipitated with a polyclonal antiserum to the IL-2 receptor, and subjected to electrophoresis on an 8.75% SDS–polyacrylamide gel. Reproduced from Leonard *et al.* (1984b) with permission of *Nature.*

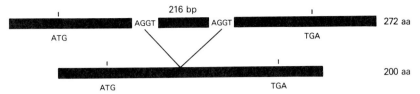

FIG. 3. Schematic diagram of the inserts of pIL2R3 (top) and pIL2R4 (bottom). The translation initiation start and stop sites are indicated (ATG and TGA sequences, respectively). Further, the 216-base pair segment present in clone 3 but absent in clone 4 is indicated. aa, Amino acids.

into M13 phage and then using dideoxy sequencing (Sanger and Coulson, 1975), as previously described (Leonard *et al.*, 1984b). The sequences of the two clones differ in two major ways. First, clone 3 is longer and extends further 3'. Second, clone 3 contains a 216-base pair segment not contained in clone 4. This region is bounded by typical donor and acceptor mRNA splice signals. Thus, the clone 4 cDNA encoded a protein 72 amino acids shorter but which shared both N- and C-termini with clone 3 (Fig. 3). It was therefore critical to determine which cDNA encoded a functional IL-2 receptor. The insert of each clone was therefore subcloned in the correct orientation into the *Eco*RI site of pcEXV-I, an SV40 expression vector (prepared and generously provided by J. Miller and R. Germain, NIH). These constructs were then used to transfect COS-1 cells. Both radiolabeled anti-Tac and IL-2 binding studies were then performed on the transfected cells. As indicated in Fig. 4, only the longer clone (clone 3) was able to direct the synthesis of IL-2 receptors, as determined by IL-2 or anti-Tac binding, even though both clone 3 and clone 4 constructs were transcriptionally active. Clone 4 is the result of alternative mRNA splicing of exon 4 (see Section IV) but has no known function at present.

Using low stringency hybridization studies with human IL-2 receptor cDNAs, the murine IL-2 receptor has also been cloned (Miller *et al.*, 1985; Shimizu *et al.*, 1985). The mouse receptor shares 72% DNA and 61% amino acid homology with the human receptor (see Cosman *et al.* as well as Miller *et al.*, this volume).

IV. Structure of the IL-2 Receptor Gene

Using IL-2 receptor cDNAs, genomic phage clones spanning the IL-2 receptor gene (except part of the first intron) were isolated (Leonard *et al.*, 1985d) from libraries prepared in the laboratories of P. Leder and T. Maniatis. All exons and exon–intron splice junctions were sequenced. As

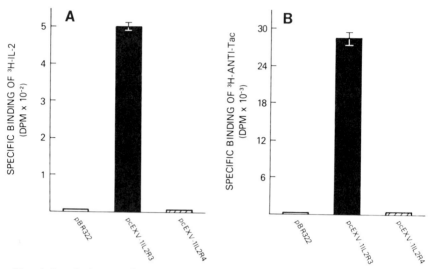

F IG. 4. Interleukin 2 and anti-Tac binding. The unspliced cDNA encodes a functional IL-2 receptor. Five micrograms of either pBR322 or the SV40 expression vector, pcEXV-1, containing the insert from either pIL2R3 or the pIL2R4 was precipitated with calcium phosphate and used to transfect COS-1 cells. The cells were grown overnight, the media changed, and the cells cultured for another 48 hr. Cells were then washed, incubated at 4°C for 90 min in RPMI 1640 medium containing 3% fetal bovine serum and either 45,000 dpm of ³H-labeled IL 2 or 194,000 dpm of ³H-labeled anti-Tac, with or without excess unlabeled IL-2 or anti-Tac, respectively. Cells were washed, dissolved in 0.1 M NaOH, and associated radioactivity was determined. Specific IL-2 and anti-Tac binding are indicated. (A) IL-2 binding; (B) anti-Tac binding.

shown in Fig. 5, the IL-2 receptor consists of 8 exons and 7 introns, spanning more than 25 kilobases (Leonard *et al.*, 1985d). The length of intron 1 exceeds 15 kb, but its precise length is unknown since the phage clone that contains the first exon does not extend far enough 3' to overlap any of the other phage clones isolated. J. Miller and R. N. Germain (personal communication) have isolated cosmid clones for the murine IL-2 receptor and have data to suggest that intron 1 in mouse exceeds 15 kb, and may exceed 30 kb.

Exon 1 contains the signal peptide and the 5' nontranslated region. The second exon contains the N-terminal part of the mature protein. Exons 2 and 3 contain clusters of serines and threonines and therefore may contain O-linked carbohydrate addition sites. Exons 2 and 3 each contain one N-linked carbohydrate addition site. Exons 2 and 4 share significant homology, suggesting an historical gene-duplication event, also noted in the murine IL-2 receptor (Miller *et al.*, 1985). Exons 2 and 4 also share statistically significant homology to complement factor B, Ba

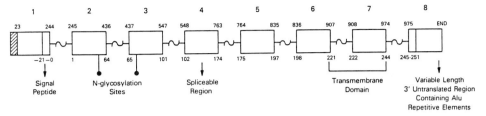

FIG. 5. Structure of the human interleukin 2 receptor gene. The gene consists of eight exons and seven introns. The diagram indicates the location of the signal peptide, spliceable region, transmembrane domains. The locations of N-linked carbohydrate addition sites are also noted. Exons are numbered at the top. The numbers above the boxes correspond to the numbering scheme of the DNA sequence of pIL2R3 (Leonard *et al.*, 1984b). The numbers below the boxes correspond to the amino acids of the IL-2 receptor.

fragment. This is the binding (recognition) domain of complement factor B and has been reported to have DNA binding activity (Leonard *et al.*, 1985d). As noted above, exon 4 corresponds precisely to the 216-base pair segment that may be alternatively spliced. Exons 5 and 6 correspond to the domain of the protein located immediately outside the cell membrane. Like exons 2 and 3, these exons encode clusters of serines or threonines, suggesting that they may contain potential O-linked carbohydrate addition sites. Exon 7 encodes the hydrophobic transmembrane crossing region, and exons 7 and 8 together encode the cytoplasmic domain. Exon 8 also contains the 3' untranslated region and unexpectedly contains repetitive alu sequences.

Although the IL-2 receptors expressed on normal activated T cells and HuT 102B2 cells differ slightly in their apparent M_rs on SDS–polyacrylamide gels, comparison of the sequences of the HuT 102B2 cDNA to the normal gene indicated that the DNA and, therefore, protein sequences are identical.

V. One Gene but Multiple mRNA Species

When IL-2 receptor cDNAs were hybridized to a Southern blot of genomic DNA digested with *Bam*HI or *Eco*RI, the relatively simple pattern of hybridization suggested the existence of a single gene. *In situ* hybridization experiments, performed by Dr. T. A. Donlon, demonstrated that this gene is on chromosome 10, bands p14 →15 (see Leonard *et al.*, 1985b).

In contrast, mRNA of two principal sizes, approximately 1500 and 3500 bases long, are identified on Northern blots using mRNAs from activated T cells (Fig. 6). It is of interest that both of these hybridizing

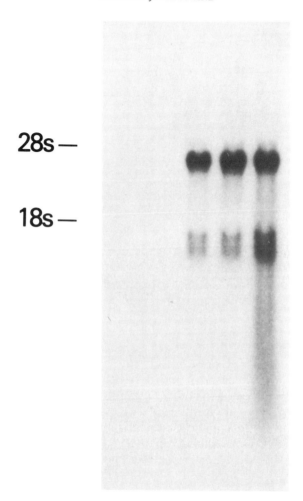

FIG. 6. Northern blot using IL-2 receptor cDNAs. Northern blot of 10 µg mRNA, from the indicated cell types, hybridized to IL-2 receptor cDNA. Ribonucleic acid from B cells (lane A), resting T cells (lane B), T cells activated with phytohemagglutinin (PHA) (lane C), T cells activated phorbol 12-myristate 13-acetate (PMA) (lane D), and T cells activated with PHA plus PMA (lane E).

regions clearly contain functionally active IL-2 receptor mRNA. When HuT 102B2 mRNA was size fractionated on a methyl mercuric hydroxide agarose gel, the gel sliced, and mRNAs from all regions of the gel translated, it was possible to precipitate the same primary translation product from both the 1500 and 3500 base regions of the gel. Careful analysis of the sequence of the insert of pIL2R3 revealed that it contained two internal polyadenylation signal sequences (ATTAAA and AATAAA) in the 3' untranslated region. When Northern blots were hybridized with a radiolabeled probe from the part of the cDNA 3' to these sequences, only the 3500-base mRNA species was identified (Leonard *et al.*, 1984b). This confirmed that the 3500-base mRNAs had utilized a more distal polyadenylation signal not contained in the cDNA. S1 nuclease protection assays definitively proved that there are IL-2 receptor mRNA species that were polyadenylated at at least three different sites (Kronke *et al.*, 1985a; Leonard *et al.*, 1985c). The smaller signal on the Northern blots (1500-base mRNAs) actually represents a combination of mRNAs that utilizes the two polyadenylation signals contained within pIL2R3.

In addition to the variable polyadenylation, S1 nuclease assays have also been used to demonstrate that the 216-base pair segment missing from pIL2R4 results from alternative mRNA splicing (Kronke *et al.*, 1985a; Leonard *et al.*, 1985c). Combining three different polyadenylation sites and alternative mRNA splicing suggests to this point that there may be at least six mRNA species generated from the IL-2 receptor gene.

However, the situation is even more complex. In order to evaluate whether the 5' end of the cDNA corresponded to the 5' end of IL-2 receptor mRNA, primer extension experiments were performed. A synthetic oligonucleotide probe, complementary to mRNA near the 5' end of the cDNA, was synthesized and generously provided by Dr. R. M. Belagaje, Lilly Research Laboratories. This synthetic primer was end labeled with [γ-32P]ATP and polynucleotide kinase, annealed to mRNA, and then extended using reverse transcriptase. The studies indicated that there were two major transcription initiation sites in both normal activated T cells and in HuT 102B2 cells. However, a third additional initiation site was identified only in the HuT 102B2 cells (Leonard *et al.*, 1985d).

In order to confirm these findings, S1 nuclease protection assays were performed using a genomic DNA fragment that overlapped the 5' end of the cDNA and extended almost 500 bp further 5'. As in the primer extension experiments, two major transcription initiation sites (and therefore two distinct principal promoters) were identified. In HuT 102B2 cells a third additional site was identified. This third site was also clearly identified when experiments were performed using mRNA from four other HTLV-I-infected adult T cell leukemia (ATL) cell lines (Leonard et al., 1985d). Thus, it is a finding apparently associated with ATL. It should be noted that the third site is also present in .5B4 cells, an Epstein–Barr virus-transformed B cell line that expressed IL-2 receptors (Waldmann et al., 1984); thus, the finding is not unique to ATL.

Taken together, the combination of alternative mRNA splicing, multiple polyadenylation sites, and multiple transcription initiation sites suggests that perhaps as many as 18 mRNAs may be generated from this one gene.

As noted above (see Fig. 1), resting T cells do not express IL-2 receptors, but they are rapidly expressed following activation with phytohemagglutinin (PHA). Nuclear run off experiments indicate that this induction is regulated at the level of transcription (Leonard et al., 1985c) and temporally precedes induction of the IL-2 gene (Kronke et al., 1985b).

VI. Analysis of IL-2 Receptor Protein

The amino acid sequence of the IL-2 receptor was deduced from the nucleic acid sequence (Leonard et al., 1984b; Nikaido et al., 1984; Cosman et al., 1984) (see Fig. 7). The receptor is synthesized as a precursor protein of 272 amino acids that is processed to a mature receptor of 251 amino acids. There are 13 cysteine residues, at least some of which form intrachain disulfide bonds as indicated by the fact that the mature protein has faster mobility on SDS gels electrophoresed under nonreducing conditions than on SDS gels electrophoresed under reducing conditions. There are two potential N-linked carbohydrate addition sites, both of which are utilized as indicated by earlier studies of the protein that demonstrate two N-linked precursors with apparent M_rs of 35,000 and 37,000 (Leonard et al., 1983, 1985a). The receptor also contains multiple potential O-linked carbohydrate addition sites.

Near the C-terminus, there is a long hydrophobic region that, Kyte–Doolittle plots predict, represents an α helical transmembrane crossing. There is a short cytoplasmic domain containing six positively charged amino acids that presumably serves a cytoplasmic-anchoring function. This region also contains one serine and one threonine as potential phosphorylation sites, at least one of which is utilized (Shackleford and Trowbridge, 1984; Leonard et al., 1985a). The cytoplasmic region is so small that it would seem unlikely that it contains an enzymatic function. It is therefore puzzling to hypothesize the mechanism of signal transduction for the IL-2/IL-2 receptor system or of receptor-mediated endo-

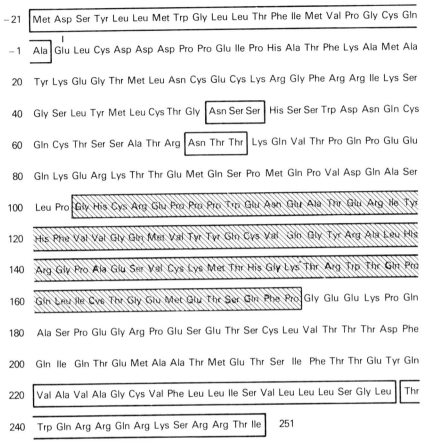

FIG. 7. Deduced amino acid sequence of the human IL-2 receptor. Boxed are the signal peptide (amino acids −21 to −1), two potential N-linked glycosylation sites (Asn-Ser-Ser and Asn-Thr-Thr), the hydrophobic transmembrane region (beginning Val-Ala-Val-Ala), and the cytoplasmic domain (beginning Thr-Trp-Gln). The cross-hatched area corresponds to the 72 amino acids that are absent when alternative mRNA splicing occurs.

cytosis of IL-2. It is conceivable that a receptor complex exists and that other critical subunits of the IL-2 receptor remain to be identified. Above, only the binding protein for IL-2 has been considered.

VII. Summary

Herein, I have reviewed some aspects of the cDNA and genomic cloning of the human interleukin 2 receptor. The IL-2 receptor serves as an interesting example of a protein whose gene generates multiple mRNA species, as determined by differential transcription initiation and polyadenylation, in addition to alternative mRNA splicing. The availability of these IL-2 receptor cDNA and genomic clones should help to elucidate the unanswered questions regarding IL-2 receptor regulation, in normal T cells and HTLV-I-infected leukemic cells, and the mechanisms of signal transduction.

REFERENCES

Cosman, D., Ceretti, D. P., Larsen, A., Park, L., March, C., Dower, S., Gillis, S., and Urdal, D. (1984). *Nature (London)* **312**, 768.

Coutinho, A., Larsson, E. L., Gronvik, K. O., and Andersson, J. (1979). *Eur. J. Immunol.* **9**, 587–592.

Depper, J. M., Leonard, W. J., Kronke, M., Waldmann, T. A., and Greene, W. C. (1984). *J. Immunol.* **311**, 626–631.

Devos, R., Plaetinck, G., Cheroutre, H. *et al.* (1983). *Nucleic Acids Res.* **11**, 4307–4322.

Fujita, T., Takaoka, C., Matsui, H., and Taniguchi, T. (1983). *Proc. Natl. Acad. Sci. U.S.A.* **80**, 7437–7441.

Gillis, S., Baker, P. E., Ruscetti, F. W., and Smith, K. A. (1978). *J. Exp. Med.* **148**, 1093–1098.

Holbrook, N. J., Smith, K. A., Fornace, A. J., Jr., Comeau, C. M., Wiskocil, R. L., and Crabtree, G. R. (1984). *Proc. Natl. Acad. Sci. U.S.A.* **81**, 1634–1638.

Kronke, M., Leonard, W. J., Depper, J. M., and Greene, W. C. (1985a). *Science* **228**, 1215.

Kronke, M., Leonard, W. J., Depper, J. M., and Greene, W. C. (1985b). *J. Exp. Med.* **161**, 1593–1598.

Leonard, W. J., Depper, J. M., Uchiyama, T., Smith, K. A., Waldmann, T. A., and Greene, W. C. (1982). *Nature (London)* **300**, 267–269.

Leonard, W. J., Depper, J. M., Robb, R. J., Waldmann, T. A., and Greene, W. C. (1983). *Proc. Natl. Acad. Sci. U.S.A.* **80**, 6957–6961.

Leonard, W. J., Depper, J. M., Waldmann, T. A., and Greene, W. C. (1984a). *Recept. Recognition Ser. B* **17**, 45–66.

Leonard, W. J., Depper, J. M., Crabtree, G. R., Rudikoff, S., Pumphrey, J., Robb, R. J., Kronke, M., Svetlik, P. B., Peffer, N. J., Waldmann, T. A., and Greene, W. C. (1984b). *Nature (London)* **311**, 626–631.

Leonard, W. J., Depper, J. M., Kronke, M., Robb, R. J., Waldmann, T. A., and Greene, W. C. (1985a). *J. Biol. Chem.* **260**, 1872.

Leonard, W. J., Donlon, T. A., Lebo, R. V., and Greene, W. C. (1985b). *Science* **228**, 1547.

Leonard, W. J., Kronke, M., Peffer, N. J., Depper, J. M., and Greene, W. C. (1985c). *Proc. Natl. Acad. Sci. U.S.A.* **82**, 6281.

Leonard, W. J., Depper, J. M., Kanehisa, M., Kronke, M., Peffer, N. J., Svetlik, P. B., Sullivan, M., and Greene, W. C. (1985d). *Science*, in press.

Miller, J., Malek, T. R., Leonard, W. J., Greene, W. C., Shevach, E. M., and Germain, R. N. (1985). *J. Immunol.* **134**, 4212.

Morgan, D. A., Ruscetti, F. W., and Gallo, R. C. (1976). *Science* **193**, 1007–1008.

Nikaido, T., Shimizu, A., Ishida, N., Sabe, H., Teshigawara, K., Maeda, M., Uchiyama, T., Yodoi, J., and Honjo, T. (1984). *Nature (London)* **311**, 631–635.

Robb, R. J., and Greene, W. C. (1983). *J. Exp. Med.* **158**, 1332–1337.

Robb, R. J., Kutny, R. M., and Chowdhry, V. (1983). *Proc. Natl. Acad. Sci. U.S.A.* **80,** 5990–5994.

Sanger, F., and Coulson, A. R. (1975). *J. Mol. Biol.* **94,** 414.

Shackleford, D. A., and Trowbridge, I. S. (1984). *J. Biol. Chem.* **259,** 11706.

Shimizu, A., Kondo, S., Takeda, S., Yodoi, J., Ishida, N., Sabe, H., Osawa, H., Diamantstein, T., Nikaido, T., and Honjo, T. (1985). *Nucleic Acids Res.* **13,** 1505–1516.

Siegel, L. J., Harper, M. E., Wong Staal, F., Gallo, R. C., Nash, W. G., and O'Brien, S. J. (1984). *Science* **223,** 174–178.

Taniguchi, T., Matsui, H., Fujita, T., Takaoka, C., Kashima, N., Yoshimoto, R., and Hamura, J. (1983). *Nature (London)* **302,** 205–209.

Uchiyama, T., Broder, S., and Waldmann, T. A. (1981). *J. Immunol.* **126,** 1393.

Waldmann, T. A. *et al.* (1984). *J. Exp. Med.* **160,** 1450.

Wano, Y., Uchiyama, T., Fukui, K., Maeda, M., Uchino, H., and Yodoi, J. (1984). *J. Immunol.* **132,** 3005–3010.

Watson, J. (1979). *J. Exp. Med.* **150,** 1510–1519.

Cloning and Expression of Human and Mouse IL-2 Receptor cDNAs

DAVID COSMAN, JANIS WIGNALL, ANDREW LEWIS, ALAN ALPERT,
KATE McKEREGHAN, DOUGLAS PAT CERRETTI, STEVEN GILLIS,
STEVEN DOWER, AND DAVID URDAL

Immunex Corporation, Seattle, Washington 98101

I. Introduction

When resting T cells are stimulated by antigen or mitogens, they synthesize the growth factor interleukin-2 (IL-2) as well as the receptor for IL-2 (IL-2-R) (Morgan *et al.*, 1976; Gillis and Smith, 1977; Robb *et al.*, 1984). The interaction of IL-2 with its receptor is necessary for the proliferation of the activated T cells. Two forms of the IL-2 receptor on activated T cells can be distinguished by the affinity with which they bind IL-2 (Robb *et al.*, 1984). In general, approximately 10% of the receptors bind IL-2 with a K_a of $1 \times 10^{11}/M$, and the remaining receptors with a K_a of 1×10^7. In contrast, monoclonal antibodies directed to the IL-2 receptor detect a single class of molecules, the number of which equals the sum of the high- and low-affinity sites detected by IL-2. As yet, no biochemical differences have been defined between the two classes of receptors; both are transmembrane glycoproteins with a molecular weight of approximately 55,000. However, it is thought that the biological effects of IL-2 are mediated by its interaction with the high-affinity receptors.

We have undertaken the cloning and expression of the IL-2 receptor in order to understand the molecular basis for the interaction of IL-2 with its receptor and the subsequent generation of a mitogenic signal for T cells.

II. Materials and Methods

A. cDNA Library Construction and Screening

Construction of cDNA libraries from HuT 102 cells and mitogen-activated peripheral blood T cells has been described (Cosman *et al.*, 1984; Cantrell *et al.*, 1985). Ribonucleic acid was isolated from CTLL-2 cells in the same way, and a cDNA library of 120,000 transformants was constructed as described in March *et al.* (1985). Low stringency hybridization and washing conditions were as described in Cantrell *et al.* (1985).

B. Plasmid Constructions

pN1/N4-S, containing the coding region of the IL-2 receptor cDNA isolated from HuT 102 cells under transcriptional control of the SV40 promoter, has been described (Cosman *et al.*, 1984). The mature coding region is contained in a 750-bp SstI–XbaI fragment. This fragment was replaced by the corresponding fragment from pTC to put the T cell-derived lL-2 receptor cDNA under SV40 transcriptional control in plasmid pMLSV-TC.

To replace the codon for serine 247 in pN1/N4-S with an alanine codon, the plasmid was digested with BclI and XbaI. The larger of the two fragments was purified by agarose gel electrophoresis and ligated to a synthetic 65-bp fragment incorporating the desired alanine codon to construct pN4Ala. The change was verified by nucleotide sequencing as described in Cosman *et al.* (1984).

The mouse IL-2 receptor cDNA pMrec-1 was digested with Sau3A, and the 923-bp fragment containing the entire coding region was cloned into the BglII site of pMLSV in the correct orientation for expression from the SV40 promoter to give pMLSV-MREC-1. In order to express the four IL-2 receptor cDNAs, each of the plasmids, pN1/N4-S, pMLSV-Tc, pN4Ala, and pMLSV-MREC-1, were digested with BamHI. The fragment containing the SV40 promoter, the cDNA, and SV40 splicing and polyadenylation signals was purified and ligated to BamHI-digested p1-8, resulting in the four plasmids pN4/1-8, pTc/1-8, pN4-Ala/1-8, and pMrec-1/1-8.

p1-8 was the kind gift of Nava Sarver and has been described in Sarver *et al.* (1985). In each case, the transcriptional orientation of the IL-2 receptor cDNAs was the same as that of the bovine papilloma virus (BPV) early region (Heilman *et al.*, 1982).

C. Transfection of C127 Cells

One million murine mammary epithelial cells (C127 cells) were transfected with 5 μg of plasmid DNA and 20 μg of carrier salmon sperm DNA as described in Sarver *et al.* (1981). After 4 hr the cells were given a 15% glycerol shock (Frost and Williams, 1978). The following day the cultures were trypsinized and replated at a 1:4 dilution in medium containing 2 mg/ml G418 (Gibco). G418-resistant cell lines were maintained in medium containing 500 μg/ml G418.

D. Analysis and Fluorescence-Activated Sorting of Cells

Analysis and sorting of C127 cells expressing the human IL-2 receptor were performed using monoclonal antibody 2A3 (Dower *et al.*, 1985) directly conjugated to biotin. Cells ($1–2 \times 10^7$) were incubated with a saturating amount of biotinyl-2A3 for 30 min at 4°C. After two washes and centrifugation with PBS/1% BSA, the cells were further incubated with FITC-avidin (Zymed Labs, Burlingame, California) for 30 min at 4°C. The samples were washed and centrifuged two times, resuspended in PBS/BSA, and propidium iodide was added at a final concentration of 5 μg/ml to aid in gating out nonviable cells. Unconjugated 2A3 and MOPC-21 (an IgG_1, κ antibody used as an isotypic control) were used to assess antibody specificity. For the detection of mouse IL-2 receptors, the cells were stained with the monoclonal antibody 7D4 (Malek *et al.*, 1983), using FITC-goat anti-rat IgM (Zymed Lab, Burlingame, CA) as a second-step antibody.

Samples were run on an EPICS-C flow cytometer (Coulter Corp., Hialeah, Florida), utilizing an argon laser at 488-nm excitation and a constant power of 300 mw. The top 1.0% of the viable 2A3-stained cells were collected at each sort and cultured in G418-containing media until the next sort. After the sixth cycle of sorting, 2A3-positive cells were cloned at 1 and 3 cells per well (96-well Costar culture dishes) using a Coulter autoclone.

E. Binding of ^{125}I-labeled Antibody and ^{125}I-labeled IL-2 to Cells

Monoclonal antibody 2A3 was radiolabeled as previously described (Dower *et al.*, 1985). The specific activity of the ^{125}I-labeled 2A3 preparation was 4.77×10^{15} cpm/mmol. Recombinant human IL-2 was expressed in, and purified from, *Escherichia coli* and provided via a collaborative arrangement between Immunex Corporation and Hoffman-La Roche. It was radiolabeled as previously described (Cosman *et al.*, 1984) with the enzymobead reagent from BioRad. The specific activity of the radiolabeled IL-2 preparation was 1.6×10^{15} cpm/mmol.

C127 cells expressing the recombinant IL-2 receptors were grown to confluence on 10-cm dishes. The plates were washed with phosphate-buffered saline containing 0.5 mM EDTA and incubated for 5 min at 37°C in the same solution. The cells were then scraped from the plates and washed twice with RPMI 1640 containing 10% fetal bovine serum. Clumps of cells were removed by filtering the cell suspension through 44-μm nylon mesh (Small Parts, Inc., Miami, Florida). Meanwhile, a nonadherent murine B cell line (NS1) that does not express IL-2 receptors was harvested from cultures to serve as a carrier cell for the binding experiments. C127 cells (2×10^6) and carrier cells (3.6×10^7) were mixed together and pelleted. The cells were then resuspended in 1 ml of binding medium (RPMI 1640 containing 2.5% BSA, 0.1% NaN_3, and

0.02 *M* HEPES, pH 7.2) and equilibrium binding experiments performed, as previously described (Dower *et al.*, 1985; Cosman *et al.*,
1984), for 2 hr at 4°C.

C127 cells were surface labeled with ^{125}I by the lactoperoxidase–
glucose oxidase technique. Cells were grown to confluence on 10-cm
tissue culture plates. The cells were washed on the plate several times
with 10-ml aliquots of PBS. The plates were then incubated with 1 ml of
PBS containing 20 µg lactoperoxidase (Sigma), 0.25 µg glucose oxidase
(Sigma), 20 m*M* glucose, and 2.5 mCi[^{125}I]NaI (NEN, low pH) for 15
min at room temperature. The plates were then washed with a solution
of PBS:0.15 *M* NaI (1:1) 3 times. Finally the cells were scraped from the
plate into 1 ml of PBS containing 1% (w/v) Triton X-100, 2 m*M* phe-
nylmethylsulfonyl fluoride (PMSF). Nuclei and cell debris were removed from the detergent-extracted cells by centrifugation in a micro-
fuge (Beckman) for 10 min at 4°C.

Immunoprecipitations and electrophoresis were performed as described in Urdal *et al.* (1984) and Dower *et al.* (1985) with Affigel-10
beads (BioRad) to which the 2A3 monoclonal antibody or a control antibody (MOPC-21) had been coupled (Urdal *et al.*, 1984).

III. Results

A. cDNA Cloning of Human IL-2 Receptors

The strategy used for cloning cDNAs encoding the Il-2 receptor has
been described (Cosman *et al.*, 1984). Briefly, the IL-2 receptor was
purified from HuT 102 cells (an HTLV-I-transformed T cell lymphoma)
and mitogen-activated peripheral blood T cells by immunoaffinity chromatography using a monoclonal antibody (2A3) specific for the receptor.
The N-terminal amino acid sequence of the receptor from both sources
was identical and was used to derive oligonucleotide probes. Screening
of a HuT 102 cDNA library led to the isolation of cDNA clones. These
were sequenced and shown to encode a protein of 251 amino acids,
including a 21-amino acid signal sequence, a 21-amino acid transmembrane domain, and a short, 11-amino acid cytoplasmic domain. The
coding sequence was subcloned into an SV40-based expression vector
and transfected into COS monkey kidney cells. The transfected cells
were shown to express human IL-2 receptors by their ability to bind both
labeled IL-2 and 2A3. Similar results have been reported by two other
groups (Leonard *et al.*, 1984; Nikaido *et al.*, 1984).

The apparent molecular weight of the IL-2 receptor on HTLV-I-transformed cells is about 5000 smaller than on peripheral blood T cells (Urdal

et al., 1984; Leonard *et al.*, 1985). The abnormal molecular weight, together with the very high numbers of IL-2 receptors on HTLV-I-transformed cells, has led to speculation that the IL-2 receptors on these cells may be aberrant and somehow involved in the transformed phenotype (Leonard *et al.*, 1985). Accordingly, we wished to isolate an IL-2 receptor cDNA from a normal T cell library in order to compare its sequence with the cDNAs isolated from HTLV-transformed cells. A cDNA library prepared from peripheral blood T cells stimulated with concanavalin A and phorbol myristic acetate was screened by hybridization with a 750-bp *Sst*I–*Xba*I probe from pN4 containing the mature coding region of the HuT 102-derived IL-2 receptor. One hybridizing cDNA clone, pTC, was characterized by nucleotide sequencing as shown in Fig. 1. The mature coding sequence showed four amino acid differences when compared to pN4. However, comparison with the sequence of IL-2 receptor cDNAs isolated from other HTLV-I-transformed cells (Table I) showed that only two of these amino acid changes were unique to the T cell-derived cDNA, Arg-105 to Lys and Arg-242 to Gln.

It has been suggested that the IL-2 receptor is phosphorylated by protein kinase C (Farrar and Anderson, 1985; Shackelford and Trowbridge, 1984). Inspection of the predicted amino acid sequence of the IL-2 receptor shows a stretch of amino acids surrounding serine 247 that conforms closely to a consensus protein kinase C phosphorylation site. In order to analyze the biological importance of this phosphorylation event, we replaced the codon for serine 247 with an alanine codon by replacing the 65-base pair *Bcl*I–*Xba*I fragment of pN4 with a synthetic fragment incorporating the altered codon.

B. EXPRESSION OF RECOMBINANT IL-2 RECEPTORS

We wished to express recombinant IL-2 receptors in sufficient quantities that we could examine their biochemical properties. In order to do this, the three IL-2 receptor cDNAs were placed under the transcriptional control of the SV40 early promoter and in front of SV40-derived RNA processing signal sequences as has been described for pN4 (Cosman *et al.*, 1984). The transcriptional unit was then inserted into a bovine papilloma virus (BPV)-derived vector, p1-8 (Fig. 2). This vector incorporates the entire BPV genome, the ampicillin resistance gene and origin of DNA replication from pML2d, and the neomycin resistance gene from Tn5 under control of the mouse metallothionein promoter and Moloney sarcoma virus enhancer. The vector thus confers resistance to the drug G418 on mammalian cells. The resulting plasmids, pN4/1-8, pTC/1-8, and pN4Ala/1-8, encoding, respectively, the HuT 102-derived and T cell-derived IL-2 receptors, and the receptor with serine 247

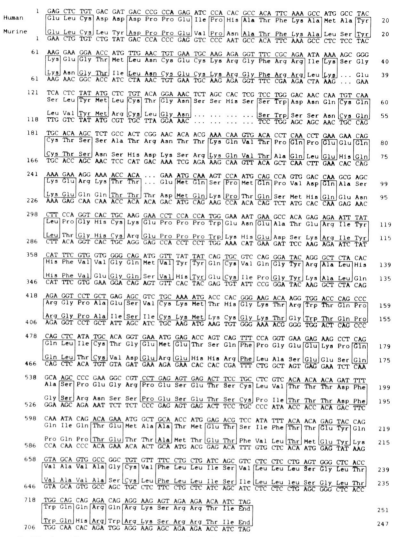

FIG. 1. Nucleotide sequences and predicted amino acid sequences of human and murine IL-2 receptors. Only the mature coding sequence of pTC (top) and pMrec-1 (bottom) are shown. Amino acids and nucleotides are numbered starting at the mature N-terminus and refer to the human sequence. Homologous amino acid residues are boxed.

changed to alanine, were transfected into C127 mouse mammary epithelial cells. Cells that were resistant to G418 were selected, pooled, and analyzed by fluorescence-activated cell sorting using biotinylated 2A3 and FITC-conjugated avidin. The brightest cells were sorted, grown, and resorted a total of six times, then single-cell cloned. In parallel, the

TABLE I

AMINO ACID SEQUENCE DIFFERENCES BETWEEN HUMAN
IL-2 RECEPTOR cDNA CLONES[a]

cDNA	Amino acid position				
	29	87	88	105	242
pN4	Glu	Lys	Ile	Arg	Arg
pTC	Glu	Glu	Met	Lys	Gln
pN1	Lys	Glu	Met	—	Arg
pIL2R3	Glu	Glu	Met	Arg	Arg
pTaC-2	Glu	Glu	Met	Arg	Arg

[a]pTC is described here; the others have been described previously (Leonard *et al.*, 1984; Nikaido *et al.*, 1984; Cosman *et al.*, 1984).

number of IL-2 receptors expressed per cell was determined by binding of ^{125}I-labeled 2A3. The results for the HuT 102-derived receptor, encoded by P1-8/N4, are shown in Fig. 3 and Table II. It can be seen that with each round of sorting there was an increase in the mean fluorescence of the cells as well as an increase in the number of receptors per

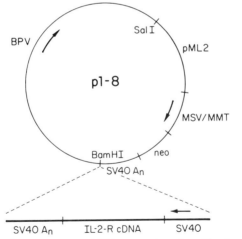

FIG. 2. Structure of IL-2 receptor cDNA expression plasmids. Arrows show the transcriptional orientation of the following: BPV, bovine papilloma virus; MoSV/MMT, the Moloney sarcoma virus enhancer linked to the mouse metallothionein promoter; and SV40, the simian virus 40 early promoter. pML2 contains sequences derived from the plasmid pBR322, neo refers to the neomycin resistance gene from Tn5, SV40 A$_n$ refers to SV40-derived sequences containing RNA splice donor and acceptor sites and a polyadenylation site, and IL-2-R cDNA designates the four IL-2 receptor cDNAs described here. p1-8 is described in more detail elsewhere (Sarver *et al.*, 1985).

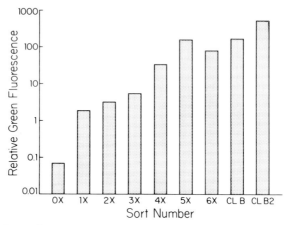

FIG. 3. Analysis of C127 cells transfected with the Hut 102-derived IL-2 receptor cDNA expression vector (pN4/1-8) during repetitive cycles of fluorescence-activated cell sorting. The relative green fluorescence (on a logarithmic scale) is shown for the starting population of cells and at each of six sorts. Also shown are two single cell clones derived after the sixth sort. Background fluorescence, determined using a control monoclonal antibody, has been subtracted from the fluorescence values obtained with 2A3, a monoclonal antibody specific for the human IL-2 receptor.

cell calculated from 2A3 binding. The final cloned cells expressed approximately 2–6×10^6 receptors per cell, whereas the starting population averaged 9×10^3 receptors per cell. Similar results were obtained with pTC/1-8 and pN4Ala/1-8, and clones were derived expressing 4×10^6 receptors per cell (data not shown). The high-level expression of the IL-2 receptor in these cells was stable.

It was of interest to determine the affinity with which IL-2 bound to the recombinant IL-2 receptors. Accordingly, cloned C127 cells expressing high levels of the three different IL-2 receptors were mixed with different amounts of ^{125}I-labeled IL-2 in a standard binding experiment. The results are shown in Fig. 4 and Table III. In each case there was a single class of receptors binding IL-2 with an affinity of $10^7/M$. This corresponds to the low-affinity class of receptors observed on HuT 102 cells or mitogen-activated peripheral blood T cells (Robb et al., 1984).

C. MOLECULAR WEIGHTS OF RECOMBINANT IL-2 RECEPTOR

The molecular weight of the recombinant IL-2 receptors was examined by immunoprecipitation of ^{125}I-surface-labeled proteins with 2A3. In each case, a band of about 55,000 Da was specifically immunoprecipitated by the antibody (Fig. 5). The three recombinant IL-2 receptors had very similar molecular weights, although the mobility of the T cell-derived receptor was slightly slower than that of the other two.

TABLE II
QUANTITATION OF THE NUMBER OF IL-2
RECEPTORS PER CELL[a]

Cells (C127/pN4/1-8)	Number of 2A3 binding sites per cell
Unsorted	9×10^3
First sort	4.6×10^4
Second sort	7.8×10^4
Third sort	1.6×10^5
Fourth sort	8.0×10^5
Fifth sort	7.4×10^5
Sixth sort	8.7×10^5
Clone B	2.7×10^6
Clone B2	4.5×10^6

[a]Quantitation, using ^{125}I-2A3 binding on C127 cells transfected with pN4/1-8, is of cells that were analyzed in Fig. 3.

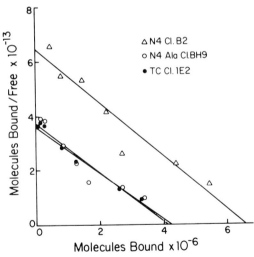

FIG. 4. Binding of ^{125}I-labeled IL-2 to C127 cells that express recombinant IL-2 receptor. Binding of ^{125}I-labeled IL-2 to cells was performed as described in Section II. The curves described by the data obtained from the equilibrium binding experiments were fitted using RS/1, a commercially available scientific processing package operating on a Vax 11/750 computer under VMS operating system. These curves were then replotted in the Scatchard coordinate system depicted in the figure. Binding to cells expressing the HuT receptor (△), cells expressing the Ser-Ala HuT receptor (○), and cells expressing the normal T cell receptor (●) is represented in the figure.

TABLE III

NUMBER OF IL-2 BINDING SITES AND AFFINITY OF IL-2 BINDING BY
C127 CELLS TRANSFECTED WITH IL-2 RECEPTOR cDNAs[a]

Cell line	Number of IL-2 binding sites per cell	Affinity constant (K_a)
C127/N4 C1.B2	6.6×10^6	$9.8 \times 10^6/M$
C127/N4A1a C1.BH9	4.2×10^6	$8.6 \times 10^6/M$
C127/TC C1.1E2	4.1×10^6	$9.0 \times 10^6/M$

[a]Data calculated from Fig. 4.

D. CLONING OF MURINE IL-2 RECEPTOR cDNA

In order to determine which regions of the IL-2 receptor were evolutionarily conserved, we isolated cDNAs encoding the murine IL-2 receptor. A cDNA library was constructed from CTLL cells, an IL-2-dependent murine T cell line, and screened by hybridization with the human IL-2 receptor cDNA probe under conditions of reduced stringency. One of the hybridizing cDNAs was purified and characterized by nucleotide sequencing. The sequence is shown in Fig. 1. It contains an open-reading frame of 268 amino acids that is 60% homologous to that of the human IL-2 receptor. In order to prove that this cDNA encoded the murine IL-2 receptor, a 923-base pair *Sau*3A fragment containing the entire open-reading frame was inserted into the *Bgl*II site of pMLSV (Cosman *et al.*, 1984). This construction places the murine IL-2 receptor under the transcriptional control of the SV40 early promoter followed by SV40 RNA processing signals. The entire cassette was then inserted into the *Bam*HI site of p1-8 to give pMrec-1/1-8, a construction analogous to that used to express the human IL-2 receptor cDNAs. Transfection into C127 cells, selection of G418 resistant cells, and multiple rounds of fluorescence-activated cell sorting using a monoclonal antibody (7D4) against the mouse IL-2 receptor (Malek *et al.*, 1983) allowed the generation of cell lines expressing high levels of the mouse IL-2 receptor (data not shown). Preliminary experiments indicate that, like the human receptor, the recombinant mouse IL-2 receptors were all of low affinity for IL-2.

IV. Discussion

The molecular cloning of the IL-2 receptor has led to the resolution of some basic questions concerning its structure and function.

First, there are only two amino acid sequence differences between the

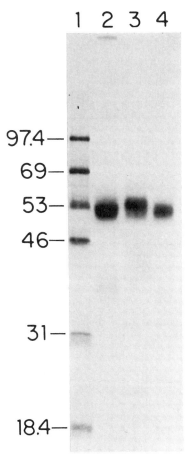

FIG. 5. Immunoprecipitation of ¹²⁵I-surface-labeled C127 cells that express recombinant IL-2 receptor. Lane 1, C127 cells expressing the Ser → Ala HuT 102 receptor; lane 2, C127 cells expressing the normal T cell receptor; lane 3, C127 cells expressing the HuT 102 cell receptor. Immunoprecipitations were performed with 2A3 coupled to Affigel-10 as described in Section II. Control antibody, MOPC-21, coupled to beads did not precipitate Arg proteins (data not shown).

normal cDNA and three HuT 102-derived cDNAs, and these are conservative amino acid substitutions. The 5000 Da difference observed between the two types of receptors is not found when both are expressed in a recombinant system. Therefore, the differences must be posttranslational as has been suggested previously (Leonard et al., 1985).

Second, we and others have shown that expression of the single small polypeptide chain encoded by the cDNA clones is sufficient to confer IL-2 binding ability upon a non-T cell (Cosman et al., 1984; Leonard et *al.*, 1984; Nikaido *et al.*, 1984; Greene *et al.*, 1985). This is an unusually small size for a receptor molecule. However, the IL-2 binding sites that are expressed in these heterologous cells are uniformly of low affinity despite the large number of receptors found on the cell surface. This raises the question of what is different about a high-affinity IL-2 receptor. Since high-affinity receptors have been observed only in lymphocytes, it may be that there is a lymphocyte-specific second subunit of the receptor or a lymphocyte-specific modification of the protein that confers the ability to bind IL-2 with high affinity. We are currently testing this hypothesis by expressing IL-2 receptor cDNAs in T cell lines using retroviral vectors.

The ability to clone IL-2 receptor cDNAs from other species by cross-hybridization under reduced stringency has allowed us and others to isolate mouse IL-2 receptor cDNAs (Shimizu *et al.*, 1985; Miller *et al.*, 1985). Comparison of IL-2 receptor sequences allows for identification of evolutionarily conserved regions which presumably have important functional properties. Surprisingly, the most highly conserved regions between the human and mouse receptors are the transmembrane and cytoplasmic domains. This suggests that the transmembrane domain has a role other than just as a stretch of hydrophobic amino acids spanning the lipid bilayer. Perhaps it interacts with other proteins within the membrane. The cytoplasmic domain is very short but contains a conserved protein kinase C phosphorylation site at Ser-247. We have shown that this is the site at which the receptor is phosphorylated in response to PMA treatment of cells (Gallis *et al.*, 1986). Whether IL-2 itself induces phosphorylation of the receptor at this site is under investigation.

We have begun to analyze the functionally important regions of the IL-2 receptor by site-directed mutagenesis. The substitution of Ser-247 by alanine does not affect the affinity of the receptors expressed in C127 cells for IL-2, but it does abolish the phosphorylation of the receptor in response to PMA. Future work will examine the effects of this change on IL-2 receptors expressed in T cells as well as the effect of other mutations.

ACKNOWLEDGMENTS

We thank Steven Gimpel, Tami Parr, and Sue Call for technical assistance, Linda Park for ^{125}I-labeled IL-2, Judy Byce for preparation of the manuscript, and Nava Sarver for the generous gift of p1-8.

REFERENCES

Cantrell, M. A. *et al.* (1985). *Proc. Natl. Acad. Sci. U.S.A.* **82**, 6250–6254.
Cosman, D. *et al.* (1984). *Nature (London)* **312**, 768–771.
Dower, S. K. *et al.* (1985). *Mol. Immunol.* **22**, 937–947.
Farrar, W. L., and Anderson, W. B. (1985). *Nature (London)* **315**, 233–235.

Frost, E., and Williams, J. (1978). *Virology* **91**, 39–50.
Gallis, B. *et al.* (1986). *J. Biol. Chem.* **261**, 5075–5080.
Gillis, S., and Smith, K. S. (1977). *Nature (London)* **268**, 154–156.
Greene, W. C. *et al.* (1985). *J. Exp. Med.* **162**, 363–368.
Heilman, C. H. *et al.* (1982). *Virology* **119**, 22–34.
Leonard, W. J. *et al.* (1984). *Nature (London)* **311**, 626–631.
Leonard, W. J. *et al.* (1985). *J. Biol. Chem.* **260**, 1872–1880.
Malek, T. *et al.* (1983). *Proc. Natl. Acad. Sci. U.S.A.* **80**, 5694–5698.
March, C. J. *et al.* (1985). *Nature (London)* **315**, 641–647.
Miller, J. *et al.* (1985). *J. Immunol.* **134**, 4212–4217.
Morgan, D. A. *et al.* (1976). *Science* **193**, 1007–1008.
Nikaido, T. *et al.* (1984). *Nature (London)* **311**, 631–635.
Robb, R. J. *et al.* (1984). *J. Exp. Med.* **160**, 1126–1146.
Sarver, N. *et al.* (1981). *Mol. Cell. Biol.* **1**, 486–496.
Sarver, N. *et al.* (1985). *In* "Papilloma Viruses: Molecular and Clinical Aspects" (P. M. Howley and T. R. Broker, eds.), Liss, New York, in press.
Shackelford, D. A., and Trowbridge, I. S. (1984). *J. Biol. Chem.* **259**, 11706–11712.
Shimizu, A. *et al.* (1985). *Nucleic Acids Res.* **13**, 1505–1516.
Urdal, D. L. *et al.* (1984). *Proc. Natl. Acad. Sci. U.S.A.* **81**, 6481–6485.

Molecular Analysis of the Murine Interleukin 2 Receptor

JIM MILLER, THOMAS R. MALEK,[1] ETHAN M. SHEVACH, AND RONALD N. GERMAIN

Laboratory of Immunology, National Institute of Allergy and Infectious Diseases, National Institutes of Health, Bethesda, Maryland 20892

I. Introduction

Polypeptide growth factors constitute a diverse family of regulatory hormones which interact with highly specific cell surface receptors and stimulate cellular proliferation (for review see James and Bradshaw, 1984). The interleukin 2 (IL-2) hormone–receptor system is the principle growth signal for antigen-activated T lymphocytes (Smith, 1984). In addition, IL-2 may play an important role in B cell activation and proliferation (Zubler *et al.*, 1984; Waldmann *et al.*, 1984), although B cell-specific factors (Kishimoto, 1985) are also involved in these processes.

Binding studies using radiolabeled IL-2 have demonstrated the presence of two classes of IL-2 receptors on the cell surface (Robb *et al.*, 1984). A small fraction (5–10%) has a high affinity for IL-2 ($K_D = 10^{-10}$ to 10^{-11} M), while the remainder is of much lower affinity ($K_D = 10^{-8}$ to 10^{-9} M). Based on concentrations of IL-2 which are biologically active, it appears that only the high-affinity component is involved in signal transduction (Robb *et al.*, 1981, 1984). Similar data have been presented for epidermal growth factor (EGF), nerve growth factor (NGF), and insulin receptors. In all cases the exact role of the low-affinity receptor is unknown.

Whereas most growth hormone receptors are constitutively expressed on the appropriate target cells, the IL-2 receptor is only present on activated, but not resting, lymphocytes (Bonnard *et al.*, 1979; Robb *et al.*, 1981). This induction of ligand and receptor is necessary for the clonal stimulation of antigen-specific cells. Other lymphocytes which do not recognize the antigen will not express IL-2 receptors and will not respond to IL-2 in the local environment. This is a crucial step in immune regulation, as polyclonal activation of lymphocytes may interfere with antigen-specific responses.

In addition to its prominent role in stimulating T cell proliferation, IL-2 has been shown to increase the number of IL-2 receptors expressed

---

[1]Present address: Department of Microbiology and Immunology, University of Miami, Miami, Florida 33101.

on the cell surface, with a corresponding increase in stable mRNA concentrations (Malek and Ashwell, 1985). This phenomenon is unlike other peptide hormones which down-regulate their receptors. The continued expression of IL-2 receptor may be important in expanding small numbers of antigen-specific cells during a primary immune response. Interestingly, this up-regulation by IL-2 only induces the low-affinity IL-2 receptor (Smith and Cantrell, 1985), whereas antigen or mitogen induces both forms. This suggests that the two forms of the IL-2 receptor can be independently regulated, which may be important in controlling autocrine growth.

In order to better understand the structure and function of the IL-2 receptor, we have isolated a cDNA clone that contains the complete coding region of the murine IL-2 receptor. When this cDNA clone is transfected into mouse L cells, only the low-affinity form of the receptor is expressed. This report focuses on the possible tissue-specific mechanisms for generating high-affinity IL-2 receptor and their implications for the mechanism of signal transduction.

II. Sequence Analysis

The cDNA clone, pcEXV-mIL2R8 (Miller et al., 1985a), was isolated from a CTLL library after identification by cross-species hybridization with the human IL-2 receptor cDNA clone, pIL2R3 (Leonard et al., 1984). A comparison of the deduced protein sequences of the mouse and human IL-2 receptors is shown in Fig. 1. Although the overall homology is only 61%, there are distinct regions which are more highly conserved. For example, amino acids 6–38 are 79% identical, with mostly conservative changes. Other stretches of high local homology are also present, notably 18/21 matches in the transmembrane region and 9/11 matches in the intracytoplasmic portion. This latter region contains two conserved sites of potential phosphorylation (see Fig. 1). These subregions with higher-than-average homology may play important roles in determining the function of the receptor.

III. Expression of pcEXV-mIL2R8 in L Cells

Inserted into the cDNA expression vector pcEXV-3 (Miller et al., 1985a), the murine IL-2 receptor cDNA clone was cotransfected with pTK (Enguist et al., 1979) into the mouse L cell line, DAP-3. After selecting transfectants with HAT medium, cells expressing the IL-2 receptor on the cell surface were purified by preparative flow micro-

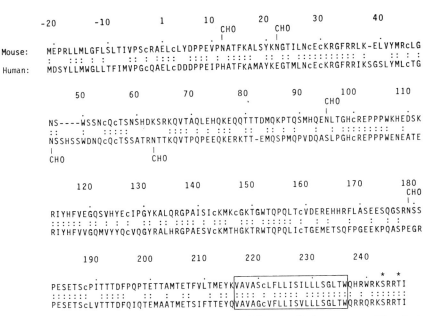

FIG. 1. Sequence comparison of the mouse and human IL-2 receptors. The single amino acid code is shown for the mouse sequence (above) and the human sequence (below). Identical amino acids are indicated by a colon between the sequences. Dashes indicate deletions introduced to maximize homology. Amino acid positions of the predicted mature protein are numbered consecutively from the glutamic acid residue at position 1 to the carboxy-terminal residue at position 247 and to position −21 for the hydrophobic leader sequence. Possible N-linked glycosylation sites (CHO) and the potential phosphorylation sites in the intracytoplasmic region (asterisks) are marked. The hydrophobic transmembrane region is boxed and the cysteine residues are shown in lowercase letters. The sequences shown here are from Miller *et al.* (1985a; mouse) and Leonard *et al.* (1984; human). Sequences for the IL-2 receptor have also been published independently for the human (Nikaido *et al.*, 1984) and the mouse (Shimuzu *et al.*, 1985).

fluorimetry after staining with the monoclonal antibody, 7D4 (Malek *et al.*, 1983). After repeated enrichment for bright cells, a subline, DAP-mIL2R8hp4, which expressed large amounts of the receptor on the cell surface (Table I), was isolated. When these cells were analyzed for their ability to bind radiolabeled IL-2 (Table I), only the low-affinity form was evident (Miller *et al.*, 1985b). As expected, the IL-2-dependent T cell line, HT-2, which was assayed in parallel with DAP-mIL2R8hp4, demonstrated both high- and low-affinity binding. Similarly, only the low-affinity form was expressed when the human IL-2 receptor was transfected into L cells (Greene *et al.*, 1985). The large number of IL-2 receptors on the cell surface of DAP-mIL2R8hp4 suggests that high-

TABLE I
EXPRESSION OF ONLY THE LOW-AFFINITY IL-2
RECEPTOR FOLLOWING TRANSFECTION INTO L CELLS[a]

	HT-2	DAP-mIL2R8hp4
High affinity		
Sites/cell	8,100	Undetectable
K_D	$1.3 \times 10^{-11}\ M$	Undetectable
Low affinity		
Sites/cell	150,000	310,000
K_D	$2.3 \times 10^{-8}\ M$	$2.8 \times 10^{-8}\ M$

[a]The affinity and number of IL-2 receptor molecules were determined by Scatchard analysis following binding with radiolabeled IL-2 (Robb et al., 1984). For complete analysis, see Miller et al. (1985b).

affinity IL-2 receptor is not simply the result of positive cooperativity following interaction of individual receptor molecules on the cell surface.

IV. A Single IL-2 Receptor Gene

Analysis of Southern blots containing mouse genomic DNA revealed multiple restriction enzyme fragments hybridizing to the cDNA clone, mIL2R8 (Miller et al., 1985a). In order to analyze the structure of the IL-2 receptor gene, genomic clones were isolated. When DNA from a single cosmid clone containing most of the IL-2 receptor gene was digested, blotted, and hybridized in parallel with genomic DNA using probes derived from various subregions of mIL2R8, identical patterns were detected (Fig. 2). In addition, the hybridizing fragments mapped in the same relative position as the homologous regions in mIL2R8 (Fig. 3), consistent with a single IL-2 receptor gene containing multiple introns. When mIL2R8 was hybridized under extremely reduced stringency to Southern blots containing genomic DNA, no additional fragments were detected. Therefore, there appears to be only a single IL-2 receptor gene homologous to mIL2R8. If the high-affinity IL-2 receptor was encoded in a separate gene, it would probably contain enough nucleic acid homology to cross-hybridize to mIL2R8, because both the high- and low-affinity IL-2 receptor molecules share the 3C7 (Ortega et al., 1984) and 7D4 (Malek et al., 1983) monoclonal antibody determinants and the ability to bind IL-2. Thus, the inability to generate high-affinity IL-2 receptors in L cells is probably not due to separate genes encoding the two affinity forms.

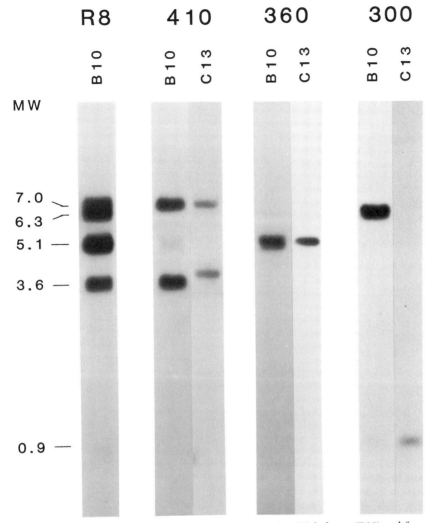

FIG. 2. A single IL-2 receptor gene. DNA from C57BL/10 kidneys (B10) and from a cosmid clone containing the mouse IL-2 receptor gene (C13) were digested with BamHI, electrophoresed on a 0.8% agarose gel, and blotted. Identical lanes were hybridized to ^{32}P-labeled fragments containing the entire mIL2R8 cDNA insert (R8) or subfragments derived from it (410, 360, and 300—see Fig. 3). The sizes in kilobases (MW) of the hybridizing fragments are given on the left. The cosmid clone, C13, does not contain the entire 3' end of the IL-2 receptor gene and therefore does not contain the 6.3-kb fragment evident in B10 DNA (see Fig. 3). The faint hybridization of the 410 probe to the 5.1-kb fragment in B10 DNA is due to contamination of the gel-purified fragment used as a probe. The apparent difference in the molecular weight of the 3.6-kb fragment in C13 DNA compared to B10 DNA is due to differences in the duration of electrophoresis.

mIL2R8

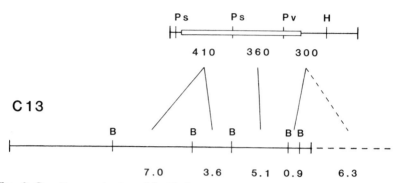

FIG. 3. Genetic organization of the IL-2 receptor gene. The cDNA clone, mIL2R8, is shown at the top. The open bar represents the coding region sequence. The restriction enzyme sites (Ps, *Pst*I; Pv, *Pvu*I; H, *Hind*III) were utilized to generate the three fragments (410, 360, and 300) used as probes in the experiment shown in Fig. 2. A map of the *Bam*HI (B) sites within the cosmid clone, C13, is shown below. The sizes in kilobases of the internal *Bam*HI fragments are given below the map of C13. Lines between the cDNA and cosmid maps indicate the positions of the fragments which hybridize to the various probes derived from mIL2R8. The dotted line corresponds to the presumed location of the 6.3-kb fragment present in B10 DNA but absent from the cosmid clone, C13. The cosmid library utilized to isolate this clone was generously provided by Dr. David Margulies.

V. Multiple mRNA Transcripts

When RNA from cells expressing the IL-2 receptor was analyzed on Northern blots, five distinct mRNA transcript lengths were identified following hybridization to mIL2R8 (Miller *et al.*, 1985a). Because the cDNA clone used to transfect the L cells was derived from only one of these molecules, it was possible that a different mRNA transcript encoded high-affinity IL-2 receptors. To examine this issue, RNA from the T cell tumor, 5.1.2 (Rosenberg, *et al.*, 1985), which only expresses low-affinity IL-2 receptors (Miller *et al.*, 1985b), was analyzed (Fig. 4). The same pattern of mRNA expression was detected regardless of the presence or absence of high-affinity IL-2 receptors. Thus, there was no obvious correlation between a specific transcript size and the expression of high-affinity receptors.

Nonetheless, it was possible that the distinct mRNA transcript sizes detected on Northern blots could contain alternatively spliced mRNA molecules. In fact, the human IL-2 receptor does contain two alternatively processed forms of mRNA which comigrate within the two major size classes of mRNA present in both HuT 102B cells (Leonard *et al.*,

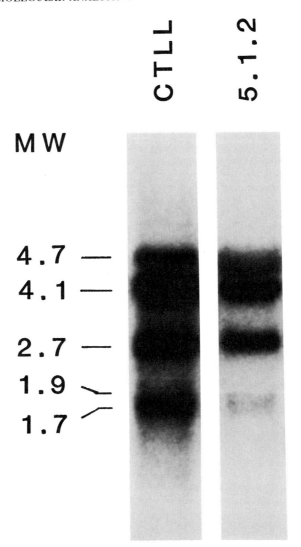

FIG. 4. The high-affinity IL-2 receptor does not correspond to a distinct mRNA species. Total cytoplasmic RNA from CTLL (1.0 μg) and from 5.1.2 (10.0 μg) was denatured and electrophoresed on a formaldehyde/agarose gel. The RNA was transferred to nitrocellulose and hybridized to the mIL2R8 cDNA insert. The sizes in kilobases (MW) of the multiple mRNA species are given in the left. The very faint 1.9-kb transcript was more evident in a longer exposure.

1984) and in normal T lymphocytes (Leonard *et al.*, 1985b). This alternative splicing event results in mRNA molecules which produce polypeptides differing by the presence or absence of an internal 70-amino acid segment. However, these forms do not represent the high- and low-affinity IL-2 receptors. When cDNA clones encoding each of these two polypeptides were transfected into COS cells, only the larger polypeptide was capable of binding IL-2 and the monoclonal antibody, anti-Tac (Leonard *et al.*, 1984). Furthermore, nuclease protection experiments with the mouse cDNA clone, mIL2R8, revealed no evidence for alternative splicing within the coding region (Miller *et al.*, 1985b). The heterogeneity in mRNA molecules probably results from multiple polyadenylation sites, generating mRNA molecules which differ only in the length of their 3' untranslated regions. Thus, because all the murine IL-2 receptor transcripts produced from the unique IL-2 receptor gene appear to encode identical primary translation products, the distinction between high- and low-affinity forms is likely to be the result of posttranslational modification of this single translation product.

VI. Glycosylation

Extensive biochemical analysis of the IL-2 receptor (Leonard *et al.*, 1983, 1985a; Malek and Korty, 1985) has not revealed any structural differences between the two affinity forms. This may be due in part to the low frequency of the high-affinity form (only 5–10% of total) and to the overall heterogeneity of the receptor. When analyzed following immunoprecipitation or on Western blots, the IL-2 receptor appears as a heterogeneous band with an apparent molecular weight of 50,000–65,000. In addition, the average molecular weight differs considerably between cell lines, with no obvious correlation with the affinity of the receptor. This heterogeneity probably derives from differential glycosylation at both O- and N-linked sites (Leonard *et al.*, 1985a) and could mask specific glycosylation events that produce the minor, high-affinity component. Thus, even though immunoprecipitation or Western blot analysis does not distinguish the IL-2 receptor expressed in DAP-mIL2R8hp4 cells from that produced by concanavalin A-activated T cells (Miller *et al.*, 1985b), tissue-specific glycosylation could explain the difference between high- and low-affinity receptors. The monoclonal antibody, EGR/G49 (Gregoriou and Rees, 1984), which is specific for the low-affinity EGF receptor expressed on the A-431 tumor cell, appears to detect a carbohydrate determinant. However, because this antibody does not bind to the EGF receptor present on normal cells, this differential glycosylation might be tumor specific and may not represent a general mechanism for generating high- and low-affinity growth hormone receptors in normal cells.

VII. Phosphorylation

Tumor-promoting phorbol esters induce the phosphorylation of the receptors for insulin (Jacobs *et al.*, 1983) and EGF (Cochet *et al.*, 1984) and result in decreased binding for ligand and a concomitant inhibition of receptor-associated tyrosine kinase activity. Scatchard analysis has shown that the decrease in ligand binding to the EGF receptor results from a specific loss of the high-affinity component (Friedman *et al.*, 1984). Analysis of isolated membrane fractions and reconstitution experiments with purified protein kinase C (Fearn and King, 1985) suggest that all these effects are mediated through phosphorylation of the EGF receptor by protein kinase C. Thus, the enhanced calcium influx and phosphatidylinositol turnover (yielding diacylglycerol) induced by EGF (Sawyer and Cohen, 1981) may activate protein kinase C, resulting in EGF receptor phosphorylation and down-regulation.

The identification of the site of phorbol ester-induced phosphorylation at threonine-654 of the EGF receptor (Hunter *et al.*, 1984; Davis and Czech, 1985) suggests that addition of a phosphate group to the intracytoplasmic side of the receptor can greatly affect the affinity of ligand binding to the extracytoplasmic portion. Threonine-654 is located 9 amino acids from the predicted transmembrane region, within the cluster of basic residues which typically follow the transmembrane region. Introduction of a phosphate group could affect the interaction of this basic region with phospholipids or other molecules within the membrane. Interestingly, the IL-2 receptor has two potential sites for phosphorylation within the 11-amino acid intracytoplasmic region (see Fig. 1). Thus, phosphorylation at one of these sites could affect the affinity for IL-2.

Although the phorbol ester, PMA, has been shown to induce IL-2 receptor phosphorylation (Shackelford and Trowbridge, 1984), its effect on ligand binding is not known. In contrast to the down-regulation of the EGF receptor, phorbol esters have been shown to induce the expression of IL-2 receptors in T lymphocytes (Depper *et al.*, 1984; Leonard *et al.*, 1985b). Although this effect may not be mediated directly through phosphorylation of the IL-2 receptor itself, it suggests that the IL-2 receptor may be regulated differently from other growth hormone receptors.

VIII. Multiple Subunits

In addition to differential posttranslational modification, another explanation for the tissue specificity of high-affinity IL-2 receptor ex-

pression involves interactions with other components. Although there is
no evidence for other peptides linked to the IL-2 receptor via covalent
disulfide bonds, additional polypeptides do coimmunoprecipitate [110
kDa in the mouse (Ortega *et al.*, 1984) and 180 and 113 kDa in the
human (Leonard *et al.*, 1982)]. However, recent data suggest that the
murine high-molecular-weight component which is detectable on Western blots with the anti-IL-2 receptor monoclonal antibody, 7D4, represents a homodimer of the IL-2 receptor (Malek and Korty, 1985). In
addition, this high-molecular-weight component is also present in the L
cells transfected with pcEXV-mIL2R8 (DAP-mIL2R8hp4) which only
express low-affinity IL-2 receptor (see above). Therefore, although this
component cannot represent the high-affinity IL-2 receptor, other molecules could interact with the IL-2 receptor and affect its affinity. If these
molecules are easily dissociated during detergent solubilization, they
would not be evident in immunoprecipitations.

IX. Membrane Events

One model for growth hormone receptor-mediated signal transduction
is that ligand binding induces activation of a second messenger generator
which transmits the signal into the cell. The association of some hormone
receptors with adenylate cyclase and the production of cAMP ex-
emplifies this model. The observation that the receptors for many growth
hormones, including EGF (Ushiro and Cohen, 1980), platelet-derived
growth factor (Ek *et al.*, 1982; Nishimura *et al.*, 1982), and insulin (Kasuga *et al.*, 1983), are associated with a tyrosine kinase activity is consistent with this hypothesis. The relationship between this activity and
the *src* family of oncogenes has suggested a generalized mode for the
induction of cellular proliferation (for a review see Heldin and Westermark, 1984). Analysis of the structure of the IL-2 receptor suggests that it
may not belong within this family of growth hormone receptors. Whereas the EGF and insulin receptors have large intracytoplasmic domains
which encode these kinase activities, the IL-2 receptor has an 11-amino
acid intracytoplasmic region, which is too small to constitute a kinase.
Thus, in order to fit the EGF receptor paradigm, the IL-2 receptor
would have to interact with a second component which would encode a
kinase activity. In fact, the ligand binding and kinase activities associated
with the insulin receptor are present on separate polypeptide chains.
Although the two chains of the insulin receptor are derived from the
same primary translation product, it is possible that the IL-2 receptor
interacts with a protein kinase that is separately encoded within the
genome. Because the IL-2 receptor lacks a tyrosine residue in the intra-

cytoplasmic region to serve as an autophosphorylation site, this putative associated kinase may not be a tyrosine-specific enzyme.

X. Receptor Clustering

Even though most growth hormones appear to bind monovalently to their receptors, rapid receptor clustering usually follows ligand binding. To distinguish between the roles in signal transduction of receptor binding and subsequent clustering, Fab fragments (Schreiber *et al.*, 1983) of a monoclonal antibody (Schreiber *et al.*, 1981) that mimics the action of EGF were analyzed. Although the Fab fragments could still bind to the EGF receptor and activate the associated kinase, they did not stimulate receptor clustering or cellular proliferation. Complete triggering was reconstituted when a secondary antibody to mouse immunoglobulin was added, suggesting that cross-linking and receptor clustering were necessary for activation. An alternative explanation is that binding of the secondary antibody affected the apparent affinity of the Fab fragment for the EGF receptor and so induced the conformational change of the EGF receptor necessary for complete triggering (Schreiber *et al.*, 1983). In either case, induction of the kinase activity alone was not sufficient to induce cellular proliferation. Thus, the proposed association of the IL-2 receptor with a protein kinase subunit (see above), may be insufficient to explain biological signal transduction. Additional activities may be intrinsic to the ligand binding or kinase subunits, or the putative complex may contain multiple polypeptide chains with different functions.

XI. Ligand–Receptor Internalization

After ligand binding and receptor clustering, most growth hormone receptor complexes are rapidly internalized and degraded. This may play the major role in the observed down-regulation of receptor by ligand, although the role of protein kinase C in the down-regulation of the EGF receptor (see above) may also be important. The fact that antibodies to the EGF receptor can mimic the effects of ligand binding (Schreiber *et al.*, 1981) suggests that the biological activity resides in the receptor itself. However, these results cannot distinguish between activation of the cell at the plasma membrane or production of stimulatory peptides resulting from degradation of the receptor itself. It is intriguing to note that purified EGF receptor may be associated with ATP-dependent, DNA topoisomerase activity, which is independent of EGF binding and the protein kinase activity (Mroczkowski *et al.*, 1984).

Although early studies showed that, following binding to the cell surface, radiolabeled IL-2 was internalized and degraded, a role for internalization in signal transduction has not been documented. Although monoclonal antibodies to the IL-2 receptor, which mimic the function of IL-2, have not been described, this may reflect the screening methods utilized rather than the biology of IL-2. Nevertheless, a role for internalized IL-2 in signal transduction cannot be excluded.

XII. Summary and Discussion

Although most cells expressing the IL-2 receptor produce both a high- and low-affinity form, when a cDNA clone for the mouse IL-2 receptor was transfected into L cells only the low-affinity component was produced. Molecular analysis has not revealed any genetic explanation for this discrepancy. Thus, there appears to be a single IL-2 receptor gene which, although multiple species of mRNA molecules are transcribed, appears to generate a single, unique primary translation product. Therefore, the tissue specificity of high-affinity IL-2 receptor expression must occur posttranslationally. Based on comparisons to other polypeptide growth hormone receptors, the high-affinity IL-2 receptor could be generated by differential posttranslational modification, including glycosylation and phosphorylation.

Alternatively, the IL-2 receptor may interact with other membrane component(s) to generate a biologically active, high-affinity IL-2 receptor complex. The relative abundance of the individual components and their affinities for each other would account for the ratio of high- vs low-affinity receptors. The high degree of conservation in the transmembrane and intracytoplasmic regions between the mouse and human IL-2 receptors (see Fig. 1) suggests that at least some of these interactions may occur at or near the cell membrane. The two conserved potential sites for phosphorylation in the intracytoplasmic portion suggest a role for a protein kinase in IL-2 receptor activity. As with other growth hormone receptors, ligand binding to the IL-2 receptor could result in activation of the protein kinase and autophosphorylation. However, the relative importance in signal transduction of this and possible subsequent phosphorylation events, and the resultant clustering and internalization of the ligand-receptor complex, is not known.

The multisubunit model could also explain the observation that up-regulation of the IL-2 receptor by ligand is limited to the low-affinity form. If the individual subunits are independently regulated, antigen induction of all the subunits could generate both affinity forms, whereas IL-2 induction of a subset of the polypeptides involved could result in low-affinity receptors only. However, this does not explain the biological role of IL-2-receptor up-regulation. One possibility is that the low-affinity form acts as a pool of spare receptors. After ligand binding to the high-affinity receptors, the subunits may dissociate, allowing ligand-bound receptor to be internalized and degraded and the secondary components to interact with a low-affinity IL-2 receptor to regenerate the high-affinity complex. IL-2 up-regulation could replace the pool of low-affinity, spare receptors, so that during clonal expansion of antigen-specific cells, the surface expression of biologically relevant, high-affinity IL-2 receptors would remain relatively constant regardless of the local concentration of IL-2. This would provide for continuous cell growth and expansion of antigen-specific clones during an immune response. Autocrine growth would be regulated by the requirement for continued exposure to antigen to maintain the expression of the other components necessary to generate a high-affinity, biologically active IL-2 receptor complex.

If the secondary components necessary for the generation of the high-affinity IL-2 receptor are indeed tissue specific, then transfection of the IL-2 receptor cDNA construct into lymphoid cells may produce both high- and low-affinity IL-2 receptors. Identification of this recipient cell, in conjunction with site-specific mutagenesis, may provide insights into the possible mechanisms of high-affinity IL-2 receptor expression. In addition, if the recipient cell utilized in the transfection is responsive to IL-2, these same mutant molecules can be assayed in parallel for their ability to transmit biological signals. By determining the structural features necessary for the generation of high-affinity IL-2 receptors and/or biological signal transduction, the relative roles for glycosylation and phosphorylation on subunit interaction may be addressed. These results could lead toward a clearer understanding of the mechanisms of IL-2 receptor function and, therefore, the control of lymphocyte growth.

NOTE ADDED IN PROOF. After this article was written, Hatakeyama *et al.* [1985, *Nature (London)* **318**, 467–470] and Kondo *et al.* [1986, *Nature (London)* **320**, 75–77] reported that a human IL-2 receptor cDNA clone, which produces only low-affinity receptor in mouse L cells, will generate a functionally active high-affinity IL-2 receptor after transfection into murine T cells. These data are consistent with the mechanisms of tissue-specific, high-affinity IL-2 receptor expression presented in this report.

REFERENCES

Bonnard, G., Yasaka, K., and Jacobson, D. (1979). *J. Immunol.* **123**, 2704–2708.
Cochet, C., Gill, G., Meisenhelder, J., Cooper, J., and Hunter, T. (1984). *J. Biol. Chem.* **259**, 2553–2558.
Davis, R., and Czech, M. (1985). *Proc. Natl. Acad. Sci. U.S.A.* **82**, 1974–1978.

Depper, J., Leonard, W., Kronke, M., Noguchi, P., Cunningham, R., Waldmann, T., and Greene, W. (1984). *J. Immunol.* **133**, 3054–3061.

Ek, B., Westermark, B., Wasteson, A., and Heldin, C. (1982). *Nature (London)* **295**, 419–420.

Enguist, L., Vande Wonde, G., Wagner, M., Smiley, J., and Summers, W. (1979). *Gene* **7**, 335–342.

Fearn, J., and King, A. C. (1985). *Cell* **40**, 991–1000.

Friedman, B., Frackelton, A. R., Ross, A., Connors, J., Fujiki, H., Sugimura, T., and Rosner, M. (1984). *Proc. Natl. Acad. Sci. U.S.A.* **81**, 3034–3038.

Greene, W., Robb, R., Svetlik, P., Rusk, C., Depper, J., and Leonard, W. (1985). *J. Exp. Med.* **162**, 363–368.

Gregoriou, M., and Rees, A. (1984). *EMBO J.* **3**, 929–937.

Heldin, C., and Westermark, B. (1984). *Cell* **37**, 9–20.

Hunter, T., Ling, N., and Cooper, J. (1984). *Nature (London)* **311**, 480–483.

Jacobs, S., Sahyoun, N., Saltiel, A., and Cuatrecasas, P. (1983). *Proc. Natl. Acad. Sci. U.S.A.* **80**, 6211–6213.

James, R., and Bradshaw, R. (1984). *Annu. Rev. Biochem.* **53**, 259–292.

Kasuga, M., Fujita-Yamaguchi, Y., Blithe, D., and Kahn, C. R. (1983). *Proc. Natl. Acad. Sci. U.S.A.* **80**, 2137–2141.

Kishimoto, T. (1985). *Annu. Rev. Immunol.* **3**, 133–157.

Leonard, W., Depper, J., Uchiyama, T., Smith, K., Waldmann, T., and Greene, W. (1982). *Nature (London)* **300**, 267–269.

Leonard, W., Depper, J., Robb, R., Waldmann, T., and Greene, W. (1983). *Proc. Natl. Acad. Sci. U.S.A.* **80**, 6957–6961.

Leonard, W., Depper, J., Crabtree, G., Rudikoff, S., Pumphrey, J., Robb, R., Kronke, M., Svetlik, P., Pefter, N., Waldmann, T., and Greene, W. (1984). *Nature (London)* **311**, 626–631.

Leonard, W., Depper, J., Kronke, M., Robb, R., Waldmann, T., and Greene, W. (1985a). *J. Biol. Chem.* **260**, 1872–1880.

Leonard, W., Kronke, M., Pefter, N., Depper, J., and Greene, W. (1985b). *Proc. Natl. Acad. Sci. U.S.A.* **82**, 6281–6285.

Malek, T., and Ashwell, J. (1985). *J. Exp. Med.* **161**, 1575–1580.

Malek, T., and Korty, P. (1985). *J. Immunol.* **136**, 4092–4098.

Malek, T., Robb, R., and Shevach, E. (1983). *Proc. Natl. Acad. Sci. U.S.A.* **80**, 5694–5698.

Miller, J., Malek, T., Leonard, W., Greene, W., Shevach, E., and Germain, R. (1985a). *J. Immunol.* **134**, 4212–4217.

Miller, J., Germain, R., Robb, R., Shevach, E., and Malek, T. (1985b). In preparation.

Mroczkowski, B., Mosig, G., and Cohen, S. (1984). *Nature (London)* **309**, 270–273.

Nikaido, T., Shimuzu, A., Ishida, N., Sebe, H., Teshigawara, K., Maeda, M., Uchiyama, T., Yodoi, J., and Honjo, T. (1984). *Nature (London)* **311**, 631–635.

Nishimura, J., Huang, J., and Deuel, T. (1982). *Proc. Natl. Acad. Sci. U.S.A.* **79**, 4303–4307.

Ortega, G., Robb, R., Shevach, E., and Malek, T. (1984). *J. Immunol.* **133**, 1970–1975.

Robb, R., Munck, A., and Smith, K. (1981). *J. Exp. Med.* **154**, 1455–1474.

Robb, R., Greene, W., and Rusk, C. (1984). *J. Exp. Med.* **160**, 1126–1146.

Rosenberg, Y., Malek, T., Schaffer, D., Santoro, T., Mark, G., Steinberg, A., and Mountz, J. (1985). *J. Immunol.* **134**, 3120–3123.

Sawyer, S., and Cohen, S. (1981). *Biochemistry* **20**, 6280–6286.

Schreiber, A., Lax, I., Yarden, Y., Eshhar, Z., and Schlessinger, J. (1981). *Proc. Natl. Acad. Sci. U.S.A.* **78,** 7535–7539.

Schreiber, A., Liberman, T., Lax, I., Yarden, Y., and Schlessinger, J. (1983). *J. Biol. Chem.* **258,** 846–853.

Shackelford, D., and Trowbridge, I. (1984). *J. Biol. Chem.* **259,** 11706–11712.

Shimuzu, A., Kondo, S., Takedo, S., Yodoi, J., Ishida, N., Sabe, H., Osawa, H., Diamantstein, T., Nikaido, T., and Honjo, T. (1985). *Nucleic Acids Res.* **13,** 1505–1516.

Smith, K. (1984). *Annu. Rev. Immunol.* **2,** 319–333.

Smith, K., and Cantrell, D. (1985). *Proc. Natl. Acad. Sci. U.S.A.* **82,** 864–868.

Ushiro, H., and Cohen, S. (1980). *J. Biol. Chem.* **255,** 8363–8365.

Waldmann, T., Goldman, C., Robb, R., Depper, J., Leonard, W., Sharrow, S., Bongiovanni, K., Korsmeyer, S., and Greene, W. (1984). *J. Exp. Med.* **160,** 1450–1466.

Zubler, R., Lowenthal, J., Erard, F., Hashimoto, N., Devos, R., and MacDonald, H. R. (1984). *J. Exp. Med.* **160,** 1170–1183.

Cloning and Expression of Murine, Human, and Rabbit Interleukin 1 Genes

PETER T. LOMEDICO, UELI GUBLER, AND STEVEN B. MIZEL*

*Department of Molecular Genetics, Hoffmann-La Roche Inc., Roche Research Center, Nutley, New Jersey 07110, and *Department of Microbiology and Immunology, Bowman Gray School of Medicine, Wake Forest University, Winston-Salem, North Carolina 27103*

I. Introduction

Interleukin 1 (IL-1) is a polypeptide hormone synthesized and secreted by activated macrophages. This protein has previously been termed lymphocyte activating factor (LAF), B cell activating factor (BAF), leukocyte endogeneous mediator (LEM), endogeneous pyrogen (EP), and mononuclear cell factor (MCF). As indicated by its previous pseudonyms, IL-1 acts on many different cells to modulate a variety of biologic activities including lymphocyte activation, fever, liver cell function, production and release of neutrophils from the bone marrow, and connective tissue cell activation and proliferation (Dinarello, 1984). Through these diverse activities, IL-1 is viewed as a "stress hormone" (Gery and Lepe-Zuniga, 1984) which helps to stimulate immune and inflammatory responses in the body's defense against infection and other forms of trauma. In addition to its role in normal physiological homeostasis, IL-1 is believed to contribute to the pathology observed in certain inflammatory conditions.

Biochemical studies have revealed that IL-1 activity produced by stimulated macrophages is associated with a single polypeptide chain with a molecular weight between 12,000 and 19,000. Most IL-1 preparations show evidence of polypeptide size and charge heterogeneity; for example, multiple pI species have been described for both human and rabbit IL-1 (Ihrie and Wood, 1985; Murphy et al., 1980), and microheterogeneity on both tris-glycinate and SDS–polyacrylamide gels has been documented for mouse IL-1 preparations (Mizel and Mizel, 1981). Since it has been difficult to prepare sufficient amounts of IL-1 protein for structural studies, until recently it was not clear how the different IL-1 forms are related or whether all the activities ascribed to IL-1 are contained within one molecule.

II. Murine IL-1

Mizel and co-workers have studied mouse IL-1 produced by a macrophage-like tumor cell line, $P388D_1$, following superinduction with phorbol ester, cycloheximide, and actinomycin D. The activity of P388D$_1$-derived IL-1, measured in the murine thymocyte proliferation assay, can not be destroyed by urea, SDS, reduction and alkylation, trypsin, chymotrypsin, or papain; inactivation can be affected by proteinase K or by treatment with papain in the presence of 8 M urea (Mizel, 1979). Mizel and Mizel (1981) were able to purify small amounts of P388D$_1$-derived IL-1 and show that this material exhibits size and charge microheterogeneity. Mizel et al. (1983) were able to purify the major IL-1 species and generate an antiserum in a goat against this protein. The goat antibody completely neutralized mouse IL-1 activity secreted from stimulated normal and cell-line macrophages. In addition, a goat anti-IL-1 immunoadsorbent was used to purify a population of IL-1 molecules which demonstrated the same size and charge heterogeneity seen in conventionally purified samples. These results suggest that differential processing of a single primary protein may explain murine IL-1 polypeptide chain microheterogeneity.

The availability of the goat anti-murine IL-1 antibody has permitted a detailed analysis of the biosynthesis and structual characterization of mouse IL-1. Cell-free synthesis experiments using mRNA prepared from superinduced P388D$_1$ cells have demonstrated that a 33,000 MW polypeptide reacts specifically with the anti-IL-1 antibody (Lomedico et al., 1984; Giri et al., 1985) and hence represents the primary translation product of IL-1 mRNA. Pulse-labeling experiments have indicated that the 33,000 MW polypeptide is synthesized by stimulated normal and cell-line macrophages, and is the precursor to the heterogeneous collection of low-molecular-weight IL-1 polypeptides found in the culture supernatant of stimulated cells (Giri et al., 1985). Using a mRNA hybrid selection/translational analysis (Parnes et al., 1981), we have cloned a cDNA copy of the mRNA coding for the mouse IL-1 precursor (Lomedico et al., 1984). The nucleotide sequence of the cDNA predicts a protein of 270 amino acids (Fig. 1) with a calculated molecular weight of 31,026. It is estimated that ~0.005% of the poly(A)+ RNA from superinduced P388D$_1$ cells codes for this IL-1 precursor. Partial amino acid sequence studies on P388D$_1$-derived IL-1 (Lomedico et al., 1984) confirmed that the protein sequence predicted by nucleotide sequencing is correct and suggested that the carboxy-terminal region (beginning at amino acid 115) of the 270-amino acid precursor contained the information encoding IL-1 activity. To prove this point, the carboxy-terminal 156 amino acids (that is, amino acids 115–270) were expressed in Escherichia coli yielding the expected size protein (17,400 MW). This recombinant protein reacts with the goat anti-IL-1 antibody and is active in the murine thymocyte proliferation assay with a specific activity identical

```
                              10                                        20
Met Ala Lys Val Pro Asp Leu Phe Glu Asp Leu Lys Asn Cys Tyr Ser Glu Asn Glu Asp

                              30                                        40
Tyr Ser Ser Ala Ile Asp His Leu Ser Leu Asn Gln Lys Ser Phe Tyr Asp Ala Ser Tyr

                              50                                        60
Gly Ser Leu His Glu Thr Cys Thr Asp Gln Phe Val Ser Leu Arg Thr Ser Glu Thr Ser

                              70                                        80
Lys Met Ser Asn Phe Thr Phe Lys Glu Ser Arg Val Thr Val Ser Ala Thr Ser Ser Asn

                              90                                       100
Gly Lys Ile Leu Lys Lys Arg Arg Leu Ser Phe Ser Glu Thr Phe Thr Glu Asp Asp Leu

                             110                ↓                      120
Gln Ser Ile Thr His Asp Leu Glu Glu Thr Ile Gln Pro Arg Ser Ala Pro Tyr Thr Tyr

                             130                                      140
Gln Ser Asp Leu Arg Tyr Lys Leu Met Lys Leu Val Arg Gln Lys Phe Val Met Asn Asp

                             150                                      160
Ser Leu Asn Gln Thr Ile Tyr Gln Asp Val Asp Lys His Tyr Leu Ser Thr Thr Trp Leu

                             170                                      180
Asn Asp Leu Gln Gln Glu Val Lys Phe Asp Met Tyr Ala Tyr Ser Ser Gly Gly Asp Asp

                             190                                      200
Ser Lys Tyr Pro Val Thr Leu Lys Ile Ser Asp Ser Gln Leu Phe Val Ser Ala Gln Gly

                             210                                      220
Glu Asp Gln Pro Val Leu Leu Lys Glu Leu Pro Glu Thr Pro Lys Leu Ile Thr Gly Ser

                             230                                      240
Glu Thr Asp Leu Ile Phe Phe Trp Lys Ser Ile Asn Ser Lys Asn Tyr Phe Thr Ser Ala

                             250                                      260
Ala Tyr Pro Glu Leu Phe Ile Ala Thr Lys Glu Gln Ser Arg Val His Leu Ala Arg Gly

                             270
Leu Pro Ser Met Thr Asp Phe Gln Ile Ser
```

FIG. 1. Predicted amino acid sequence of murine IL-1 precursor protein. The nucleotide sequence of murine IL-1 cDNA predicts a single open-reading frame coding for a protein of 270 amino acids (Lomedico *et al.*, 1984). This sequence, in three-letter amino acid code, is shown with corresponding numbering above the line. The arrow points to the Ser at position 115 which is the amino-terminus of a subset of the IL-1 molecules secreted from $P388D_1$ cells and the beginning of the biologically active carboxy-terminal fragment synthesized in *E. coli* (Lomedico *et al.*, 1984).

with purified "natural" murine IL-1. In other IL-1 test systems (stimulation of fibroblast proliferation and synovial cell prostaglandin/collagenase production, fever, hepatocyte responses, *in vivo* humoral immune responses, etc.) recombinant mouse IL-1 is active, hence proving that many of the activities previously ascribed to IL-1 are exhibited by a single molecule.

III. Human IL-1

Human IL-1 preparations exhibit charge heterogeneity, with the major species possessing a *pI* ~6.8 and several minor species between p*I* 5 and 6. The explanation for this charge heterogeneity is provided by gene-cloning experiments which prove that a human IL-1 gene family exists. The nomenclature suggested by March *et al.* (1985) will be followed.

A. HUMAN IL-1β

This first human IL-1 cDNA cloning and sequencing was accomplished by Auron *et al.* (1984). Starting with poly(A)+ RNA isolated from endotoxin-stimulated human peripheral blood monocytes, they demonstrated that this mRNA programmed the cell-free synthesis of a 35,000 MW polypeptide that was immunologically related to IL-1. This mRNA also directed the synthesis of biologically active IL-1 in *Xenopus laevis* oocytes. Auron *et al.* (1984) were able to isolate cDNA clones by differential hybridization with stimulated and unstimulated monocyte probes. Positive clones, but not control clones, were able to hybrid-select mRNA which directed the synthesis of the 35,000 molecular weight IL-1 precursor *in vitro* and biologically active IL-1 in oocytes. The nucleotide sequence of the Auron *et al.* (1984) cDNA predicts a protein of 269 amino acids (Fig. 2) with a calculated molecular weight of 30,747.

Confirmation of the sequence predicted by Auron *et al.* (1984) was provided by Van Damme *et al.* (1985) who were the first to purify and sequence human IL-1. Van Damme *et al.* (1985) isolated a 17,000 MW protein with IL-1 activity from culture supernatants of human peripheral blood mononuclear cell suspensions stimulated with concanavalin A. Amino-terminal sequence analysis of this protein showed some heterogeneity, but the major sequence matched the predicted sequence of Auron *et al.* (1984) beginning at amino acid 117. Hence the 17 kDa Van Damme *et al.* IL-1 protein probably represents the carboxy-terminal 153 amino acids (amino acids 117–269) of the 269-amino acid IL-1 precursor described by Auron *et al* (1984).

March *et al.* (1985) provided final proof for the identity of the Auron *et al.* gene product. They were able to purify (Kronheim *et al.*, 1985) an IL-1 protein with a molecular weight of 17,500 secreted from human peripheral blood mononuclear cell suspensions stimulated with *Staphylococcus aureus*. Amino-terminal sequence analysis of this protein confirmed the Van Damme *et al.* (1985) sequence. Using synthetic oligonucleotide hybridization probes based on their amino acid sequencing work, March *et al.* (1985) were able to identify a cDNA clone [generated to a mRNA from lipopolysaccharide (LPS)-stimulated human monocytes] the sequence of which predicted the same 269-amino acid protein postulated by Auron *et al.* (1984). March *et al.* (1985) engineered expression of the carboxy-terminal 153 amino acids (beginning at amino acid 117) of the 269-amino acid polypeptide in *E. coli*, resulting in high levels of IL-1 activity. March *et al.* (1985) have termed the 17 kDa IL-1

```
                                        10                                      20
Met Ala Glu Val Pro Lys Leu Ala Ser Glu Met Met Ala Tyr Tyr Ser Gly Asn Glu Asp
                   ‾

                                        30                                      40
Asp Leu Phe Phe Glu Ala Asp Gly Pro Lys Gln Met Lys Cys Ser Phe Gln Asp Leu Asp

                                        50                                      60
Leu Cys Pro Leu Asp Gly Gly Ile Gln Leu Arg Ile Ser Asp His His Tyr Ser Lys Gly

                                        70                                      80
Phe Arg Gln Ala Ala Ser Val Val Val Ala Met Asp Lys Leu Arg Lys Met Leu Val Pro

                                        90                                     100
Cys Pro Gln Thr Phe Gln Glu Asn Asp Leu Ser Thr Phe Phe Pro Phe Ile Phe Glu Glu

                                       110                      ↓              120
Glu Pro Ile Phe Phe Asp Thr Trp Asp Asn Glu Ala Tyr Val His Asp Ala Pro Val Arg

                                       130                                     140
Ser Leu Asn Cys Thr Leu Arg Asp Ser Gln Gln Lys Ser Leu Val Met Ser Gly Pro Tyr

                                       150                                     160
Glu Leu Lys Ala Leu His Leu Gln Gly Gln Asp Met Glu Gln Gln Val Val Phe Ser Met

                                       170                                     180
Ser Phe Val Gln Gly Glu Glu Ser Asn Asp Lys Ile Pro Val Ala Leu Gly Leu Lys Glu

                                       190                                     200
Lys Asn Leu Tyr Leu Ser Cys Val Leu Lys Asp Asp Lys Pro Thr Leu Gln Leu Glu Ser

                                       210                                     220
Val Asp Pro Lys Asn Tyr Pro Lys Lys Lys Met Glu Lys Arg Phe Val Phe Asn Lys Ile

                                       230                                     240
Glu Ile Asn Asn Lys Leu Glu Phe Glu Ser Ala Gln Phe Pro Asn Trp Tyr Ile Ser Thr

                                       250                                     260
Ser Gln Ala Glu Asn Met Pro Val Phe Leu Gly Gly Thr Lys Gly Gly Gln Asp Ile Thr

                         269
Asp Phe Thr Met Gln Phe Val Ser Ser
```

FIG. 2. Predicted amino acid sequence of human IL-1β precursor protein. The nucleotide sequence of human IL-1β cDNA predicts a single open-reading frame coding for a protein of 269 amion acids (Auron *et al.*, 1984). Auron *et al.* (1984) predict a Lys at position 6 (1 clone sequenced?), while March *et al.* (1985) predict a Glu at this position (2 clones sequenced). The arrow points to the Ala at position 117 which is the amino-terminus of the majority of the IL-1β population (Van Damme *et al.*, 1984) and the beginning of the biologically-active carboxy-terminal fragment synthesized in *E. coli* by March *et al.* (1985).

protein contained within the 269-amino acid precursor "IL-1β" and estimated the abundance of its mRNA to be ~0.1% of the poly(A)+ RNA from stimulated macrophages. One assumes, given the abundance of both the IL-1β mRNA and its product, that IL-1β corresponds to the p*I* 6.8 human IL-1 species.

B. HUMAN IL-1α

March *et al.* (1985) were able to measure IL-1 activity in rabbit reticulocyte lysates programmed with poly(A)+ RNA from LPS-stimulated human peripheral blood monocytes. Using this assay together with hybrid selection, they identified a cDNA clone which codes for a protein

```
                              10                                        20
Met Ala Lys Val Pro Asp Met Phe Glu Asp Leu Lys Asn Cys Tyr Ser Glu Asn Glu Glu

                              30                                        40
Asp Ser Ser Ser Ile Asp His Leu Ser Leu Asn Gln Lys Ser Phe Tyr His Val Ser Tyr

                              50                                        60
Gly Pro Leu His Glu Gly Cys Met Asp Gln Ser Val Ser Leu Ser Ile Ser Glu Thr Ser

                              70                                        80
Lys Thr Ser Lys Leu Thr Phe Lys Glu Ser Met Val Val Val Ala Thr Asn Gly Lys Val

                              90                                       100
Leu Lys Lys Arg Arg Leu Ser Leu Ser Gln Ser Ile Thr Asp Asp Asp Leu Glu Ala Ile

                             110              ↓                         120
Ala Asn Asp Ser Glu Glu Glu Ile Ile Lys Pro Arg Ser Ala Pro Phe Ser Phe Leu Ser
                                            ―――          ―――
                             130                                       140
Asn Val Lys Tyr Asn Phe Met Arg Ile Ile Lys Tyr Glu Phe Ile Leu Asn Asp Ala Leu

                             150                                       160
Asn Gln Ser Ile Ile Arg Ala Asn Asp Gln Tyr Leu Thr Ala Ala Ala Leu His Asn Leu

                             170                                       180
Asp Glu Ala Val Lys Phe Asp Met Gly Ala Tyr Lys Ser Ser Lys Asp Asp Ala Lys Ile

                             190                                       200
Thr Val Ile Leu Arg Ile Ser Lys Thr Gln Leu Tyr Val Thr Ala Gln Asp Glu Asp Gln

                             210                                       220
Pro Val Leu Leu Lys Glu Met Pro Glu Ile Pro Lys Thr Ile Thr Gly Ser Glu Thr Asn

                             230                                       240
Leu Leu Phe Phe Trp Glu Thr His Gly Thr Lys Asn Tyr Phe Thr Ser Val Ala His Pro

                             250                                       260
Asn Leu Phe Ile Ala Thr Lys Gln Asp Tyr Trp Val Cys Leu Ala Gly Gly Pro Pro Ser

                             271
Ile Thr Asp Phe Gln Ile Leu Glu Asn Gln Ala
```

FIG. 3. Predicted amino acid sequence of human IL-1α precursor protein. The nucleotide sequence of human IL-1α cDNA predicts a single open-reading frame coding for a protein of 271 amino acids (March *et al.*, 1985). The amino acids at positions 110 and 114 are underlined to reflect the differences noted at these positions by different investigators as follows (number of clones analyzed in parenthesis). Position 110, Lys (1) and Asn (1) (March *et al.* 1985); Lys (4) (Gubler *et al.* 1986); Lys (1) (Furutani *et al.* 1985). Position 114, Ala (2) (March *et al.* 1985); Ala (2) and Ser (2) (Gubler *et al.* 1986); Ser (1) (Furutani *et al.* 1985). The arrow points to the Ser at position 113 which was selected, by homology from the murine IL-1 protein sequencing, as the beginning of the biologically active carboxy-terminal fragment synthesized in *E. coli* by March *et al.* (1985).

of 271 amino acids (Fig. 3) which is highly homologous to the 270-amino acid murine IL-1 precursor (Lomedico *et al.*, 1984). Based upon the murine IL-1 sequencing and expression studies in *E. coli* (Lomedico *et al.*, 1984), March *et al.* (1984) engineered expression of the carboxy-terminal 159 amino acids (beginning at amino acid 113) of the 271-amino acid polypeptide in *E. coli*, resulting in high levels of IL-1 activity. March *et al.* (1985) have termed the IL-1 protein contained within this precursor "IL-1α." Given the 10-fold lower abundance (March *et al.*, 1984) of the IL-1α mRNA (relative to the IL-1β mRNA) and the acidic nature of its homolog, murine IL-1, one assumes that IL-1α corresponds to the relatively minor IL-1 species observed between pI 5 and 6.

Recently, we used the murine IL-1 cDNA as a hybridization probe to isolate cDNA clones generated to LPS-stimulated human mononuclear cell mRNA (Gubler *et al.*, 1986). Nucleotide sequence analysis of these clones confirm the sequence of the 271-amino acid IL-1α precursor (see Fig. 3). The carboxy-terminal 154 amino acids of IL-1α have been expressed in *E. coli*, and this protein has been purified to homogeneity and evaluated in various IL-1 assays.

IV. Rabbit IL-1

Furutani *et al.* (1985) have cloned rabbit IL-1 cDNA by using hybrid selection and IL-1 expression in *X. laevis* oocytes to screen a library prepared to stimulated rabbit alveolar macrophage mRNA. The nucleotide sequence of this cDNA predicts a protein of 267 amino acids (Fig. 4) highly related to the murine IL-1 precursor. This rabbit IL-1

```
                                10                                  20
Met Ala Lys Val Pro Asp Leu Phe Glu Asp Leu Lys Asn Cys Phe Ser Glu Asn Glu Glu
                                30                                  40
Tyr Ser Ser Ala Ile Asp His Leu Ser Leu Asn Gln Lys Ser Phe Tyr Asp Ala Ser Tyr
                                50                                  60
Glu Pro Leu His Glu Asp Cys Met Asn Lys Val Val Ser Leu Ser Thr Ser Glu Thr Ser
                                70                                  80
Val Ser Pro Asn Leu Thr Phe Gln Glu Asn Val Val Ala Val Thr Ala Ser Gly Lys Ile
                                90                                 100
Leu Lys Lys Arg Arg Leu Ser Leu Asn Gln Pro Ile Thr Asp Val Asp Leu Glu Thr Asn
                               110                                 120
Val Ser Asp Pro Glu Glu Gly Ile Ile Lys Pro Arg Ser Val Pro Tyr Thr Phe Gln Arg
                               130                                 140
Asn Met Arg Tyr Lys Tyr Leu Arg Ile Ile Lys Gln Glu Phe Thr Leu Asn Asp Ala Leu
                               150                                 160
Asn Gln Ser Leu Val Arg Asp Thr Ser Asp Gln Tyr Leu Arg Ala Ala Pro Leu Gln Asn
                               170                                 180
Leu Gly Asp Ala Val Lys Phe Asp Met Gly Val Tyr Met Thr Ser Glu Asp Ser Ile Leu
                               190                                 200
Pro Val Thr Leu Arg Ile Ser Gln Thr Pro Leu Phe Val Ser Ala Gln Asn Glu Asp Glu
                               210                                 220
Pro Val Leu Leu Lys Glu Met Pro Glu Thr Pro Arg Ile Ile Thr Asp Ser Glu Ser Asp
                               230                                 240
Ile Leu Phe Phe Trp Glu Thr Gln Gly Asn Lys Asn Tyr Phe Lys Ser Ala Ala Asn Pro
                               250                                 260
Gln Leu Phe Ile Ala Thr Lys Pro Glu His Leu Val His Met Ala Arg Gly Leu Pro Ser
                267
Met Thr Asp Phe Gln Ile Ser
```

FIG. 4. Predicted amino acid sequence of rabbit IL-1 precursor protein. The nucleotide sequence of rabbit IL-1 cDNA predicts a single open-reading frame coding for a protein of 267 amino acids (Furutani *et al.* 1985).

polypeptide is likely to be the homolog of both murine IL-1 and human IL-1α. Presumably rabbit IL-1β exists, given the evidence of charge heterogeneity in rabbit IL-1 preparations.

V. IL-1 Gene Family Evolution

Nucleotide sequence analysis of the cloned IL-1 cDNAs and their expression in *E. coli* clearly demonstrate that biologically active IL-1 is liberated from the carboxy-terminus of a larger molecular-weight precursor. While evaluation of recombinant IL-1 is continuing, it is obvious that there exists a family of at least two independently evolving genes whose dissimilar protein products have similar biological activities. One member of the gene family codes for murine, rabbit, and human IL-1α; these gene products are all between 61 and 65% homologous with one another (Table I and Fig. 5). The differences between the IL-1α gene products represent divergence during the past 90 million years since the start of the mammalian radiation. The other member of the IL-1 gene family is represented by human IL-1β which is between 27 and 33% homologous with the different IL-1α proteins (Table I and Fig. 6). The sequence homology between α and β gene products is statistically significant and mainly restricted to the carboxy-terminal portions of the proteins (i.e., the regions responsible for biological activity). Given the other similarities between the α and β precursors (see below), it is likely that there was a gene duplication before or during vertebrate evolution that created two genes that began to diverge independently of one another. Whether IL-1α and IL-1β have separate activities is still an open question. However, since these proteins interact with the same cell-surface receptor (Kilian *et al.*, 1986) we feel that this possibility is unlikely, and hence there probably is no selection for the maintenance of two distinct genes. This view may help to rationalize why the relative

TABLE I

SEQUENCE HOMOLOGY PERCENTAGE BETWEEN DIFFERENT IL-1 PRECURSORS[a]

	Mouse	Rabbit α	Human α	Human β
Mouse	—	61[b]	61	28
Rabbit α	61	—	65	33
Human α	61	65	—	27
Human β	28	33	27	—

[a] For each IL-1 precursor pair the best sequence alignment was determined (Wilbur and Lipman, 1983).

[b] The numbers represent sequence homology percentages. Sequence homology percentage = (number of amino acid identities/total number of amino acids) × 100.

```
X        10        20        30        40        50        60
MAKVPDLFEDLKNCFSENEEYSSAIDHLSLNQKSFYDASYEPLHEDCMNKVVSLSTSETS         RABBIT
:: ::::: : ::::::: :: :: :::::::::: :: :::: :: :::: ::::
MAKVPDMFEDLKNCYSENEEDSSSIDHLSLNQKSFYHVSYGPLHEGCMDQSVSLSISETS         HUMAN α
:: ::::: :: ::::::::: :: ::: ::: : :: ::::
MAKVPDLFEDLKNCYSENEDYSSAIDHLSLNQKSFYDASYGSLHETCTDQFVSLRTSETS         MOUSE
X        10        20        30        40        50        60


         70        80        90       100       110       120
VSPNLTFQENVVAVTA---SGKILKKRRLSLNQPITDVDLETNVSDPEEGIIKPRSVPYTFQR       RABBIT
: : : : ::  :: ::::::::: : ::: ::: : :: :::::: : :
KTSKLTFKESMVVVAT---NGKVLKKRRLSLSQSITDDDLEAIANDSEEEIIKPRSAPFSFLS       HUMAN α
: : : : ::: ::::::: :: ::: : ::: :::: :
KMSNFTFKESRVTVSATSSNGKILKKRRLSFSETFTEDDLQSITHDLEETIQ-PRSAPYTYQS       MOUSE
         70        80        90       100       110       120


        130       140       150       160       170       180
NMRYKYLRIIKQEFTLNDALNQSLVRDTSDQYLRAAPLQNLGDAVKFDMGVYMTSEDSIL         RABBIT
: :  :::: :: ::::::::: : :::: :: : ::  :::::::: : :
NVKYNFMRIIKYEFILNDALNQSIIRAN-DQYLTAAALHNLDEAVKFDMGAYKSSKDDAK         HUMAN α
: :  :: ::: :  :: ::::: :: :: : : :
DLRYKLMKLVRQKFVMNDSLNQTIYQDVDKHYLSTTWLNDLQQEVKFDMYAYSSGGDDSK         MOUSE
        130       140       150       160       170       180


        190       200       210       220       230
P-VTLRISQTPLFVSAQNEDEPVLLKEMPETPRIITDSESDILFFWETQGNKNYFKSAAN         RABBIT
:: ::::: :: :: ::::::::: : :: ::::: : :::: : :
ITVILRISKTQLYVTAQDEDQPVLLKEMPEIPKTITGSETNLLFFWETHGTKNYFTSVAH         HUMAN α
: : : : :  ::::::::: :: ::::: :: ::::: :
YPVTLKISDSQLFVSAQGEDQPVLLKELPETPKLITGSETDLIFFWKSINSKNYFTSAAY         MOUSE
        190       200       210       220       230       240


        250       260       267
PQLFIATKPEHLVHMARGLPSMTDFQIS         RABBIT
: : :::::: ::: : :
PNLFIATKQDYWVCLAGGPPSITDFQILENQA         HUMAN α
: : :::::: :: :::::
PELFIATKEQSRVHLARGLPSMTDFQIS         MOUSE
        250       260       270
```

FIG. 5. Amino acid sequence comparison of IL-1α precursors. The analysis was performed using the Wilbur and Lipman (1983) alignment algorithm.

```
X        10        20        30        40        50
MAKVPDMFEDLKNCYSENEEDSSSIDHLSLNQK-SFYHVSYGPLHEGCMDQSVSLSISET         HUMAN α
:: :  : :: ::  : :  : :: : ::
MAEVPKLASEMMAYYSGNEDDLFFEADGPKQMKCSFQDLDLCPLDGGIQ-----LRISDH         HUMAN β
X        10        20        30        40        50


         70        80        90       100
SKTSKLTFKESMVVVATNGKVLKKRRLSLSQSITDDDL----------EAIANDSEEEII         HUMAN α
::      :::: : :  :: :::
HY-SKGFRQAASVVVAMDK--LRKMLVPCPQTFQENDLSTFFPFIFEEEPIFFDTWDNEA         HUMAN β
         60        70        80        90       100       110


        120       130       140       150       160
KPRSAPFSFLSNVKYNFMRIIKYEFILNDALNQSIIRANDQYLTAAALHNLDEA--VKFD         HUMAN α
::  :  : :  : ::: :: :  : :
YVHDAPVRSLNCT------------LRDSQQKSLVMSGPYELKALHLQGQDMEQQVVFS         HUMAN β
        120       130       140       150


170       180       190       200       210       220
MGAYKSSKDDAKITVILRISKTQLYVTAQDEDQPVLLKEMPEIPKTITGS--ETNLLFFW       HUMAN α
:      :: ::: :::  :: :: :  : :
MSFVQGEESNDKIPVALGLKEKNLYLSCVLKDDKPTLQLESVDPKNYPKKKMEKRFVFNK       HUMAN β
        170       180       190       200       210


        230       240       250       260       271
ETHGTKNYFTSVAHPNLFIATKQDYW--VCLAG--GPPSITDFQILENQA         HUMAN α
: : : : :::: :: :: ::::
IEINNKLEFESAQFPNWYISTSQAENMPVFLGGTKGGQDITDFTMQFVSS         HUMAN β
        230       240       250       260       269
```

Score=6, Matched=73, Mismatched=170, Unmatched=40, Gaps=10
Window=20, Word-size=1, Density=Less, Gap-Penalty=2

FIG. 6. Amino acid sequence comparison of human IL-1 precursors.

abundance of the IL-1α and IL-1β gene products differ in related organisms [i.e., β is more abundant in humans, but α and β are present in
roughly equal amounts in pigs (Saklatvala *et al.*, 1985)].

VI. IL-1 Precursor Structure and Function

The primary structures of the IL-1 precursors predicted by cDNA
cloning have several common features (see Figs. 5 and 6). In addition to
being approximately the same size (267–271 amino acids) and having
IL-1 activity map to the carboxy-terminal half, the IL-1α and β precursors do not appear to possess a classic signal sequence. There is no
sizable hydrophobic region in any of the sequenced precursors. Since
there is no evidence for low-molecular-weight (i.e., 15–17 kDa) IL-1
molecules inside macrophages (Giri *et al.*, 1985), we feel it is likely that
IL-1 precursor processing occurs extracellularly or at the cell membrane.
How the IL-1 precursor is secreted is nevertheless a mystery. Possibly
the extreme amino-terminus of the IL-1 precursor plays some role in
cellular compartmentalization and/or secretion because this region is
well conserved among the IL-1α family members (Fig. 5). The sug-
gestion has been made that IL-1 is really stored within the macrophage
and only released upon significant cellular insult resulting in cell death
(Gery and Lepe-Zuniga, 1984).

The human IL-1α precursor synthesized in rabbit reticulocyte lysates
is biologically active (March *et al.*, 1985), as is the murine IL-1 precursor
synthesized in *E. coli* (C. P. Hellmann and P. T. Lomedico, unpublished). It is not clear if the IL-1α precursor is intrinsically active, or
whether local proteolysis in the assay creates active fragments. March *et
al.* (1985) infer that the human IL-1β precursor is biologically inactive (or
resistant to proteolysis during assay), although Auron *et al.* (1984) were
able to detect activity secreted from *X. laevis* oocytes with hybrid-se-
lected mRNA.

It is not known how the IL-1 precursor is processed, however a
tetrabasic region, Lys-Lys-Arg-Arg, is conserved among the IL-1α family
members around position 85. We have suggested a model (Lomedico *et
al.*, 1984) which predicts that this highly charged region is a primary
processing site. Proteases released by the macrophage may be responsible for cleaving at this site, resulting in the release of an ~180-amino acid
carboxy-terminal fragment which possesses a protease-resistant core.
Subsequent proteolytic attack at the newly exposed amino-terminus
would generate a heterogeneous population of molecules with "ragged"
amino-termini. Amino-terminal end heterogeneity, as revealed by sequencing studies (Lomedico *et al.*, 1984; Van Damme *et al.*, 1985; March
et al., 1985), supports this model. In addition, evaluation of recombinant

murine IL-1 proteins created by site-directed mutagenesis demonstrates that the integrity of the carboxy-terminus of the 270-amino acid precursor is important for activity, while different amino-termini can be utilized to generate molecules with equivalent specific activities (DeChiara *et al.*, 1986).

VII. Appendix

Gray *et al.* (1986) recently used the human IL-1β cDNA as a hybridization probe to isolate a mouse IL-1β cDNA clone from a cDNA library prepared from the macrophage-like cell line PU5-1.8. The nucleotide sequence of this cDNA predicts a protein of 269 amino acids (see Fig. 7) which is ~67% homologous with the human IL-1β precursor and ~30% homologous with the different IL-1α precursors.

```
              10        20        30        40        50        60
    MAKVPDLFEDLKNCFSENEEYSSAIDHLSLNQK-SFYDASYEPLHEDCMNKVVSLSTSET   RABBIT α
    ::::::  ::::::::::: ::: :: :::: ::  :::: ::::::::
    MAKVPDMFEDLKNCYSENEEDSSSIDHLSLNQK-SFYHVSYGPLHEGCMDQSVSLSISET   HUMAN α
    :::::  ::::::::::::  :::::::::::: ::::: ::::  ::  :::  ::::
    MAKVPDLFEDLKNCYSENEDYSSAIDHLSLNQK-SFYDASYGSLHETCTDQFVSLRTSET   MOUSE α
    :: ::: ::  ::  :  ::   ::  :  :    ::::    :    :    :::  ::
    MAEVPKLASEMMAYYSGNEDDLFFEADGPKQMKCSFQDLDLCPL-----DGGIQLRISDH   HUMAN β
    :: :  :: :::  ::::: :::  ::: :: :: :    :::        : :::: :
    MATVPELNCEMPPFDSD-ENDLFFEVDGPQKMKGCFQTFDLGCP-----DESIQLQISQQ   MOUSE β
    **  ** **              *  *        *      *           *   *

              70        80        90       100       110
    SVSPNLTFQENVVAVTA---SGKILKKRRLSLNQPITDVDL--ETNVSDPEEGIIKPRSV   RABBIT α
    :   :: ::::: :::    ::::::::::: : : :::::   :    ::::::::::::
    SKTSKLTFKESMVVVAT---NGKVLKKRRLSLSQSITDDDL--EAIANDSEEEIIKPRSA   HUMAN α
    : :   ::::: :: ::   :: ::::::: : :: :::::  :: :  :::: ::: ::
    SKMSNFTFKESRVTVSATSSNGKILKKRRLSFSETFTEDDL--QSITHDLEETIQ-PRSA   MOUSE α
    :  :::  :  ::::::     :: :::   : : :::::   ::: ::::::::: ::::
    HYSKGFRQAASVVVAM------DKLRKMLVPCPQTFQENDLSTFFPFIFEEEPIFFDTWD   HUMAN β
    :  : :::: :: :::      :  : ::   :  :    :: ::::::::::: :  ::
    HINKSFRQAVSLIVAV------EKLWQLPVSFPWTFQDEDMSTFFSFIFEEEPILCDSWD   MOUSE β
                                 *                 ** *

             120       130       140       150       160       170
    PYTFQRNMRYKYLRIIKQEFTLNDALNQSLVRDTSDQYLRAAPL--QNLGDAVKFDMGVY   RABBIT α
    :  :  :::  ::  :: :::::::::::::  :: ::: :  :   ::::::::::::: :
    PFSFLSNVKYNFMRIIKYEFILNDALNQSIIRAN-DQYLTAAAL--HNLDEAVKFDMGAY   HUMAN α
    :  :  ::: :  :: ::: :::::::::: :  : ::: :  :    ::: :::::::: :
    PYTYQSDLRYKLMKLVRQKFVMNDSLNQTIYQDVDKHYLSTTWL--NDLQQEVKFDMYAY   MOUSE α
    :  :  :  :::  :::   :  :: :  ::   ::: :::   :   ::  :::: :::::
    NEAY------VHDAPVRSLNCTLRDSQQKSLVMSGPYELKALHLQGGQDMEQQVVFSMSFV   HUMAN β
    :   :::::  :: ::::::::: :::: :::::::: :::::::::::::  :::::::::
    DDDNLL----VCDVPIRQLHYRLRDEQQKSLVLSDPYELKALHLNGQNINQQVIFSMSFV   MOUSE β
                *         *  *  ****   *        *    *  * *

             180       190       200       210       220
    MTSEDSILP-VTLRISQTPLFVSAQNEDEPVLLKEMPETPRIITDS--ESDILFFWETQG   RABBIT α
    :  :    :   ::  :: :: :::  :::::::::::: ::  ::   :  ::::::::
    KSSKDDAKITVILRISKTQLYVTAQDEDQPVLLKEMPEIPKTITGS--ETNLLFFWETHG   HUMAN α
    :  ::   :   ::  ::  :: :::  :::::::::::: :: ::   ::  :::::: :
    SSGGDDSKYPVTLKISDSQLFVSAQGEDQPVLLKELPETPKLITGS--ETDLIFFWKSIN   MOUSE α
    :    :::    :: ::::  :::: ::  ::::::::::::: ::  ::: ::: :::::
    QGEESNDKIPVALGLKEKNLYLSCVLKDDKPTLQLESVDPKNYPKKKMEKRFVFNKIEIN   HUMAN β
    :::  :::::::::::::::::::::::: ::::::::::::  ::::::::::::::: :
    QGEPSNDKIPVALGLKGKNLYLSCVMKDGTPTLQLESVDPKQYPKKKMEKRFVFNKIEVK   MOUSE β
               **     *       *          *       *         *   *

             240       250       260
    NKNYFKSAANPQLFIATK--PEHLVHMAR--GLPSMTDFQIS   RABBIT α
    : ::::  : :: ::::::  :::   :    :::: ::::
    TKNYFTSVAHPNLFIATK--QDYWVCLAG--GPPSITDFQILENQA   HUMAN α
    : ::::: :  :: ::::::  :: ::  :    :::: :::::
    SKNYFTSAAYPELFIATK--EQSRVHLAR--GLPSMTDFQIS   MOUSE α
    : ::: : :::::::::::  :::::::::: :::: ::::::::
    NKLEFESAQFPNWYISTSQAENMPVFLGGTKGGQDITDFTMQFVSS   HUMAN β
    : :::::: :::::::::::::::  :::: ::::: ::::::
    SKVEFESAEFPNWYISTSQAEHKPVFLGNNSG-QDIIDFTMESVSS   MOUSE β
      *  *   *    * *       *        *      **
```

FIG. 7. Amino acid sequence comparison of IL-1 precursors. Homologies between sequences are marked with a double dot; homologies extending to all of the sequences are marked with an asterisk.

ACKNOWLEDGMENTS

We thank Laurie Bowen for excellent secretarial assistance.

REFERENCES

Auron, P. E., Webb, A. C., Rosenwasser, L. J., Mucci, S. F., Rich, A., Wolff, S. M., and Dinarello, C. A. (1984). *Proc. Natl. Acad. Sci. U.S.A.* **81**, 7907–7911.

DeChiara, T. M., Young, D., Semionow, R., Stern, A. S., Batula-Bernardo, C., Fielder-Nagy, C., Kaffka, K., Kilian, P. L., Yamazaki, S., Mizel, S. B., and Lomedico, P. T. (1986). *Proc. Natl. Acad. Sci. U.S.A.* **83**, 8303–8307.

Dinarello, C. A. (1984). *Rev. Infect. Dis.* **6**, 51–95.

Furutani, Y., Notake, M., Yamayoshi, M., Yamagishi, J.-I., Nomura, H., Ohue, M., Furuta, R., Fukui, T., Yamada, M., and Nakamura, S. (1985). *Nucleic Acids Res.* **13**, 5869–5882.

Gery, I., and Lepe-Zuniga, J. L. (1984). *Lymphokines* **9**, 109–125.

Giri, J., Lomedico, P. T., and Mizel, S. (1985). *J. Immunol.* **134**, 343–349.

Gray, P. W., Glaister, D., Chen, E., Goeddel, D. V., and Pennica, D. (1986). *J. Immunol.*, in press.

Gubler, U., Chua, A. O., Hellmann, C. P., Vitek, M. P., Benjamin, W. R., Collier, K. J., Dukovich, M., Familletti, P. C., Fiedler-Nagy, C., Jenson, J., Kaffka, K., Kilian, P. L., Stern, A. S., Stremlo, D., Wittreich, B. H., Woehle, D., Mizel, S. B., and Lomedico, P. T. (1986). *J. Immunol.* **136**, 2492–2497.

Ihrie, E. J., and Wood, D. D. (1985). *Lymphokine Res.* **4**, 169–181.

Kilian, P. L., Kaffka, K. L., Stern, A. S., Woehle, D., Benjamin, W. R., DeChiara, T. M., Gubler, U., Farrar, J. J., Mizel, S. B., and Lomedico, P. T. (1986). *J. Immunol.* **136**, 4509–4514.

Kronheim, S. R., March, C. J., Erb, S. K., Conlon, P. J., Mochizuki, D. Y., and Hopp, T. P. (1985). *J. Exp. Med.* **161**, 490–502.

Lomedico, P. T., Gubler, U., Hellmann, C. P., Dukovich, M., Giri, J. G., Pan, Y.-C. E., Collier, K., Semionow, R., Chua, A. O., and Mizel, S. B. (1984). *Nature (London)* **312**, 458–462.

March, C. J., Mosley, B., Larsen, A., Cerretti, D. P., Braedt, G., Price, V., Gillis, S., Henney, C. S., Kronheim, S. R., Grabstein, K., Conlon, P. J., Hopp, T. P., and Cosman, D. (1985). *Nature (London)* **315**, 641–647.

Mizel, S. B. (1979). *J. Immunol.* **122**, 2167–2172.

Mizel, S. B., and Mizel, D. (1981). *J. Immunol.* **126**, 834–837.

Mizel, S. B., Dukovich, M., and Rothstein, J. (1983). *J. Immunol.* **131**, 1834–1837.

Murphy, P. A., Simon, P. L., and Willoughby, W. F. (1980). *J. Immunol.* **124**, 2498–2501.

Parnes, J. R., Velan, B., Felsenfeld, A., Ramanathan, L., Ferrini, U., Appella, E., and Seidman, J. G. (1981). *Proc. Natl. Acad. Sci. U.S.A.* **78**, 2253–2257.

Saklatvala, J., Sarsfield, S. J., and Townsend, Y. (1985). *J. Exp. Med.* **162**, 1208–1222.

Van Damme, J., De Ley, M., Opdenakker, G., Billiau, A., and De Somer, P. (1985). *Nature (London)* **314**, 266–268.

Wilbur, W. J., and Lipman D. J. (1983). *Proc. Natl. Acad. Sci. U.S.A.* **80**, 726–730.

Molecular Biology of Interferon-Gamma

PATRICK W. GRAY AND DAVID V. GOEDDEL

Department of Molecular Biology, Genentech, Inc., South San Francisco, California 94080

I. Introduction

Interferon-γ (IFN-γ) was first identified by its potent antiviral activity (Wheelock, 1965) and was recognized to be distinct from virally induced IFN-α and IFN-β by virtue of its sensitivity to pH 2. Falcoff (1972) proposed the name "immune IFN" based on its synthesis by sensitized T lymphocytes following exposure to the sensitizing antigen. Youngner and Salvin (1973) demonstrated that IFN-γ was antigenically distinct from IFN-α and IFN-β and proposed the term "Type II IFN" to distinguish IFN-γ from the Type I IFNs.

IFN-γ can be further distinguished from the Type I IFNs by biological and chemical properties. IFN-β and the IFN-α gene family are structurally related and closely linked genetically (reviewed by Weissman and Weber, 1985). Furthermore, IFN-α and IFN-β are recognized by the same receptor, which is distinct from the IFN-γ receptor (Raziuddin *et al.*, 1984). IFN-γ appears to have greater immunomodulatory properties than IFN-α or IFN-β (Sonnenfeld *et al.*, 1978). The antiproliferative effect of IFN-γ on tumor cells *in vitro* was originally reported to be 10–100 times that of IFN-α and IFN-β (Rubin and Gupta, 1980; Blalock *et al.*, 1980), but this greater activity may be due to synergistic activity with other lymphokines such as lymphotoxin and tumor necrosis factor.

The lack of pure IFN-γ precluded the absolute determination of its physical and biological properties. Once the cDNA for IFN-γ was cloned and expressed, recombinant IFN-γ became available for biological testing. This has allowed the identification of numerous activities and has revealed the importance of this lymphokine in the regulation of the immune system.

II. Identification of IFN-γ cDNA Clones

The cDNA for human IFN-γ was first isolated and characterized in 1981 (Gray *et al.*, 1982) by our group at Genentech. Cultures of human peripheral blood lymphocytes were stimulated with mitogens for 24 hr and then used for the preparation of mRNA. The mRNA was fractionated by acid urea–agarose gel electrophoresis, and eluted fractions were injected into *Xenopus* oocytes for bioassay. The active fractions corre-

151

sponded to 18 S in size and were enriched approximately 20-fold. A cDNA library of 8300 clones was prepared from this mRNA fraction by insertion into the *Pst*I site of pBR322. Duplicate copies of the cDNA library were prepared on nitrocellulose filters and screened with two probes. The "induced probe" was radiolabeled cDNA prepared using 18 S mRNA from an induced culture (the same mRNA used in the preparation of the library), and the "uninduced probe" was radiolabeled cDNA prepared using 18 S mRNA from an unstimulated culture containing no active IFN-γ in the culture supernatant).

Approximately 1% of the cDNA clones hybridized weakly with the induced probe but undetectably with the uninduced probe. These "induced clones" were further characterized by cross-hybridization studies and restriction endonuclease analysis. Surprisingly, all of these induced clones appeared to be related. The clone containing the plasmid with the longest cDNA insert, p69, was chosen for DNA sequence analysis (Fig. 1).

The longest open-reading frame of the cDNA insert of p69 predicted a protein length of 166 amino acids. This size corresponds to about half that observed for natural IFN-γ as determined by gel filtration experiments (Langford *et al.*, 1979; de Ley *et al.*, 1980; Yip *et al.*, 1981; Nathan *et al.*, 1981). The amino-terminal coding portion of the cDNA had several features in common with typical eukaryotic signal sequences. The amino-terminal methionine is followed by a single basic amino acid and 18 residues which are mostly hydrophobic (Fig. 1). In addition, sequence identity with several IFN-α sequences was observed at positions 18–21 (Ser-Leu-Gly-Cys), where Gly was the last signal residue and Cys the first residue of secreted mature IFN-α. Consequently, the first cysteine residue was thought to be the first amino acid of the protein encoded by this induced cDNA and was chosen for engineered expression in *Escherichia coli*. Synthetic DNA was utilized to construct an expression plasmid containing the *E. coli trp* promoter, an introduced methionine codon, and the coding sequences for the mature protein. The cDNA was also engineered for expression in yeast (Derynck *et al.*, 1983) and mammalian (COS) cells (Gray *et al.*, 1982).

All three expression systems produced an antiviral activity that was characterized as IFN-γ. The activity was sensitive to pH 2, 0.1% SDS, and antibodies specific for natural IFN-γ. The activity was not neutralized by antibodies directed against IFN-α and IFN-β. Furthermore, the activity was observed on human cells but not bovine or murine cells; this species specificity is characteristic of IFN-γ but not IFN-α or IFN-β. Other investigators have shown that antibodies directed against recombinant IFN-γ will neutralize the activity of natural IFN-γ preparations

```
                                          *
1                       AGCACATTGTTCTGATCATCTGAAGATCAGCTATTAGAAGAGAAAGATCAGT

53   TAAGTCCTTTGGACCTGATCAGCTTGATACAAGAACTACTGATTTCAACTTCTTTGGCTTAATTCTCTCGGAAACG

     -23            -20                                            -10
     met lys tyr thr ser tyr ile leu ala phe gln leu cys ile val leu gly ser leu
129  ATG AAA TAT ACA AGT TAT ATC TTG GCT TTT CAG CTC TGC ATC GTT TTG GGT TCT CTT

                         1                              10
     gly cys tyr cys Gln Asp Pro Tyr Val Lys Glu Ala Glu Asn Leu Lys Lys Tyr Phe
286  GGC TGT TAC TGC CAG GAC CCA TAT GTA AAA GAA GCA GAA AAC CTT AAG AAA TAT TTT

                 20                                    30
     Asn Ala Gly His Ser Asp Val Ala Asp Asn Gly Thr Leu Phe Leu Gly Ile Leu Lys
243  AAT GCA GGT CAT TCA GAT GTA GCG GAT AAT GGA ACT CTT TTC TTA GGC ATT TTG AAG

                         40                                    50
     Asn Trp Lys Glu Glu Ser Asp Arg Lys Ile Met Gln Ser Gln Ile Val Ser Phe Tyr
300  AAT TGG AAA GAG GAG AGT GAC AGA AAA ATA ATG CAG AGC CAA ATT GTC TCC TTT TAC

                                 60                                    70
     Phe Lys Leu Phe Lys Asn Phe Lys Asp Asp Gln Ser Ile Gln Lys Ser Val Glu Thr
357  TTC AAA CTT TTT AAA AAC TTT AAA GAT GAC CAG AGC ATC CAA AAG AGT GTG GAG ACC

                                 80                                    90
     Ile Lys Glu Asp Met Asn Val Lys Phe Phe Asn Ser Asn Lys Lys Lys Arg Asp Asp
414  ATC AAG GAA GAC ATG AAT GTC AAG TTT TTC AAT AGC AAC AAA AAG AAA CGA GAT GAC

                                 100                                   110
     Phe Glu Lys Leu Thr Asn Tyr Ser Val Thr Asp Leu Asn Val Gln Arg Lys Ala Ile
471  TTC GAA AAG CTG ACT AAT TAT TCG GTA ACT GAC TTG AAT GTC CAA CGC AAA GCA ATA

                                 120
     His Glu Leu Ile Gln Val Met Ala Glu Leu Ser Pro Ala Ala Lys Thr Gly Lys Arg
528  CAT GAA CTC ATC CAA GTG ATG GCT GAA CTG TCG CCA GCA GCT AAA ACA GGG AAG CGA

     130                            140         143
     Lys Arg Ser Gln Met Leu Phe Arg Gly Arg Arg Ala Ser Gln
585  AAA AGG AGT CAG ATG CTG TTT CGA GGT CGA AGA GCA TCC CAG TAA TGGTTGTCCTGCCTGC

646  AATATTTGAATTTTAAATCTAAATCTATTTATTAATATTTAACATTATTTATATGGGGAATATATTTTTAGACTCA

722  TCAATCAAATAAGTATTTATAATAGCAACTTTTGTGTAATGAAAATGAATATCTATTAATATATGTATTATTTATA

798  ATTCCTATATCCTGTGACTGTCTCACTTAATCCTTTGTTTTCTGACTAATTAGGCAAGGCTATGTGATTACAAGGC

874  TTTATCTCAGGGGCCAACTAGGCAGCCAACCTAAGCAAGATCCCATGGTTGTGTGTGTTTATTTCACTTGATGATACA

950  ATGAACACTTATAAGTGAAGTGATACTATCCAGTTACTGCCGGTTTGAAAATATGCCTGCAATCTGAGCCAGTGCT

1026 TTAATGGCATGTCAGACAGAACTTGAATGTGTCAGGTGACCCTGATGAAAACATAGCATCTCAGGAGATTTCATGC

1102 CTGGTGCTTCCAAATATTGTTGACAACTGTGACTGTACCCAAATGGAAAGTAACTCATTTGTTAAAATTATCAATA

1178 TCTAATATATATGAATAAAGTGTAAGTTCACAACT (1212) AAAAAAAAAAAAAAAAAAAA
```

FIG. 1. Sequence of human IFN-γ cDNA. The sequence begins at the start of the mRNA (Derynck *et al.*, 1982; Gray and Goeddel, 1982) and the proposed cap site is marked with an asterisk. This sequence contains 19 residues at the 5′ end which were not identified in the original sequence (Gray *et al.*, 1982). In addition, residue 137 is Arg (CGA), which was found in more cDNAs than Gln (CAA) (Derynck *et al.*, 1982).

(Schreiber *et al.*, 1985). These studies convincingly demonstrate the isolation and expression of the human IFN-γ cDNA.

Several other investigators have subsequently reported expression of human recombinant IFN-γ. Devos *et al.* (1982) utilized a hybrid selection protocol to identify a human IFN-γ cDNA clone, which they then expressed in mammalian cell culture. Several groups have reported the construction of a synthetic gene for IFN-γ (Alton *et al.*, 1983; Tanaka *et al.*, 1983) based on the published sequence. Such a method allows rapid manipulation of the DNA sequence to produce variants of IFN-γ.

III. IFN-γ Protein Structure

The cloning and characterization of IFN-γ cDNA facilitated the understanding of IFN-γ protein structure and helped to resolve apparent problems of size heterogeneity. Most reports prior to 1982 described IFN-γ as a protein of 40,000–60,000 MW. Yip *et al.* (1982) demonstrated that natural human IFN-γ could be resolved into two bands of 20,000 and 25,000 Da on SDS–polyacrylamide gels, suggesting that the earlier estimates were probably due to dimerization. IFN-γ readily aggregates to form dimers and this is probably the biologically active form (Le *et al.*, 1984a; Chang *et al.*, 1984). Strong denaturants such as SDS are required to dissociate the IFN-γ into monomers.

Heterogeneity in size and charge is observed for natural human IFN-γ. The majority of this variability is due to differential glycosylation. There are two potential N-linked glycosylation sequences in the IFN-γ sequence (Fig. 1). The 25,000 MW IFN-γ is glycosylated at both positions, while the 20,000 MW form contains carbohydrate at only the first glycosylation site, asparagine-25 (Rinderknecht *et al.*, 1984). A small amount of nonglycosylated IFN-γ with a monomeric size of 15,500 MW has also been reported (Kelker *et al.*, 1984).

Rinderknecht *et al.* (1984) demonstrated that natural human IFN-γ differed at the amino- and carboxy-termini from the predicted cDNA structure. The amino-terminal residue of natural IFN-γ is pyroglutamate, in contrast to the cysteine predicted by the homology with human IFN-α (Gray *et al.*, 1982). This result suggested that the signal sequence for IFN-γ is 23 rather than 20 residues in length, and that the first amino acid of secreted IFN-γ is glutamine, which subsequently cyclizes to form the pyroglutamate derivative. The carboxy-terminal end of natural IFN-γ is quite variable, and six different termini were observed. Proteolysis is probably responsible for the alternate carboxyl ends since the IFN-γ sequence is quite hydrophilic with numerous basic residues at the carboxy-terminus.

Recombinant DNA methodology has been utilized to construct plasmids which direct the synthesis of IFN-γ molecules. IFN-γ containing the Cys-Tyr-Cys residues at the amino-terminus (preceded by a methionine residue) has about 10% of the antiviral activity of recombinant IFN-γ in which these three amino acids are deleted (Burton *et al.*, 1985).

Removal of 18 residues from the carboxyl-terminus reduces the specific activity to approximately 1%, whereas deletion of 12 C-terminal amino acids has no effect on activity.

A specific receptor for IFN-γ has been partially characterized. Radioiodinated recombinant IFN-γ binds to monocytes or cell lines in a saturable and reversible manner (Celada *et al.*, 1984, 1985; Anderson *et al.*, 1982; Sarkar and Gupta, 1984). There are approximately 3000–7000 binding sites per cell with an affinity of $1-5 \times 10^8$ M^{-1}. Binding can be inhibited by unlabeled IFN-γ but not significantly by IFN-α or IFN-β. The receptor appears to be a protein since trypsin or pronase treatment greatly reduces the binding affinity. Cross-linking experiments with iodinated IFN-γ suggest that the receptor has a molecular weight of approximately 70,000 (Celada *et al.*, 1985; Sarkar and Gupta, 1984).

IV. IFN-γ Gene Structure

The IFN-γ cDNA was utilized as probe to analyze the structure of the IFN-γ gene. IFN-γ is encoded by a single gene which contains three intervening sequences (Fig. 2) (Gray and Goeddel, 1982; Taya *et al.*, 1982) in contrast to the intronless IFN-α gene family and IFN-β gene. The IFN-γ gene is found on chromosome 12 in humans (Naylor *et al.*, 1983), while the Type I IFN genes are all clustered on the short arm of chromosome 9 (Owerbach *et al.*, 1981; Shows *et al.*, 1982). There is no significant DNA homology and little (if any) protein homology between IFN-γ and the Type I IFNs. The IFN-α and IFN-β genes diverged from

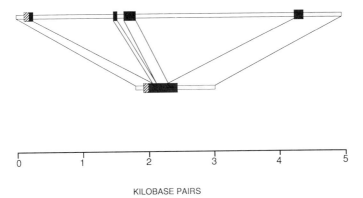

KILOBASE PAIRS

FIG. 2. Gene and message structure of IFN-γ. The structure of the primary transcript is presented at the top and the spliced mRNA is shown below. Coding sequence of the mature protein is shown in black and the signal sequence is hatched. The three introns are open boxes, and the 5' and 3' untranslated sequences are stippled.

a common ancestor some 200–300 million years ago (Weissmann and Weber, 1985), while the IFN-γ gene probably has an independent origin.

The single IFN-γ transcript (Derynck *et al.*, 1982) is preceded by characteristic promoter signals (Gray and Goeddel, 1982): a "TATA" box (TATAAATA) 28 bp upstream from the 5' end of the mRNA and "CAAT" box at −89. Although the IFN-β has an identical TATA box, no other significant homology is observed with the other IFN genes. This is not surprising in view of their independent regulatory mechanisms. Some weak promoter homology is observed between the IFN-γ gene and the interleukin-2 gene (Fujita *et al.*, 1983) and the lymphotoxin gene (Nedwin *et al.*, 1985), which might suggest common regulatory mechanisms.

V. Animal IFN-γ Sequences

Because of the strict species specificity of IFN-γ, human IFN-γ is inactive in the tumor model systems of the rat or mouse. Therefore, human IFN-γ cDNA has been utilized to identify sequences coding for IFN-γ in DNA of other organisms. The murine IFN-γ gene was isolated by screening a murine genomic-λ library with the human cDNA sequence (Gray and Goeddel, 1983). The complete murine IFN-γ gene sequence, previously unreported, is presented in Fig. 3. The overall DNA sequence homology with the human gene is 65%, and the gene structure is quite similar, with three introns of similar length in homologous positions. The murine IFN-γ gene was localized to chromosome 10 (Naylor *et al.*, 1984) which has several gene loci homologous to those found on human chromosome 12. The protein encoded by the murine IFN-γ gene shows only 40% homology with human IFN-γ and contains 10 fewer amino acids at the carboxy-terminus. Natural murine IFN-γ has been purified extensively and has an apparent molecular weight of 20,500 on SDS–polyacrylamide gel electrophoresis and 41,000 on sieving columns (Havell and Spitalny, 1982).

Sequences for bovine IFN-γ (D. Leung and D. Capon, unpublished; Rinderknecht and Burton, 1985) and rat IFN-γ (Dijkema *et al.*, 1985) have also been reported. Confirmation of these sequences as IFN-γ has been by homology with the human sequence and by expression of the

---

Fig. 3. Murine IFN-γ gene sequence. The murine IFN-γ gene was isolated and sequenced as described in Gray and Goeddel (1983). Sequences important for transcription initiation (TATA at base 86) and poly(A) addition (AATAAA at base 4943) are underlined. The putative start of transcription (based on homology with the human IFN-γ gene) is marked with a star (base 112).

```
                                                                                                   *
  1  CCCTACCTATCTGTAACCATCTTAAAAAAAAAAAAAACCAAAAAAAAACTGTGAAAATACGTAATCCCGAGGAGCCTTCGATCAGGTATAAAACTGGAAGCCAGAGAGGTGCAGGCTATAG

                                                                                                              -22    -20
                                                                                                              met asn ala
121  CTGCCATCGGCTGACCTAGAGAAGACACATCAGCTGATCCTTTGGACCCTCTGACTTGAGACAGAAGTTCTGGGCTTCTCCTCCTGCGGCCTAGCTCTGAGACA ATG AAC GCT

         thr his cys ile leu ala leu gln leu phe leu met ala val ser gly cys tyr cys His Gly Thr Val Ile Glu Ser Leu Glu Ser Leu
234  ACA CAC TGC ATC TTG GCT TTG CAG CTC TTC CTC ATG GCT GTT TCT GGC TGT TAC TGC CAC GGC ACA GTC ATT GAA AGC CTA GAA AGT CTG

     Asn Asn Tyr Phe
324  AAT AAC TAT TTT      GTAAGTATGAATTCTTAATAATGCTTGTGGTTGGTGACCGTAATTGATGTTGACTTGCTACGGTGAGCGCCAGGCTGCCGTCTCTGGTCCCCAGTCATTTT
438  GAGAAGATGGGGTGCTACGTTGCTATTTGCTGGAGAGGTGTTTATTGACTTAATGATCTCAATATCGATTTAACCCTCTGTCCAACTTACTACGGAGTTAGAGGGCAATTACCAATCTTC
558  CCAAAGATAGGCATAGTATAGGTCCAAGGTACAAAGATGCTGATTGATTTTGTGATTTGTTTATCATTTAGTTGTGATAAAAAATATCCTTACCTCAATGGTTCTTATTCCTTCAGACGTC
678  TTGAAAGTGATAGTGAGAGATGGATATTACCACCAAAACTACGCAGGGAAACAGCTTATCACTTAAAGTAATGGGAGGCAAAGTTCTTAATGTTTCTGTTTAAGAAATGCCCCCCTCCCC
798  CGAAGTTGTTTTACCCTGAGGAGTAATTTTGAAATTCTACTACAATCGAATCAAAGCCAGCCGCTTAATGAGGTTTAATGAGACTCTATATTTCTCAGAGTTTTCAGGATTTTCTCTTTT
918  GTGATTTTTTTTTTTAAATTAATGGTTAACAGAAGCAAATTTTATATCCTTAGAATTTTTATAATTTGTCCCAAATGTATATACTAGTATACACATATAGCTATTAGCATAATGTTCAAGCATC
1038 TACGGTCAATCCTCTCCTCACTGTGTAAATCAAGCTGCCTCCCGTATGTGTTTGGAGCTATTTTTTAAAGTAGCAATGAAGCCCTATTACAGCACAGACTGATGTTTCAGAGGCTTGAAC
1158 CATAAGGGGGCAGTGTGCACGGTGGGATGATTCTAATGATTTTCTCTCTCCCTTTCTTAATTTGAGAGTAAGTTTCTTTTTAGCTCACTATGGTTACTTGAGGGTACTTGAAACCTCGTC
1278 AGCTTTGTTGAGTTTATTTGTGGCCTTGCAGTTTCAAGACTGGGCCAGTACATCCTGCAGCTAAAAGAATGTAACAGTAACAGTGTTTGGCTACATGCAGTCTTTTAGGGGATACTTGTT
1398 GTTAGAAGTAAGTGGAAGGGCCCAGAAGGAAACCTGTGACCATTATCAGCACTGAATTCACAAACTTGATGATATTTTCAGGGCAATTGGTGAAATAATTACAATCAATTTTTTTCTCTT

                       20                                30
       Asn Ser Ser Gly Ile Asp Val Glu Glu Lys Ser Leu Phe Leu Asp Ile Trp Arg Asn Trp Gln Lys
1518 TTCCTCAG      AAC TCA AGT GGC ATA GAT GTG GAA GAA AAG AGT CTC TTC TTG GAT ATC TGG AGG AAC TGG CAA AAG      GTGAGTTGAATATTTCTCC

                                                                         40
                                                                         Asp Gly Asp Met Lys Ile Leu Gln Ser Gln Ile Ile
1611 TCTCCCAGTTTCCCTGTTGTTTCTAATGGGTCATTTCTTAAAATCCTCCCTTTGTGTTATTTCCCAAG      GAT GGT GAC ATG AAA ATC CTG CAG AGC CAG ATT ATC

       50                            60                            70
       Ser Phe Tyr Leu Arg Leu Phe Glu Val Leu Lys Asp Asn Gln Ala Ile Ser Asn Asn Ile Ser Val Ile Glu Ser His Ile Thr Thr
1715 TCT TTC TAC CTC AGA CTC TTT GAA GTC TTG AAA GAC AAT CAG GCC ATC AGC AAC AAC ATA AGC GTC ATT GAA TCA CAC CTG ATT ACT ACC

       80                            90
       Phe Phe Ser Asn Ser Lys Ala Lys Lys Asp Ala Phe Met Ser Ile Ala Lys Phe Glu
1805 TTC TTC AGC AAC AGC AAG GCG AAA AAG GAT GCA TTC ATG AGT ATT GCC AAG TTT GAG      GTGAGACGGCATTGCAAGTTGCTGTATTGTTGGCTTTTTATT
1904 TTTCATTGTCTCTAATTATCAAGCGGTAGAAACTAACTACTCATCAGCTGATAAAGCTAGGAGGTGAAGCAGGATCTCATGTTTCCCCACTGCAGACAGATTGGGAGGACTTTTTTTTGT
2024 GTGTGTGTCAATTTTGGAAAAACACAGACAATCAAACTATTGCCCACATGCTGGGTAAATGCACTGAGGAGGGAGGCAGAATAGGGGAGCATTGAGCAGAGCTCTTGTGGTCCCCCCTGGG
2144 TGTGTGATGGAAACTCTTGCTTAGGCTGGGAGGTTGTGTGTTAGTGGAAAGAGCAGTGGGTAGGAGGGGGTGAGAAGACTTGTATCCTCCTCCTCCTCCTCCTCCTAGTTAGGCCACAAG
2264 GAGGAACGCTGACTACAGATGACTCACACGACTGGCTGGGGTGCAACTGGGATCGCTACATAAGTTTTATCTCTTTTGTCAAAAACAAAACAAAATGAAACCTCCACAGTGTCAAGGGTA
2384 GAAGACGAGGATGAGGGAAGGAAAGGAATCAGGCTCTGAGGAGACTTCTGGGCGTCCTACCCCTCGGCTCTGGTTAGCCTCTAGTGCTATGCAGTTCGGTTTGTTTTCGGGCGAAGCAAT
2504 AGTAGACATCCTTTAAAAGGATTGCTTTATACATCTTATGAAAGGCTTGGTCAATTAACTTTCAGATATGGCGGTATTCCAGCCATTCATGCTTTATATCATGAAACTACCTTAAAAGTA
2624 CCTTTAAAGTATGGCCGTGAGAATCCAAAAGGTAACTTAAAAGCATAAAGACTATTCTCATTCTTCTAAATTTTACATAGAAGGCCAAAGGCATTCCAAACATCCTTGGGTTTTGAATGA
2744 ATGAAATGAACGTCAAAATGAAAAGGGACAGGTGTTTTGTTACATTTTGTGGCCTAATTACTCATGCTCACCTTTCAGGCTACCTGCCTCTGCCTCTAAACTAGCCTACCGCTCTCGCTC
2864 AGGAGCAGGGAGATGGTAAGCCCGTCTTAGTCCATGGACTAGAGATGGATGAAATAATCGTTTCTCACTGACTTTGCTTCTGCCTTTCCATCCTGCTCTGGCTAAGTCTCTTGGAGTCTT
2984 GACAATGTCCTGAAACACAGGAAATACATTTGTGTTCACAACACACAGTTGGGAGAAACCTGTAACTCCCCAGGCCTTGGTTTCATCTTTTTGGAAACCCTGGGTCTTGTGCTTCCTGTG
3104 GGTGACCTTGTGACAAGCTCTTAACTCTTATCCTATATTGATGCATTGTCAACATGTTTTAGGAACACACACACACACACACACACACACACACACACACACACTTTCCTTAGT
3224 AACTAGTCCTATAAACTTCTGTGTCTTTCTTGGAAATGTAGCAAGGGAGTCAGAGTATTTTCAGTATTAGAAACAAACAAACAAACAGACAGACAGACAGACAGACCCACACAGCAGTAAA
3344 TGGTCTTCATTTTACTAAGCACAAAATTGCCCAAGTGGTCCTTCTGGTTAGAATGAAAAAATCTAAGTAGTTAAATTAATGATGGAGAAAGCAGAGAAGAGGAAAATATTGTTGCACCTT
3464 CAAATTGTAACTACTCTCTGATGTCAACAAATTGATTATTACTAATCTGGTCATGATTTGTGTTTATTTTTAATCCCATCCCAGAAATGATGACACCTATCTGATTTGGGAGAAAATTGA
3584 AAATATATATTTTTTCATTTATTTTGGACTTGGGTTGTTCCTACAGTACTTAGACTGTTGGTGGCTCTCAAATTGTGGCTTGTACAGAATCTCTTGGTGGGACTTAGCTCACAAAGGCAT
3704 CTGGGTCTCTGGGCTCCTTGGTAGATATCCAAAGCATTCTGCTAGAGCAAGGGGAGCCTTGGCTAACATAAATGTTTTTCCTGGTCTGAATAGAGAGGACTAATCAAAGAAGAAGGTGGT
3824 AGACCTTGTAGATAAGAGATTATCTTGCCAATATCTTCATAAGAAAACAGGTTCCTGCAGGTTAAGTGTCTGATTCAAGTTCAGAGTTACCGTCTATTCATCCCCATTCTTTCTCCACCC
3944 CATGCCACCCAGCAGTCTCTTTAATTCTCCATTTTGAGTTTTCTGTAGCAGTTAAGGGAAAGGTAGATGTGTGATGTGTGAGGTGGCTCAGCACACTCCCTGTGGTACAACTTAGAAATC
4064 ATGATGGTCTTAACTGCTACAGAAGTGAATACCACAAGTAGAAGGAATAATTATTGCTGTACTTTTCTTAAAAGGAAGATTTCCATCTTCACTGACCATGATGTAAAAACAAAAAATAGCCC

                                                                                       100                            110
                                                                                       Val Asn Asn Pro Gln Val Gln Arg Gln Ala Phe Asn Glu Leu Ile Arg Val Val
4184 AACAACTTGTATACTTGGAATTAATTTCATTTTTTTCCCCATTAG      GTC AAC AAC CCA CAG GTC CAG CGC CAA GCA TTC AAT GAG CTC ATC CGA GTG GTC

       120                            130
       His Gln Leu Leu Pro Glu Ser Ser Leu Arg Lys Arg Lys Arg Ser Arg Cys
4283 CAC CAG CTG TTG CCG GAA TCC AGC CTC AGG AAG CGG AAA AGG AGT CGC TGC TGA      TTCGGGGTGGGGAAGAGATTGTCCCAATAAGAATAATTCTGCCAGC
4383 ACTATTTGAATTTTTAAATCTAAACCTATTTATTAATAATTTAAAACTATTTATATGGAGAATCTATTTTAGATGCATCAACCAAAGAAGTATTTATAGTAACAACTTATATGTGATAAGA
4503 GTGAATTCCTATTAATATATGTGTTATTTATAATTTCTGTCTCCTCAACTATTTCTCTTTGACCAATTAATTATTCTTTCTGACTAATTAGCCAAGACTGTGATTGCGGGGTTGTATCTG
4623 GGGGTGGGGGACAGCCAAGCGGCTGACTGAACTCAGATTGTAGCTTGTACCTTTACTTCACTGACCAATAAGAAACATTCAGAGCTGCAGTGACCCCGGGAGTGCTGCTGATGGGAGGAG
4743 ATGTCTACACTCCGGGCCAGCGCTTTAACAGCAGGCCAGACAGCACTCGAATGTGTCAGGTAGTAACAGGCTGTCCCTGAAAGAAAGCAGTGTCTCAAGAGACTTGACACTGGTCTTCCC
4863 TATACAGCTGAAAACTGTGACTACACCCGAATGACAAATAACTCGCTCATTTATAGTTTATCACTGTCTAATTGCATATGAATAAAGTATACCTTTGCAACCAATCATGCCGTGTCAGAC
4983 TTCTTCTAAGGGAAGGCTGGGTGAAT
```

```
          S1                              S10                          S20        1
Human   |met| lys tyr |thr| ser tyr ile |leu| ala phe gln |leu| cys ile val leu gly ser leu |gly| cys |tyr| cys GLN ASP PRO TYR VAL LYS GLU
Bovine  |met| lys tyr |thr| ser tyr phe |leu| ala leu leu |leu| cys gly leu leu gly phe ser |gly| ser |tyr| gly GLN GLY GLN PHE PHE ARG GLU
Murine  |met| asn ala |thr| his cys ile |leu| ala leu gln |leu| phe leu met ala val ser --- |gly| cys |tyr| cys HIS GLY THR VAL ILE GLU SER
Rat     |met| ser ala |thr| arg arg val |leu| val leu gln |leu| cys leu met ala leu ser --- |gly| cys |tyr| cys GLN GLY THR LEU ILE GLU SER

             10                            20                            30
Human   ALA |GLU| ASN |LEU| LYS LYS LYS TYR PHE ASN ALA GLY HIS SER |ASP| VAL ALA ASP ASN GLY THR |LEU| PHE LEU GLY |ILE| LEU LYS |ASN TRP| LYS
Bovine  ILE |GLU| ASN |LEU| LYS LYS TYR PHE ASN ALA SER SER PRO |ASP| VAL ALA LYS GLY GLY PRO |LEU| PHE SER GLU |ILE| LEU LYS ASN TRP LYS
Murine  LEU |GLU| SER |LEU| ASN ASN TYR PHE ASN SER SER GLY ILE |ASP| VAL GLU GLU --- LYS SER |LEU| PHE LEU ASP |ILE| TRP ARG ASN TRP GLN
Rat     LEU |GLU| SER |LEU| LYS ASN TYR PHE ASN SER SER SER MET |ASP| ALA MET GLU GLY LYS SER |LEU| LEU LEU ASP |ILE| TRP ARG ASN TRP GLN

             40                            50                            60
Human   GLU GLU SER ASP ARG |LYS ILE| MET |GLN| SER GLN ILE |VAL| SER PHE TYR PHE LYS |LEU PHE| LYS ASN PHE |LYS ASP| ASP |GLN| SER |ILE| GLN
Bovine  ASP GLU SER ASP MET |LYS ILE| ILE |GLN| SER GLN ILE |VAL| SER PHE TYR PHE LYS |LEU PHE| GLU ASN |LYS ASP| ASN |GLN| SER |ILE| GLN
Murine  LYS ASP ALA GLY ASP MET |LYS ILE| LEU |GLN| SER GLN ILE |ILE| SER PHE TYR LEU ARG |LEU PHE| GLU VAL |LYS ASP| ASN |GLN| ALA |ILE| SER
Rat     LYS ASP GLY ASN THR |LYS ILE| LEU |LEU| GLN SER GLN ILE |ILE| SER PHE TYR LEU ARG |LEU PHE| GLU VAL |LYS ASP| ASN |GLN| ALA |ILE| SER

             70                            80                            90
Human   LYS SER VAL GLU THR |ILE| LYS GLU ASP MET ASN VAL LYS |PHE| PHE ASN ASN LYS THR |LYS| ARG ASP ASP |PHE| GLU LYS LEU THR ASN
Bovine  ARG SER MET ASP ILE |ILE| LYS GLN ASP MET PHE GLN LYS |PHE| LEU ASN GLY SER SER GLU |LYS| LEU GLU ASP |PHE| LYS LYS LEU ILE GLN
Murine  ASN ASN ILE SER VAL |ILE| GLU SER HIS LEU ILE THR THR |PHE| PHE SER ASN SER LYS ALA |LYS| LYS ASP ALA |PHE| MET SER ILE ALA LYS
Rat     ASN ASN ILE SER VAL |ILE| GLU LYS SER LEU LEU THR ASN |PHE| PHE SER ASN SER LYS ALA |LYS| LYS ASP ALA |PHE| MET SER ILE ALA LYS

             100                           110                          120
Human   TYR SER |VAL| THR ASP LEU ASN VAL |GLN| ARG LYS |ALA| ILE HIS |GLU LEU ILE| GLN |VAL| MET ALA |GLU LEU| SER |PRO| ALA ALA LYS THR GLY
Bovine  ILE PRO |VAL| ASP ASP LEU GLN ILE |GLN| ARG LYS |ALA| ILE ASN |GLU LEU ILE| LYS |VAL| MET ASN ASP |LEU| SER |PRO| LYS SER ASN LEU ARG
Murine  PHE |GLU VAL| ASN ASN PRO GLN VAL |GLN| ARG GLN |ALA| PHE ASN |GLU LEU ILE| ARG |VAL| VAL HIS GLN |LEU LEU| PRO |GLU| SER SER LEU ARG
Rat     PHE |GLU VAL| ASN ASN PRO GLN ILE |GLN| HIS LYS |ALA| VAL ASN |GLU LEU ILE| ARG |VAL| ILE HIS GLN |LEU| SER |PRO| GLU SER SER LEU ARG

             130                           140
Human   LYS ARG LYS ARG SER |GLN MET LEU PHE ARG GLY ARG ARG ALA SER GLN
Bovine  LYS ARG LYS ARG SER |GLN ASN LEU PHE ARG GLY ARG ARG ALA SER MET
Murine  LYS ARG LYS ARG SER |ARG CYS
Rat     LYS ARG LYS ARG SER |ARG CYS
```

FIG. 4. Comparison of IFN-γ protein sequences. The bovine IFN-γ sequence was reported by Rinderknecht and Burton (1985), and the rat sequence was characterized by Dijkema *et al.* (1985). Human IFN-γ shares 61, 40, and 39% homology with the bovine, murine, and rat sequences, respectively. Bovine IFN-γ shares 44 and 39% homology with murine and rat IFN-γ. Murine and rat IFN-γ are 87% homologous.

recombinant proteins. The protein sequences of human, bovine, rat, and murine IFN-γ are shown in Fig. 4. The low homology seen among these sequences is probably responsible for the lack of cross-species activity of IFN-γ. Species which are more closely related, such as rat and mouse, have IFN-γ sequences which are also much more closely related (87% amino acid homology). It is therefore not surprising that rat IFN-γ exhibits antiviral activity on murine cell lines (Dijkema *et al.*, 1985).

VI. IFN-γ Biology

The cloning of IFN-γ cDNA has allowed the characterization of its gene and protein structure. More significantly, the synthesis of IFN-γ in heterologous systems has provided recombinant IFN-γ which can be prepared in large quantities and purified to homogeneity. This pure reagent has subsequently been tested by numerous investigators in many biological systems. The results demonstrate that IFN-γ exhibits an array of activities both *in vitro* and *in vivo*.

IFN-γ was originally identified on the basis of its antiviral activity (Wheelock, 1965). Recombinant murine IFN-γ has been shown to protect mice *in vivo* from a lethal encephalomyocarditis viral infection (Shalaby *et al.*, 1984). Purified IFN-γ also exhibits an antiproliferative activity on numerous cell lines *in vitro* (Czarniecki *et al.*, 1984; Shalaby *et al.*, 1984). The use of murine tumor model systems has demonstrated the *in vivo* antitumor activity of murine IFN-γ (P. L. Trown, unpublished; S. H. Lee, unpublished).

Perhaps the most important function for IFN-γ is as an immunomodulatory agent. IFN-γ induces both Class I and Class II antigens of the major histocompatibility complex (Steeg *et al.*, 1982; Basham and Merigan, 1983; King and Jones, 1983). Class II (Ia in the mouse, HLA-DR in humans) expression is important for antigen presentation by macrophages and may be responsible for the enhanced antibody production observed *in vivo* (Nakamura *et al.*, 1984). IFN-γ may also stimulate resting B cells to secrete antibody (Sidman *et al.*, 1984) and probably acts as a B cell differentiation agent (Liebson *et al.*, 1984).

Resting macrophages require a signal to exhibit cytotoxic activity toward tumor cells. Recombinant IFN-γ preparations contain potent macrophage activation factor (MAF) activity (Roberts and Vasil, 1982; Pace *et al.*, 1983; Schultz and Kleinschmidt, 1983; Schreiber *et al.*, 1983), and antibodies to recombinant IFN-γ have demonstrated that the predominant MAF activity found in activated lymphocyte cultures is due to IFN-γ (Schrieber *et al.*, 1985). In addition, IFN-γ antibodies have convincingly demonstrated that IFN-γ is produced *in vivo* in mice treated with *Leishmania* (Buchmeier and Schreiber, 1985). Mice receiving anti-IFN-γ antibodies did not effectively clear the infection after 6 days, whereas control mice did.

IFN-γ is also involved in the regulation of lymphokine action both through inducing their expression and by enhancing their biological activities. IFN-γ induces macrophages to secrete interleukin-1 (Palladino *et al.*, 1983), which is important in T cell growth regulation, antigen presentation, and inflammatory responses. IFN-γ also can directly enhance the production of interleukin-2 (T cell growth factor) and lymphotoxin by lymphocyte cultures (Svedersky *et al.*, 1985). It has been demonstrated that IFN-γ has a synergistic effect on the activity of other biological agents. A 5- to 10-fold enhancement of antiviral and antiproliferative activity is seen for the combination of IFN-γ with either IFN-α or IFN-β (Czarniecki *et al.*, 1984). IFN-γ also acts synergistically with lymphotoxin and tumor necrosis factor to produce increased tumor cell lysis *in vitro* (Stone-Wolff *et al.*, 1984; Lee *et al.*, 1984).

The characterization of IFN-γ and elucidation of its bioactivities were dependent on a source of pure, recombinant material. The isolation of a human IFN-γ cDNA and determination of its structure were the first steps in understanding the important role of IFN-γ *in vivo*. Investigators now have the challenge of broadening the understanding of the biological activities of IFN-γ and the relationship of IFN-γ with other lymphokines as additional recombinant lymphokine preparations become available.

REFERENCES

Alton, K., Stabinsky, Y., Richards, R., Ferguson, B., Goldstein, L., Altrock, B., Miller, L., and Stebbing, N. (1983). In "The Biology of the Interferon System 1983" (E. De Maeyer and H. Schellekens, eds.), pp. 119–128. Elsevier, Amsterdam.

Anderson, P., Yip, Y. K., and Vilcek, J. (1982). J. Biol. Chem. 257, 11301–11304.

Basham, T. Y., and Merigan, T. C. (1983). J. Immunol. 130, 1492–1494.

Blalock, J. E., Georgiades, J. A., Langford, M. P., and Johnson, H. M. (1980). Cell. Immunol. 49, 390–394.

Buchmeier, N. A., and Schreiber, R. D. (1985). Proc. Natl. Acad. Sci. U.S.A. 82, 7404–7408.

Burton, L. E., Gray, P. W., Goeddel, D. V., and Rinderknecht, E. (1985). In "The Biology of the Interferon System 1984" (H. Kirchner and H. Schellekens, eds.), pp. 403–409. Elsevier, Amsterdam.

Celada, A., Gray, P. W., Rinderknecht, E., and Schreiber, R. D. (1984). J. Exp. Med. 160, 55–74.

Celada, A., Allen, R., Gray, P. W., and Schreiber, R. D. (1985). J. Clin. Invest. 76, 2196–2205.

Chang, T. W., McKinney, S., Liu, V., Kung, P. C., Vilcek, J., and Le, J. (1984). Proc. Natl. Acad. Sci. U.S.A. 81, 5219–5222.

Czarniecki, C. W., Fennie, C. W., Powers, D. B., and Estell, D. A. (1984). J. Virol. 49, 490–496.

De Ley, M., Van Damme, J., Claeys, H., Weening, H., Heine, J. W., Billiau, A., Vermylen, C., and De Somer, P. (1980). Eur. J. Immunol. 10, 877–883.

Derynck, R., Leung, D. W., Gray, P. W., and Goeddel, D. V. (1982). Nucleic Acids Res. 10, 3605–3615.

Derynck, R., Singh, A., and Goeddel, D. V. (1983). Nucleic Acids Res. 11, 1819–1837.

Devos, R., Cheroutre, H., Taya, Y., DeGrave, W., Van Heuverswyn, H., and Fiers, W. (1982). Nucleic Acids Res. 10, 2487–2501.

Dijkema, R., van der Meide, P. H., Pouwels, P. H., Caspers, M., Dubbeld, M., and Schellekens, H. (1985). EMBO J. 4, 761–767.

Falcoff, R. (1972). J. Gen. Virol. 16, 251–253.

Fujita, T., Takaoka, C., Matsui, H., and Taniguchi, T. (1983). Proc. Natl. Acad. Sci. U.S.A. 80, 7437–7441.

Gray, P. W., and Goeddel, D. V. (1982). Nature (London) 298, 859–863.

Gray, P. W., and Goeddel, D. V. (1983). Proc. Natl. Acad. Sci. U.S.A. 80, 5842–5846.

Gray, P. W., Leung, D. W., Pennica, D., Yelverton, E., Najarian, R., Simonsen, C., Derynck, R., Sherwood, P. J., Wallace, D. M., Berger, S. L., Levinson, A. D., and Goeddel, D. V. (1982). Nature (London) 295, 503–508.

Havell, E. A., and Spitalny, G. L. (1982). J. Exp. Med. 156, 112–127.

Kelker, H. C., Le, J., Rubin, B. Y., Yip, Y. K., Nagler, C., and Vilcek, J. (1984). J. Biol. Chem. 259, 4301–4304.

King, D. P., and Jones, P. P. (1983). J. Immunol. 131, 315–318.

Langford, M. P., Georgiades, J. A., Stanton, G. J., Dianzani, F., and Johnson, H. M. (1979). Infect. Immun. 26, 36–41.

Le, J., Barrowclough, B. S., and Vilcek, J. (1984a). J. Immunol. Methods 69, 61–70.

Lee, S. H., Aggarwal, B. B., Rinderknecht, E., Assisi, F., and Chiu, H. (1984). *J. Immunol.* **133**, 1083–1086.

Liebson, H. J., Gefter, M., Zlotnik, A., Marrack, P., and Kappler, J. W. (1984). *Nature (London)* **309**, 799–801.

Nakamura, M., Manser, T., Pearson, G. D. N., Daley, M. J., and Gefter, M. L. (1984). *Nature (London)* **307**, 381–382.

Nathan, I., Groopman, J. E., Quan, S. G., Bersch, N., and Golde, D. W. (1981). *Nature (London)* **292**, 842–844.

Naylor, S. L., Sakaguchi, A. Y., Shows, T. B., Law, M. L., Goeddel, D. V., and Gray, P. W. (1983). *J. Exp. Med.* **157**, 1020–1027.

Naylor, S. L., Gray, P. W., and Lalley, P. A. (1984). *Somatic Cell Mol. Genet* **10**, 531–534.

Nedwin, G. E., Naylor, S. L., Sakaguchi, A. Y., Smith, D., Jarrett-Nedwin, J., Pennica, D., Goeddel, D. V., and Gray, P. W. (1985). *Nucleic Acids Res.* **13**, 6361–6373.

Owerbach, D., Rutter, W. J., Shows, T. B., Gray, P., Goeddel, D. V., and Lawn, R. M. (1981), *Proc. Natl. Acad. Sci. U.S.A.* **78**, 3123–3127.

Pace, J. L., Russell, S. W., Torres, B. A., Johnson, H. M., and Gray, P. W. (1983). *J. Immunol.* **130**, 2011–2013.

Palladino, M. A., Svedersky, L. P., Shepard, H. M., Pearlstein, K. T., Vilcek, J., and Scheid, M. P. (1983). *In* "Interferson Research: Clinical Application and Regulatory Consideration" (K. C. Zoon, ed.), pp. 139–147. Elsevier, Amsterdam.

Raziuddin, A., Sarkar, F. H., Dutkowski, R., Shulman, L., Ruddle, F. H., and Gupta, S. L. (1984). *Proc. Natl. Acad. Sci. U.S.A.* **81**, 5504–5508.

Rinderknecht, E., and Burton, L. E. (1985). *In* "The Biology of the Interferon System" (H. Kirchner and H. Schellekens, eds.), pp. 397–402. Elsevier, Amsterdam.

Rinderknecht, E., O'Connor, B. H., and Rodriguez, H. (1984). *J. Biol. Chem.* **259**, 6790–6797.

Roberts, W. K., and Vasil, A. (1982). *J. Interferon Res.* **2**, 519–532.

Rubin, B. Y., and Gupta, S. L. (1980). *Proc. Natl. Acad. Sci. U.S.A.* **77**, 5928–5932.

Sarkar, F. H., and Gupta, S. L. (1984). *Proc. Natl. Acad. Sci. U.S.A.* **81**, 5160–5164.

Schreiber, R. D., Pace, J. L., Russel, S. W., Altman, A., and Katz, D. H. (1983). *J. Immunol.* **131**, 826–832.

Schreiber, R. D., Hicks, L. J., Celada, A., Buchmeier, N. A., and Gray, P. W. (1985). *J. Immunol.* **134**, 1609–1618.

Schultz, R. M., and Kleinschmidt, W. J. (1983). *Nature (London)* **305**, 239–240.

Shalaby, M. R., Weck, P. K., Rinderknecht, E., Harkins, R. N., Frane, J. W., and Ross, M. J. (1984). *Cell. Immunol.* **81**, 380–392.

Shalaby, M. R., Hamilton, E. B., Benninger, A. H., and Marafino, B. J. (1985). *J. Interferon Res.* **5**, 339–345.

Shows, T. B., Sakaguchi, A. Y., Naylor, S. L., Goeddel, D. V., and Lawn, R. M. (1982). *Science* **218**, 373–374.

Sidman, C. L., Marshall, J. D., Schultz, L. D., Gray, P. W., and Johnson, H. M. (1984). *Nature (London)* **309**, 801–803.

Sonnenfeld, G., Mandel, A., and Merigan, T. C. (1978). *Cell. Immunol.* **40**, 285–293.

Steeg, P. G., Moore, R. N., Johnson, H. M., and Oppenheim, J. J. (1982). *J. Exp. Med.* **156**, 1780–1793.

Stone-Wolff, D. S., Yip, Y. K., Kelker, H. C., Le, J., Henriksen-DeStefano, D., Rubin, B. Y., Rinderknecht, E., Aggarwal, B. B., and Vilcek, J. (1984). *J. Exp. Med.* **159**, 828–843.

Svedersky, L. P., Nedwin, G. E., Goeddel, D. V., and Palladino, M. A. (1985). *J. Immunol.* **134,** 1604–1608.

Tanaka, S., Oshima, T., Ohsuye, K., Ono, T., MIzono, A., Ueno, A., Nakazato, H., Tsujimoto, M., Higashi, N., and Noguchi, T. (1983). *Nucleic Acids Res.* **11,** 1707–1723.

Taya, Y., Devos, R., Tavernier, J., Cherontre, H., Engler, G., and Fiers, W. (1982). *EMBO J.* **1,** 953–958.

Weissmann, C., and Weber, H. (1985). *Prog. Nucleic Acid Res.*, in press.

Wheelock, E. F. (1965). *Science* **149,** 310–311.

Yip, Y. K., Pang, R. H. L., Urban, C., and Vilcek, J. (1981). *Proc. Natl. Acad. Sci. U.S.A.* **78,** 1601–1605.

Yip, Y. K., Barrowclough, B. S., Urban, C., and Vilcek, J. (1982). *Science* **215,** 411–413.

Youngner, J. S., and Salvin, S. B. (1973). *J. Immunol.* **111,** 1914–1922.

Cloning and Characterization of the Genes for Human and Murine Tumor Necrosis Factors

DIANE PENNICA AND DAVID V. GOEDDEL

Department of Molecular Biology, Genentech, Inc., South San Francisco, California 94080

I. Introduction

Tumor necrosis factor (TNF) was first described in 1975 by Carswell *et al.* as an activity present in the serum of mice infected with bacillus Calmette-Guerin (BCG) and subsequently treated with endotoxin. TNF activity caused the necrosis of certain tumors when injected into tumor-bearing animals and was found to be cytotoxic to a number of transformed cell lines *in vitro* (Carswell *et al.*, 1975; Helson *et al.*, 1975; Green *et al.*, 1976; Matthews and Watkins, 1978; Matthews, 1981; Ruff and Gifford, 1981a,b). A detailed discussion of the history, early observations, and some of the characteristics associated with this cytotoxic activity has been reviewed by Ruff and Gifford (1981a,b) and will not be discussed here.

The purpose of this article is to describe how the techniques of modern molecular biology were used to identify and synthesize a cytotoxic factor distinct from lymphotoxin (LT). This factor, called tumor necrosis factor, has tumor-cell-killing potential *in vitro* as well as hemorraghic necrosis activity for tumors *in vivo*. The cloning and expression of cDNAs for both human (Pennica *et al.*, 1984) and murine (Pennica *et al.*, 1985) TNF allowed us to determine the sequence of the encoded proteins and also provide a source of purified proteins for studying their biological properties.

The cloning and expression of the cDNA for human lymphotoxin, a B cell-derived cytotoxic factor, were recently reported by Gray *et al.* (1984) and are the subjects of another contribution to this volume. Studies using purified human lymphotoxin from both natural and recombinant sources have shown that this protein can also cause the hemorrhagic necrosis of certain tumors when administered to mice. Due to the fact that TNF and LT have many common structural characteristics and because they share cytotoxic effects *in vitro* and tumor necrosis ability *in vivo*, we now refer to tumor necrosis factor as TNF-α and to lymphotoxin as TNF-β. In order to avoid confusion in this chapter, however, the old nomenclature of tumor necrosis factor (TNF) and lymphotoxin (LT) will be used.

In this paper we present a summary of the strategy used in the cloning and expression of the cDNAs for both human and murine TNF. We also

163

discuss the structure and chromosomal localization of the genes for human TNF and lymphotoxin. Finally, in an attempt to elucidate the mechanism of action and *in vivo* function(s) of human TNF, we have included some recent studies describing the diverse biological activities associated with purified recombinant human TNF.

II. Cellular Sources of Tumor Necrosis Factor

Our first attempt at finding a suitable cell source for human TNF (HuTNF) involved a number of induction schemes using various mitogens on peripheral blood leukocyte (PBL) cultures (Pennica *et al.*, 1984). BCG and lipopolysaccharide (LPS) addition to unfractionated PBLs resulted in the induction of a low but detectable cytotoxic activity when assayed on murine L-929 fibroblasts as described previously (Aggarwal *et al.*, 1984). This activity could not be neutralized by anti-LT antiserum and was therefore attributed to TNF. In an attempt to further increase this activity, other mitogens were tested. The combination of *Staphylococcus* enterotoxin B, desacetyl-thymosin-α_1, and the tumor-promoting agent 4β-phorbol 12β-myristate 13α-acetate (PMA) provided the most significant increase in cytotoxic activity. Antibody neutralization experiments revealed, however, that only a portion of the induced cytotoxic activity was TNF; the remainder was due to LT.

After fractionating the PBLs we were able to show that the adherent cells (containing primarily monocytes) produced a cytotoxic activity which could not be neutralized by antibodies to LT, whereas the non-adherent cells (containing primarily lymphocytes) secreted the activity neutralized by anti-LT antibodies. This seemed to be in agreement with earlier studies which suggested that the macrophage was the cellular source of TNF (Carswell *et al.*, 1975; Matthews and Watkins, 1978; Hoffman *et al.*, 1978; Mannel *et al.*, 1980). Partially purified TNF prepared from the adherent cell fraction of PBLs was used for immunizations in order to obtain anti-TNF antiserum. Due to the difficulty in obtaining sufficient quantities of adherent cells from PBLs, however, we screened several transformed monocytic and macrophage cell lines to find a TNF producer. The human promyelocytic leukemia cell line, HL-60, gave the highest titer of cytotoxic activity (approximately 100–300 U/ml following induction with PMA). This activity was completely neutralized by the anti-TNF antibodies but not by anti-LT antibodies.

III. Purification and Characterization

The availability of a cell line that synthesized sufficient quantities of human TNF provided a convenient source for purification and characterization of the natural protein (Aggarwal *et al.*, 1985a). Serum-free cultures of HL-60 cells were induced with PMA and the medium collected 18 hr after induction. The purification of TNF from HL-60 cell supernatants involved sequential steps of controlled pore glass chromatography, DEAE-cellulose chromatography, and Mono Q fast protein liquid chromatography. This was followed by reverse phase high performance liquid chromatography (HPLC) (Aggarwal *et al.*, 1985a). The specific activity of the purified TNF was calculated to be approximately 10^8 units/mg with a 6% recovery and an approximately 4100-fold purification (Aggarwal *et al.*, 1985a).

When analyzed by SDS–polyacrylamide gel electrophoresis (PAGE) under both reducing and nonreducing conditions, purified TNF migrated as a single protein band at an apparent molecular weight of 17,000. A single peak of activity having a molecular weight of 45,000 ±6,000 was observed following TSK-HPLC under nondenaturing conditions. This discrepancy in molecular weights suggests that TNF may occur naturally in an SDS-dissociable oligomeric form.

The primary structure of TNF was determined by sequence analysis of peptides generated after cleavage with the proteolytic enzymes trypsin, *Staphylococcus aureus* V8 protease, and chymotrypsin. The first of the nine tryptic peptides analyzed (TD6) yielded the preliminary sequence Glu-Thr-Pro-Glu-Gly-Ala-Glu-Ala-Lys-Pro-Trp-Tyr-Glu-Lys, which was subsequently used for the design of a synthetic 42-base-long deoxyoligonucleotide as a hybridization probe. Amino acid analysis of the remaining peptides revealed that HuTNF contains no methionines but does contain two cysteine residues involved in a single disulfide bond. In contrast to lymphotoxin, TNF is not a glycoprotein (Aggarwal *et al.*, 1985a).

Some additional physicochemical properties of HuTNF include an isoelectric point of 5.3, stability to heating at 56°C for 30 min, relative insensitivity to pH and organic solvents, and, unlike LT, a fairly high sensitivity to proteolytic enzymes (Aggarwal *et al.*, 1985a). This suggests a less rigid conformation for the TNF molecule compared to LT.

IV. Human TNF cDNA

In addition to providing a source of TNF for protein purification, the HL-60 cells were also used for the isolation of mRNA for cloning. Since considerable activity was observed 4 hr after PMA induction, this time was chosen for the isolation of HL-60 RNA. A λgt10 cDNA library of approximately 200,000 clones was obtained using oligo(dT)-primed poly(A)+ RNA from the induced HL-60 cells.

In order to screen the cDNA library, a unique 42-base-long deoxyoligonucleotide (42-mer) was synthesized which could code for the amino acid sequence of tryptic peptide TD6 (Fig. 1). The primary screen using this 42-mer yielded nine positive clones, seven of which hybridized to a PMA-induced, but not uninduced, ^{32}P-labeled cDNA probe prepared from HL-60 mRNA. The cDNA sequence of the longest clone, λ42-4, was determined and it was found that the sequence of the region hybridizing with the 42-mer probe had an overall homology of 81% and included a stretch of 17 consecutive homologous nucleotides (Fig. 1). The first 13 amino acids of peptide TD6 were in agreement with the amino acids encoded by the cDNA. Inspection of the open-reading frame of λ42-4 revealed matches with the amino acid sequence of several additional proteolytic peptides of purified TNF, confirming that we had in fact isolated a cDNA clone encoding human TNF. The first amino acid of mature TNF was determined by amino-terminal sequence analysis of HL-60-derived TNF. Clone λ42-4 was found to contain the entire mature TNF coding region but lacked the complete signal peptide. Therefore, a second clone was isolated from a specifically primed cDNA library and found to contain the missing 5' sequence.

The complete 1643-bp cDNA sequence (Fig. 2) predicts an open-reading frame of 233 amino acids. The NH_2-terminal amino acid sequence of natural TNF showed that the mature polypeptide of 157 amino acids was preceded by a presequence of 76 residues. From the cDNA sequence a molecular weight of 17,356 was calculated for the mature protein, which is in close agreement with the value obtained for the naturally derived TNF monomer on SDS gels.

To provide further evidence that the isolated DNA sequence encodes HuTNF, an expression plasmid (pTNF*trp*) was constructed which should direct the synthesis in *Escherichia coli* of mature TNF preceded by a methionine residue necessary for translation initiation (Pennica *et al.*, 1984). Extracts of *E. coli* transformed with pTNF*trp* contained a promi-

```
TD6        glu–thr–pro–glu–gly–ala–glu–ala–lys–pro–trp–tyr–glu–lys

Probe      GAA ACC CCT GAA GGG GCT GAA GCC AAG CCC TGG TAT GAA AAG
           **  *** **  **  *** *** **  *** *** *** *** *** **
Actual     GAG ACC CCA GAG GGG GCT GAG GCC AAG CCC TGG TAT GAG CCC
                                                               pro
```

FIG. 1. Homology of the synthetic 42-base deoxyoligonucleotide probe with the HuTNF cDNA sequence. TD6 refers to the amino acid sequence of one of nine tryptic peptides of HuTNF. The probe sequence shown, which could code for this amino acid sequence, was chosen on the basis of published human codon usage frequencies. The DNA sequence listed below the synthetic 42-mer probe is the actual sequence of nucleotides 690–731 (Fig. 2) of HuTNF as determined by DNA sequencing. The asterisks indicate identical matches between the probe sequence and actual TNF sequence.

```
GCAGAGGACCAGCTAAGAGGGAGAGAAGCAACTACAGACCCCCCCTGAAAACAACCCTCAGACGCCACATCCCCTGACAAGCTGCCAGGCAGGTTCTCTTCCTCTCACATACTGACCCAC
T                               50                                                              100
```

```
                         -76                        -70                                  -60
                         met ser thr glu ser met ile arg asp val glu leu ala glu glu ala leu pro lys lys thr
GGCTCCACCCTCTCTCCCCTGGAAAGGACACC ATG AGC ACT GAA AGC ATG ATC CGG GAC GTG GAG CTG GCC GAG GAG GCG CTC CCC AAG AAG ACA
                      150                                                             200
```

```
        -50                                  -40                                  -30
        gly gly pro gln gly ser arg arg cys leu phe leu ser leu phe ser phe leu ile val ala gly ala thr thr leu phe cys leu leu
        GGG GGG CCC CAG GGC TCC AGG CGG TGC TTG TTC CTC AGC CTC TTC TCC TTC CTG ATC GTG GCA GGC GCC ACC ACG CTC TTC TGC CTG CTG
                                    250                                                              300
```

```
        -20                                  -10                                  1
        his phe gly val ile gly pro gln arg glu glu phe pro arg asp leu ser leu ile ser pro leu ala gln ala Val Arg Ser Ser Ser
        CAC TTT GGA GTG ATC GGC CCC CAG AGG GAA GAG TTC CCC AGG GAC CTC TCT CTA ATC AGC CCT CTG GCC CAG GCA GTC AGA TCA TCT TCT
                                    350
```

```
        10                                  20                                  30
        Arg Thr Pro Ser Asp Lys Pro Val Ala His Val Val Ala Asn Pro Gln Ala Glu Gly Gln Leu Gln Trp Leu Asn Arg Arg Ala Asn Ala
        CGA ACC CCG AGT GAC AAG CCT GTA GCC CAT GTT GTA GCA AAC CCT CAA GCT GAG GGG CAG CTC CAG TGG CTG AAC CGC CGG GCC AAT GCC
        400                                         450
```

```
        40                                  50                                  60
        Leu Leu Ala Asn Gly Val Glu Leu Arg Asp Asn Gln Leu Val Val Pro Ser Glu Gly Leu Tyr Leu Ile Tyr Ser Gln Val Leu Phe Lys
        CTC CTG GCC AAT GGC GTG GAG CTG AGA GAT AAC CAG CTG GTG GTG CCA TCA GAG GGC CTG TAC CTC ATC TAC TCC CAG GTC CTC TTC AAG
                        500                                         550
```

```
        70                                  80                                  90
        Gly Gln Gly Cys Pro Ser Thr His Val Leu Leu Thr His Thr Ile Ser Arg Ile Ala Val Ser Tyr Gln Thr Lys Val Asn Leu Leu Ser
        GGC CAA GGC TGC CCC TCC ACC CAT GTG CTC CTC ACC CAC ACC ATC AGC CGC ATC GCC GTC TCC TAC CAG ACC AAG GTC AAC CTC CTC TCT
                                    600                                         650
```

```
        100                                 110                                 120
        Ala Ile Lys Ser Pro Cys Gln Arg Glu Thr Pro Glu Gly Ala Glu Ala Lys Pro Trp Tyr Glu Pro Ile Tyr Leu Gly Gly Val Phe Gln
        GCC ATC AAG AGC CCC TGC CAG AGG GAG ACC CCA GAG GGG GCT GAG GCC AAG CCC TGG TAT GAG CCC ATC TAT CTG GGA GGG GTC TTC CAG
                                    700                                                     750
```

```
        130                                 140                                 150
        Leu Glu Lys Gly Asp Arg Leu Ser Ala Glu Ile Asn Arg Pro Asp Tyr Leu Asp Phe Ala Glu Ser Gly Gln Val Tyr Phe Gly Ile Ile
        CTG GAG AAG GGT GAC CGA CTC AGC GCT GAG ATC AAT CGG CCC GAC TAT CTC GAC TTT GCC GAG TCT GGG CAG GTC TAC TTT GGG ATC ATT
                                    800
```

```
        157
        Ala Leu OP
        GCC CTG TGA GGAGGACGAACATCCAACCTTCCCAAACGCCTCCCCTGCCCCAATCCCTTTATTACCCCCTCCTTCAGACACCCTCAACCTCTTCTGGCTCAAAAAGAGAATTGGGGG
        850                                 900                                             950
```

```
CTTAGGGTCGGAACCCAAGCTTAGAACTTTAAGCAACAAGACCACCACTTCGAAACCTGGGATTCAGGAATGTGTGGCCTGCACAGTGAATTGCTGGCAACCACTAAGAATTCAAACTGG
                        1000                                            1050
```

```
GGCCTCCAGAACTCACTGGGGCCTACAGCTTTGATCCCTGACATCTGGAATCTGGAGACCAGGGAGCCTTTGGTTCTGGCCAGAATGCTGCAGGACTTGAGAAGACCTCACCTAGAAATT
            1100                                            1150                                            1200
```

```
GACACAAGTGGACCTTAGGCCTTCCTCTCTCCAGATGTTTCCAGACTTCCTTGAGACACGGAGCCCAGCCCTCCCCATGGAGCCAGCTCCCTCTATTTATGTTTGCACTTGTGATTATTT
                        1250                                            1300
```

```
ATTATTTATTTATTATTTATTTATTTACAGATGAATGTATTTATTTGGGAGACCGGGGTATCCTGGGGGACCCAATGTAGGAGCTGCCTTGGCTCAGACATGTTTTCCGTGAAAACGGAG
                        1350                                            1400
```

```
CTGAACAATAGGCTGTTCCCATGTAGCCCCCTGGCCTCTGTGCCTTCTTTTGATTAGTTTTTTAAAATATTTATCTGATTAAGTTGTCTAAACAATGCTGATTTGGTGACCAACTGTCA
1450                                            1500                                            1550
```

```
CTCATTGCTGAGCCTCTGCTCCCCAGGGGAGTTGTGTCTGTAATCGCCCTACTATTCAGTGGCGAGAAATAAAGTTTGCTT
                        1600
```

FIG. 2. HuTNF cDNA sequence and predicted amino acid sequence. Numbers above each line refer to amino acid positions and numbers below each line to nucleotide positions. The amino acid labeled 1 represents the first amino acid of mature HuTNF (Aggarwal *et al.*, 1985a). The 76 amino acids preceding this position are indicated by lowercase lettering. The underlined sequence indicates the polyadenylation recognition site (Proudfoot and Brownlee, 1976). Reprinted by permission from *Nature*, Vol. 312, No. 5996, pp. 724–729, copyright (©) 1984, Macmillan Journals Limited.

nent 17,000 Da polypeptide when analyzed on SDS–polyacrylamide gels. This polypeptide comigrated with authentic TNF isolated from the HL-60 cell line and was not apparent in pBR322-transformed *E. coli* extracts, suggesting it was the translational product of the TNF cDNA sequence (Pennica *et al.*, 1984). When assayed for cytolytic activity in the L-929 assay, approximately 300,000 units of activity were detected per ml of culture, corresponding to about 3 mg per liter or 300,000 molecules of active TNF per cell. NH_2-terminal sequence analysis of TNF produced intracellularly in *E. coli* revealed that 40% of the molecules retained the NH_2-terminal initiator methionine, whereas the remaining 60% had been processed and lacked the methionine (W. J. Kohr, unpublished results).

In addition to demonstrating the *in vitro* cytotoxic activity of recombinant HuTNF (rHuTNF), we also wished to examine its ability to cause the *in vivo* necrosis of Meth A sarcomas when administered to mice (Carswell *et al.*, 1975). Using either purified natural or recombinant TNF, significant necrotic responses were observed following injection either intralesionally or intraveneously (Pennica *et al.*, 1984).

Another procedure was followed to express the cDNA insert of λ42-4 as a secreted protein (Fig. 3). The secretion plasmid pTNFSTII*trp* was constructed such that the mature TNF coding region was fused to the coding region of the signal peptide for the *E. coli* STII enterotoxin (Picken *et al.*, 1983). *E. coli* K-12 strain 294 containing either the plasmid pTNFSTII*trp* or the direct expression plasmid pTNF*trp* (Pennica *et al.*, 1984) was grown and fractionated into periplasmic and intracellular fractions and assayed for cytolytic activity. Approximately 98% of the activity was detected in the periplasm and only 2% in the intracellular fraction for pTNFSTII*trp*; whereas for pTNF*trp*, 87% of the activity was found in the intracellular fraction. These results suggest that biologically active TNF was indeed being synthesized and secreted by *E. coli* 294 /pTNFSTII*trp*. NH_2-terminal sequence analysis of purified, secreted TNF confirmed that the signal sequence had been correctly processed from the mature protein.

A comparison between the amino acid sequences of human TNF and LT (Pennica *et al.*, 1984; Gray *et al.*, 1984; Aggarwal *et al.*, 1985a) indicates that these proteins share 36% identity and, if conservative substitutions are considered, an overall homology of about 50%. The hydrophobic carboxy-terminal amino acids in particular are significantly conserved, which may indicate that this region is important for the cytotoxic activities of the two molecules. On the nucleotide level there is a 46% homology between the coding regions. Some interesting differences between TNF and LT include 18 more NH_2-terminal amino acids on LT than TNF (although these amino acids are not required for cytolytic activity) and a nonconserved region for amino acids 67–109 (TNF numbering), where only 2 of the 43 residues are identical to LT.

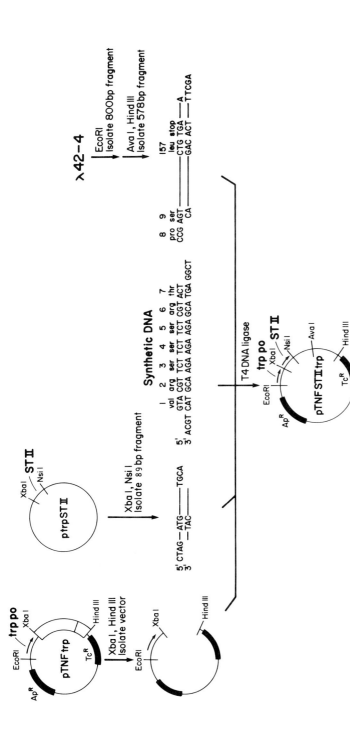

FIG. 3. Construction of a plasmid directing the synthesis of human TNF as a secreted protein in *E. coli*. To express high levels of recombinant human TNF and secrete it into the periplasm in *E. coli*, the initiation of protein synthesis occurs at an ATG codon of the STII signal sequence (Picken *et al.*, 1983), which is located 69-bp 5' of codon 1 of the mature TNF polypeptide. An *Ava*I restriction site located at codon 8 of the mature coding sequence was utilized to remove the TNF presequence coding region as described previously (Pennica *et al.*, 1984). Two synthetic deoxyoligonucleotides were designed which restore the codons for amino acids 1–7 and create an *Nsi*I cohesive terminus. The 89-bp STII signal sequence was obtained by cleavage of ptrpSTII with *Xba*I and *Nsi*I. The plasmid pTNFtrp (Pennica *et al.*, 1984) was cleaved with *Xba*I and *Hin*dIII and the large vector fragment recovered. The 89-bp *Xba*I–*Nsi*I fragment from ptrpSTII, 578-bp *Ava*I–*Hin*dIII isolated from λ42-4 fragment, and the two synthetic deoxyoligonucleotides were inserted into the *Xba*I–*Hin*dIII cut vector to give the plasmid pTNFSTIItrp.

V. Murine TNF

The availability of a human TNF cDNA clone allowed us to isolate the cDNA for murine TNF (MuTNF). A comparison of their amino acid sequences revealed highly conserved regions that could be important for the shared cytotoxic activity of these molecules. Furthermore, purification of recombinant MuTNF from *E. coli* made it possible to compare the *in vivo* and *in vitro* activities of human and murine TNFs.

After screening several murine monocyte–macrophage cell lines for their ability to produce a cytotoxic factor following PMA induction, the PU5-1.8 cell line was found to secrete the highest level of activity (~1500 U/ml; Pennica *et al.*, 1985). In order to determine whether this activity was due to MuTNF, murine LT (MuLT), or a previously uncharacterized cytotoxic factor, Northern blot analysis was performed. mRNA was isolated 5 hr after PMA induction of PU5-1.8 cells and probed with a ^{32}P-labeled fragment from either the HuTNF or human LT (HuLT) cDNAs. A band migrating at approximately 18 S hybridized strongly to the HuTNF probe, while no hybridization was seen with the HuLT probe. Since high stringency hybridization and wash conditions were used, the murine cytotoxic factor was most likely TNF.

From a λgt10 cDNA library of approximately 400,000 clones prepared from PMA-induced PU5-1.8 cell mRNA, 95 clones strongly hybridized with the HuTNF cDNA probe. After analyzing 10 of these clones, the one with the longest cDNA insert, λ6, was isolated and its 1638-bp insert was sequenced (Fig. 4). The identity of clone λ6 as MuTNF was established after comparing the encoded amino acid sequence of the open-reading frame with the amino acid sequence of HuTNF. This comparison between murine and human TNF revealed an overall amino acid homology of approximately 79% (Fig. 5). Mature MuTNF contains 156 amino acids, and the size of the mature protein is calculated to be M_r 17,260. The cDNA also encodes a 79-amino acid presequence region.

MuTNF contains two cysteine residues at positions 69 and 101 which, like HuTNF, may be involved in a disulfide bond. There exists one potential N-glycosylation site at asparagine 7, which agrees with previous reports (Green *et al.*, 1976) describing the glycoprotein nature of a partially purified murine TNF. HuTNF, on the other hand, lacks any sites for glycosylation.

MuTNF was directly expressed in *E. coli* and found to be biologically active in the murine L-929 fibroblast assay (Pennica *et al.*, 1985). *Escherichia coli* purified MuTNF was also shown to be active in the *in vivo* Meth A sarcoma tumor necrosis assay (Pennica *et al.*, 1985). The fact that unglycosylated MuTNF purified from *E. coli* exhibits potent cytotoxic

```
GCTGAGGGACTAGCCAGGAGGGAGAACAGAAACTCCAGAACATCCTGGAAATAGCTCCCAGAAAAGCAAGCAGCCAACCAGGCAGGTTCTGTCCCTTTCACTCACTGGCCCAAGGCGCCA
1                                               50                                              100
```

```
                    -79                                      -70                                      -60
                    met ser thr glu ser met ile arg asp val glu leu ala glu glu ala leu pro gln lys met gly gly phe
CATCTCCCTCCAGAAAAGACACC ATG AGC ACA GAA AGC ATG ATC CGC GAC GTG GAA CTG GCA GAA GAG GCA CTC CCC CAA AAG ATG GGG GGC TTC
                        150                                                    200
```

```
         -50                                      -40                                      -30
gln asn ser arg arg cys leu cys leu ser leu phe ser phe leu leu val ala gly ala thr thr leu phe cys leu leu asn phe gly
CAG AAC TCC AGG CGG TGC CTA TGT CTC AGC CTC TTC TCA TTC CTG CTT GTG GCA GGG GCC ACC ACG CTC TTC TGT CTA CTG AAC TTC GGG
                                        250                                                    300
```

```
         -20                                      -10                                      1
val ile gly pro gln arg asp glu lys phe pro asn gly leu pro leu ile ser ser met ala gln thr leu thr Leu Arg Ser Ser Ser
GTG ATC GGT CCC CAA AGG GAT GAG AAG TTC CCA AAT GGC CTC CTC ATC AGT TCT ATG GCC CAG ACC CTC ACA CTC AGA TCA TCT TCT
                                        350
```

```
         10                                      20                                      30
Gln Asn Ser Ser Asp Lys Pro Val Ala His Val Val Ala Asn His Gln Val Glu Glu Gln Leu Glu Trp Leu Ser Gln Arg Ala Asn Ala
CAA AAT TCG AGT GAC AAG CCT GTA GCC CAC GTC GTA GCA AAC CAC CAA GTG GAG GAG CAG CTG GAG TGG CTG AGC CAG CGC GCC AAC GCC
400                                                    450
```

```
         40                                      50                                      60
Leu Leu Ala Asn Gly Met Asp Leu Lys Asp Asn Gln Leu Val Val Pro Ala Asp Gly Leu Tyr Leu Val Tyr Ser Gln Val Leu Phe Lys
CTC CTG GCC AAC GGC ATG GAT CTC AAA GAC AAC CAA CTA GTG GTG CCA GCC GAT GGG TTG TAC CTT GTC TAC TCC CAG GTT CTC TTC AAG
                        500                                                    550
```

```
         70                                      80                                      90
Gly Gln Gly Cys Pro Asp Tyr Val Leu Leu Thr His Thr Val Ser Arg Phe Ala Ile Ser Tyr Gln Glu Lys Val Asn Leu Leu Ser Ala
GGA CAA GGC TGC CCC GAC TAC GTG CTC CTC ACC CAC ACC GTC AGC CGA TTT GCT ATC TCA TAC CAG GAG AAA GTC AAC CTC CTC TCT GCC
                                        600                                                    650
```

```
         100                                      110                                      120
Val Lys Ser Pro Cys Pro Lys Asp Thr Pro Glu Gly Ala Glu Leu Lys Pro Trp Tyr Glu Pro Ile Tyr Leu Gly Gly Val Phe Gln Leu
GTC AAG AGC CCC TGC CCC AAG GAC ACC CCT GAG GGG GCT GAG CTC AAA CCC TGG TAT GAG CCC ATA TAC CTG GGA GGA GTC TTC CAG CTG
                        700                                                    750
```

```
         130                                      140                                      150
Glu Lys Gly Asp Gln Leu Ser Ala Glu Val Asn Leu Pro Lys Tyr Leu Asp Phe Ala Glu Ser Gly Gln Val Tyr Phe Gly Val Ile Ala
GAG AAG GGG GAC CAA CTC AGC GCT GAG GTC AAT CTG CCC AAG TAC TTA GAC TTT GCG GAG TCC GGG CAG GTC TAC TTT GGA GTC ATT GCT
                                        800
```

```
156
Leu OP*
CTG TGA AGGGAATGGGTGTTCATCCATTCTCTACCCAGCCCCCACTCTGACCCCTTTACTCTGACCCCTTTATTGTCTACTCCTCAGAGCCCCCAGTCTGTGTCCTTCTAACTTAGA
850                                  900                                      950
```

```
AAGGGGATTATGGCTCAGAGTCCAACTCTGTGCTCAGAGCTTTCAACAACTACTCAGAAACACAAGATGCTGGGACAGTGACCTGGACTGTGGGCCTCTCATGCACCACCACCCACGGAA
                            1000                                    1050
```

```
TCGAGAAAGAGCTATCAATCTGGAATTCACTGGAGCCTCGAATGTCCATTCCTGAGTTCTGCAAAGGGAGAGTGGTCAGGTTGCCTCTGTCTCAGAATGAGGCTGGATAAGATCTCAGGC
            1100                                    1150                                    1200
```

```
CTTCCTACCTTCAGACCTTTCCAGACTCTTCCCTGAGGTGCAATGCACAGCCTTCCTCACAGAGCCAGCCCCCCTCTATTTATATTTGCACTTATTATTTATTATTTATTTATTATTTAT
                            1250                                    1300
```

```
TTATTTGCTTATGAATGTATTTATTTGGAAGGCCGGGGTGTCCTGGAGGACCCAGTGTGGGAAGCTGTCTTCAGACAGACATGTTTTCTGTGAAAACGGAGCTGAGCTGTCCCCACCTGG
                            1350                                    1400
```

```
CCTCTCTACCTTGTTGCCTCCTCTTTTGCTTATGTTTAAAACAAAATATTTATCTAACCCAATTGTCTTAATAACGCTGATTTGGTGACCAGGCTGTCGCTACATCACTGAACCTCTGCT
1450                                    1500                                    1550
```

```
CCCCACGGGAGCCGTGACTGTAATTGCCCTACGGGTCATTGAGAGAAATAAAGATCGCTTGGAAAAGAAAAAAAAA
                            1600
```

FIG. 4. MuTNF cDNA sequence and predicted amino acid sequence. Numbers above each line refer to amino acid positions and numbers below each line to nucleotide positions. The amino acid labeled 1 represents the first amino acid of mature MuTNF based on homology with HuTNF. The 79 amino acids preceding this position are indicated by lowercase lettering. The underlined sequence indicates the polyadenylation recognition site (Proudfoot and Brownlee, 1976). Reprinted by permission from *Proc. Natl. Acad. Sci. U.S.A.* **82**, 6060–6064.

activity both *in vitro* and *in vivo* suggests that the carbohydrate moiety is not required for its cytotoxic activity.

Kull and Cuatrecasas (1984) recently purified a cytotoxic factor, from the murine macrophage cell line J774.1, which they have called necrosin. Its similarity in chemical and biological properties to MuTNF suggests that the two factors may be identical.

FIG. 5 — Comparison of HuTNF and MuTNF sequences

	−76										−70									−60						−50				
HUMAN	met	ser	thr	glu	ser	met	ile	arg	asp	val	glu	leu	ala	glu	glu	ala	leu	pro	lys	lys	thr	gly	gly	pro	gln	gly	ser	arg	arg	cys
MURINE	met	ser	thr	glu	ser	met	ile	arg	asp	val	glu	leu	ala	glu	glu	ala	leu	pro	lys	lys	met	gly	gly	pro	gln	gly	asn	ser	arg	arg	cys
	−79										−70									−60						−50				

										−40										−30						−20				
HUMAN	leu	phe	leu	ser	leu	phe	ser	phe	leu	ile	val	ala	gly	ala	thr	thr	leu	phe	cys	leu	leu	his	phe	gly	val	ile	gly	pro	gln	arg
MURINE	leu	cys	leu	ser	leu	phe	ser	phe	leu	ile	val	ala	gly	ala	thr	thr	leu	phe	cys	leu	leu	asn	phe	gly	val	ile	gly	pro	gln	arg
										−40										−30						−20				

										−10												1								10
HUMAN	glu	glu	---	phe	pro	arg	asp	leu	ser	leu	ile	ser	pro	leu	ala	gln	ala	---	---	ala		Val	Arg	Ser	Ser	Arg	Thr	Pro	Ser	Asp	Lys
MURINE	asp	glu	lys	phe	pro	asn	gly	leu	ser	leu	ile	ser	ser	met	ala	gln	thr	leu	thr			Leu	Arg	Ser	Ser	Gln	Asn*	Ser	Ser	Asp	Lys
										−10												1								10

										20										30						40				
HUMAN	Pro	Val	Ala	His	Val	Val	Ala	Asn	Pro	Gln	Ala	Glu	Gly	Gln	Leu	Gln	Trp	Leu	Asn	Arg	Arg	Ala	Asn	Ala	Leu	Leu	Ala	Asn	Gly	Val
MURINE	Pro	Val	Ala	His	Val	Val	Ala	Asn	His	Gln	Val	Glu	Glu	Gln	Leu	Glu	Trp	Leu	Ser	Gln	Arg	Ala	Asn	Ala	Leu	Leu	Ala	Asn	Gly	Met
										20										30						40				

										50										60						70				
HUMAN	Glu	Leu	Arg	Asp	Asn	Gln	Leu	Val	Val	Pro	Ser	Glu	Gly	Leu	Tyr	Leu	Ile	Tyr	Ser	Gln	Val	Leu	Phe	Lys	Gly	Gln	Gly	Cys	Pro	Ser
MURINE	Asp	Leu	Lys	Asp	Asn	Gln	Leu	Val	Val	Pro	Ala	Asp	Gly	Leu	Tyr	Leu	Val	Tyr	Ser	Gln	Val	Leu	Phe	Lys	Gly	Gln	Gly	Cys	Pro	Asp
										50										60						70				

										80										90						100				
HUMAN	Thr	His	Val	Leu	Leu	Thr	His	Thr	Ile	Ser	Arg	Ile	Ala	Val	Ser	Tyr	Gln	Thr	Lys	Val	Asn	Leu	Leu	Ser	Ala	Ile	Lys	Ser	Pro	Cys
MURINE	Tyr	---	Val	Leu	Leu	Thr	His	Thr	Val	Ser	Arg	Phe	Ala	Ile	Ser	Tyr	Gln	Glu	Lys	Val	Asn	Leu	Leu	Ser	Ala	Val	Lys	Ser	Pro	Cys
										80										90						100				

										110										120						130				
HUMAN	Gln	Arg	Glu	Thr	Pro	Glu	Gly	Ala	Glu	Ala	Lys	Pro	Trp	Tyr	Glu	Pro	Ile	Tyr	Leu	Gly	Gly	Val	Phe	Gln	Leu	Glu	Lys	Gly	Asp	Arg
MURINE	Pro	Lys	Asp	Thr	Pro	Glu	Gly	Ala	Glu	Leu	Lys	Pro	Trp	Tyr	Glu	Pro	Ile	Tyr	Leu	Gly	Gly	Val	Phe	Gln	Leu	Glu	Lys	Gly	Asp	Gln
										110										120						130				

										140										150						157
HUMAN	Leu	Ser	Ala	Glu	Ile	Asn	Arg	Pro	Asp	Tyr	Leu	Asp	Phe	Ala	Glu	Ser	Gly	Gln	Val	Tyr	Phe	Gly	Ile	Ile	Ala	Leu
MURINE	Leu	Ser	Ala	Glu	Ile	Asn	Arg	Pro	Asp	Tyr	Leu	Asp	Phe	Ala	Glu	Ser	Gly	Gln	Val	Tyr	Phe	Gly	Val	Ile	Ala	Leu
										140										150						156

FIG. 5. Comparison of HuTNF and MuTNF sequences. Identical amino acids are boxed. The numbers above and below each row refer to amino acid positions of HuTNF and MuTNF, respectively. The presequence regions are numbered −76 to −1 and −79 to −1 for HuTNF and MuTNF, respectively, and are shown in lowercase lettering. The potential N-glycosylation site in MuTNF is indicated by an asterisk. The broken lines indicate amino acid deletions in the sequences. (Pennica et al., 1985). Reprinted by permission from Proc. Natl. Acad. Sci. U.S.A., Vol. 82, pp. 6060–6064.

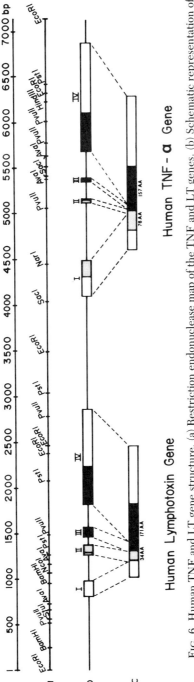

Human Lymphotoxin Gene

Human TNF - α Gene

FIG. 6. Human TNF and LT gene structure. (a) Restriction endonuclease map of the TNF and LT genes. (b) Schematic representation of the linkage of the genes for TNF and LT as determined by DNA sequencing (Nedwin et al., 1985; D. V. Goeddel, unpublished results). The mature coding region of 171 amino acids (AA) for LT and 157 amino acids for TNF is represented by solid boxes. The region encoding the putative signal sequence of 34 amino acids for LT and 76 amino acids for TNF is indicated by stippling. The 5' and 3' untranslated regions of each gene are designated by open boxes. (c) Schematic representation of the mRNAs for TNF and LT. The size of the two genes is indicated in base pairs at the top of the figure.

173

VI. TNF and LT Gene Structure

TNF and LT share similar biological activities and have a high degree of structural homology, yet are synthesized by distinct cell types. Therefore, it was of interest to compare their genomic structures in order to initiate studies on their differential regulation *in vivo*. Southern blot hybridizations of total human genomic DNA revealed that both TNF and lymphotoxin are encoded by single genes. The TNF and LT genes were isolated from recombinant λ phage–human genomic DNA libraries (Shirai *et al.*, 1985; Nedwin *et al.*, 1985). Alignment with the corresponding cDNA sequences revealed that both genes are approximately 3 kb each and contain three intervening sequences (Fig. 6). Only the third intron of TNF occurs at a homologous position with respect to the LT gene; however, none of the introns exhibits any obvious sequence homology. The most noteworthy homology between the two genes occurs in the fourth exon, which codes for 89% of the mature TNF and 80% of the mature LT proteins. Similarities do exist between the putative promoter regions for the two genes. In this area, an overall homology of 35% is observed with several areas of exact homology including the Goldberg–Hogness TATAAA sequence (Gannon *et al.*, 1979; Goldberg, 1979).

The length of the primary transcript up to the poly(A) site for TNF is 2762 bp and after processing the predicted length is 1672 bp. This is in agreement with the 18 S size of the mRNA determined by Northern analysis. LT, on the other hand, has a slightly smaller primary transcript of 2038 bp and a processed mRNA of 1420 bp (~14 S from Northern hybridization; Nedwin *et al.*, 1985).

The genes for TNF and LT have been localized to human chromosome 6, as determined by hybridization to DNA derived from human–murine somatic cell hybrids (Nedwin *et al.*, 1985). Recent data (D. V. Goeddel, unpublished results) have indicated that the two genes are closely linked on the human chromosome. These studies revealed that the genes for TNF and LT span a contiguous region of the human genome of approximately 8 kb. The two genes are separated by a spacer region of 795 bp and are oriented in the same direction with respect to transcription (Fig. 6). The fact that TNF and LT are so closely linked on the same chromosome and expressed preferentially in different cell types makes these genes an interesting system for studying their regulation and cell- or tissue-specific gene expression.

VII. *In Vitro* Response of Cell Lines to TNF

Table I summarizes the *in vitro* effect of purified HuTNF on 22 human tumor cell lines, 12 murine cell lines, and 5 cultures of normal human

TABLE I

In vitro RESPONSE OF HUMAN AND MURINE CELL LINES TO $\leq 10^4$ UNITS/ml OF rHuTNF

Human cell lines		Murine cell lines	
Growth enhancement[a]			
CCD-18Co	(normal colon)		
Detroit 551	(normal fetal skin)		
LL24	(normal lung)		
WI-38	(normal fetal lung)		
WI-1003	(normal lung)		
Null response[b]			
A549	(lung carcinoma)	B16F10	(melanoma)
Calu-3	(lung carcinoma)	CMT-93	(rectal carcinoma)
G-361	(melanoma)	S49	(lymphoma)
HeLa	(cervical carcinoma)		
HT-1080	(fibrosarcoma)		
KB	(oral epidermoid carcinoma)		
LS174T	(colon carcinoma)		
RD	(rhabdosarcoma)		
Saos-2	(osteogenic sarcoma)		
SK-CO-1	(colon carcinoma)		
SK-LU-1	(lung carcinoma)		
SK-OV-3	(ovarian carcinoma)		
SK-UT-1	(uterine carcinoma)		
T24	(bladder carcinoma)		
WI-38 VA13	(SV40-transformed WI-38)		
Antiproliferative[c]			
BT-20	(breast carcinoma)	B6MS2	(sarcoma)
BT-475	(breast carcinoma)	B6MS5	(sarcoma)
MCF-7	(breast carcinoma)	CMS4	(sarcoma)
ME-180	(cervical carcinoma)	CMS16	(sarcoma)
SK-MEL-109	(melanoma)	L-929	(fibroblast)
SK-OV-4	(ovarian carcinoma)	Meth A	(sarcoma)
WiDr	(colon carcinoma)	MMT	(breast carcinoma)
		SAC	(Maloney-transformed 3T3)
		WEHI-164	(sarcoma)

[a] Cell number increase >20%.

[b] Cytostasis/cytotoxicity <25%.

[c] Cytostasis/cytotoxicity ≥25%.

fibroblasts (Sugarman *et al.*, 1985). A 25% or greater reduction in cell viability was used as the criterion for an antiproliferative effect as determined by crystal violet staining after a 72-hr incubation with up to 10^4 U/ml HuTNF. HuTNF was found to have an antiproliferative effect on 7 human tumor cell lines and 9 murine cell lines, no effect on 15 human and 3 murine cell lines, and a growth-enhancing effect on 5 normal human fibroblast cell lines. The different responses of the cell lines do not reflect a significant difference in the number or affinity of cell-membrane binding sites for TNF (Sugarman *et al.*, 1985). It is interesting to note the growth-enhancing activity of HuTNF on normal human fibroblast cells, a property not previously ascribed to this molecule. This provides some evidence that TNF may play a role in regulating normal cell functions. Also, it is of interest that HuTNF and human interferon-γ do not synergize in this growth-enhancing activity.

Although the activity previously designated as TNF has been described as lacking species specificity [see Ruff and Gifford (1981b) review], we have observed that HuTNF has a higher specific activity on human cells as compared to murine cells. Conversely, recombinant murine TNF is more cytotoxic on cell lines of murine origin (Pennica *et al.*, 1985). Therefore, it is possible that an antiproliferative effect might be observed on some of the unresponsive murine cell lines if MuTNF were used.

VIII. Mechanism of Action

Recent studies by Hass *et al.* (1985), Aggarwal *et al.* (1985b), and Sugarman *et al.* (1985) have demonstrated the existence of specific high-affinity binding sites for TNF or LT on four cell lines: L-929, ME-180, T24, and WI-38. Despite the fact that these cell lines vary in their *in vitro* susceptibility to TNF (see Table I), approximately equal numbers of receptors (2000–3000 per cell) were found on all cell types analyzed, and their receptors appeared to have equal binding affinity for TNF or LT. TNF and LT appear to share the same receptor (Aggarwal *et al.*, 1985b). With this information, and the availability of highly purified HuTNF, it now is possible to begin studying the fate of receptor-bound TNF in an attempt to gain a better understanding of its mechanism of action.

One aspect that we chose to investigate was whether internalization of TNF or a fragment of the molecule is required for it to exert its cytolytic activity, or whether TNF can cause lysis solely by interaction with the cell surface. One approach we used to address this question was to covalently couple TNF to Sepharose beads, expose the beads to L-929 cell monolayers, and check for cell lysis. Our preliminary data (unpublished results) indicate that Sepharose-coupled TNF has no cytolytic effect on L-929 cells. This suggests that a simple interaction with the TNF receptor is insufficient for TNF to cause cell lysis. It was not possible to demonstrate that the coupling process itself did not inactivate the TNF. However, the concentration of TNF was high enough that, even assuming 99% inactivation, there would have been enough active TNF to cause significant cell killing if internalization were not required.

A second approach in attempting to localize the site of action of TNF was to microinject purified TNF directly into the cytoplasm of both TNF-sensitive L-929 cells and TNF-resistant NIH-3T3 cells. Results from these experiments (unpublished observations) indicate that injection of 10^6–10^7 molecules of TNF per cell to either cell type had no noticeable effect on cell viability. Additionally, microinjected polyclonal and monoclonal anti-TNF antibodies were not able to protect sensitive L-929 cells from killing by exogenously added TNF. Taken together, these results suggest that TNF must interact with its surface receptor and that some form of internalization of TNF is probably required for cell killing.

IX. Bioactivities of Purified rHuTNF

Purified HuTNF not only exerts cytolytic or cytostatic effects against many tumor cell lines *in vitro*, but has recently been observed to have a number of other biological effects (Table II). rHuTNF of greater than 99% purity isolated from *E. coli* and essentially free from endotoxin was used in many of these studies.

TABLE II
BIOACTIVITIES OF rHuTNF

Causes the necrosis of Meth A sarcomas when administered *in vivo*[a]
Has cytolytic or cytostatic effects against many transformed cell lines *in vitro*[b]
Enhances proliferation of normal diploid fibroblasts[b]
Stimulates osteoclastic bone resorption and inhibits bone formation[c]
Induces increased expression of neutrophil antigens[d]
Stimulates adherence of human neutrophils to human endothelial cells *in vitro*[e]
Acts synergistically with rIFN-γ causing enhanced antiproliferative effects[e]
Involved in macrophage-dependent tumor cell killing[f]
Suppresses lipoprotein lipase activity in adipocytes *in vivo* and *in vitro*[g]
Enhances polymorphonuclear neutrophil (PMN)-mediated, antibody-dependent cellular cytotoxicity[h]
Enhances PMN phagocytic ability[h]
Enhances superoxide anion production by PMNs[i]
Inhibits the transcriptional activation of adipose inducible genes[j]

[a] Pennica *et al.* (1984).
[b] Sugarman *et al.* (1985).
[c] Bertolini *et al.* (1985).
[d] Gamble *et al.* (1985).
[e] Aggarwal *et al.* (1984).
[f] H. M. Shepard (personal communication).
[g] Beutler *et al.* (1985c).
[h] Shalaby *et al.* (1985).
[i] M. R. Shalaby (personal communication).
[j] Torti *et al.* (1985).

The recent reports by Beutler *et al.* (1985a–c) describe the identity of TNF and the secreted macrophage factor cachectin. They observed that cachectin (TNF) suppresses lipoprotein lipase activity in adipocytes *in vivo* and *in vitro*, and may also play a role in the effects of endotoxin-mediated septic shock. These observations and their finding of a specific high affinity receptor for cachectin on nontumorigenic cells provides evidence that this protein also plays a role in modulating the metabolic activities of normal cells. Additional studies with cachectin by Torti *et al.* (1985) demonstrate it can inhibit the differentiation of adipocytes. Results from studies by Sugarman *et al.* (1985) also support a role for TNF in normal cell function by their observation of its growth-enhancing effect on normal diploid fibroblasts. An additional effect on normal cells is its ability to stimulate bone-resorbing activity, described by Bertolini *et al.* (1985), which implicates TNF in the control of normal bone remodeling.

TNF has been shown to modulate the immune system by enhancing the cytotoxic and phagocytic activities of polymorphonuclear neutrophils (Shalaby *et al.*, 1985). In addition, TNF was found to act synergistically in its cytotoxic action with recombinant gamma interferon (Aggarwal *et al.*, 1985b; Shalaby *et al.*, 1985). Gamble and colleagues (1985) have found that rHuTNF manifests an effect both on human peripheral blood neutrophils and human umbilical vein endothelial cells. This effect results in an enhanced *in vitro* adherence of the neutrophils to endothelial cell monolayers. They also observed a rapidly induced, increased expression of certain neutrophil surface antigens. Their findings, and the fact that neutrophils are a key component during inflammation, suggest the possibility that TNF may play a role in the regulation of inflammatory reactions.

X. Concluding Remarks

A large amount of information has accumulated since the initial description of the activity designated TNF. The picture that emerges is that this lymphokine appears to be involved in the regulation of a variety of normal cellular functions in addition to its cytotoxic properties, which were described earlier. These recent studies shed new light on the biological function and mechanism of action of TNF; however, the *in vivo* significance of many of these activities still remains to be elucidated.

The progress in human TNF research has been greatly accelerated by the availability of a source of purified protein. The large supply of purified TNF will now make it possible to study the potential antitumor activity of this factor, as well as its other activities, and should lead to a better understanding of its *in vivo* functions and clinical potential.

ACKNOWLEDGMENTS

We wish to thank all investigators for sharing preprints of their work and unpublished observations on the bioactivities of rHuTNF, H. Michael Shepard for helpful discussions and comments on the manuscript, and Jeanne Arch for preparation of the manuscript.

REFERENCES

Aggarwal, B. B., Moffat, B., and Harkins, R. N. (1984). *J. Biol. Chem.* **259**, 686–691.

Aggarwal, B. B., Kohr, W. J., Hass, P. E., Moffat, B., Spencer, S. A., Henzel, W. J., Bringman, T. S., Nedwin, G. E., Goeddel, D. V., and Harkins, R.N. (1985a). *J. Biol. Chem.* **260**, 2345–2354.

Aggarwal, B. B., Eessalu, T., and Hass, P. E. (1985b). Submitted to *Nature (London)*.

Bertolini, D. R., Nedwin, G. E., Bringman, T. S., and Mundy, G. R. (1985). Submitted to *Nature (London)*.

Beutler, B., Mahoney, J., LeTrang, N., Pekala, P., and Cerami, A. (1985a). *J. Exp. Med.* **161**, 984–995.

Beutler, B., Greenwald, D., Hulmes, J. D., Chang, M., Pan, Y.-C. E., Mathison, J., Ulevitch, R., and Cerami, A. (1985b). *Nature (London)* **316**, 552–554.

Beutler, B., Milsark, I. W., and Cerami, A. C. (1985c). *Science* **229**, 869–871.

Carswell, E. A., Old, L. J., Kassel, R. L., Green, S., Fiore, N., and Williamson, B. (1975). *Proc. Natl. Acad. Sci. U.S.A.* **72**, 3666–3670.

Gamble, J. R., Harlan, J. M., Klebanoff, S. J., Lopez, A. F., and Vadas, M. A. (1985). *Proc. Natl. Acad. Sci. U.S.A.*, in press.

Gannon, F., O'Hare, K., Perrin, F., LePennec, J. P., Benoist, C., Cochet, M., Breathnach, R., Royal, A., Garapin, A., Cami, B., and Chambon, P. (1979). *Nature (London)* **278**, 428–434.

Goldberg, M. (1979). Thesis, Stanford University.

Gray, P. W., Aggarwal, B. B., Benton, C. V., Bringman, T. S., Hensel, W. J., Jarrett, J. A., Leung, D. W., Moffat, B., Ng, P., Palladino, M. A., and Nedwin, G. E. (1984). *Nature (London)* **312**, 721–724.

Green, S., Dobrjansky, A., Carswell, E. A., Kassel, R. L., Old, L. J., Fiore, N., and Schwartz, A. (1976). *Proc. Natl. Acad. Sci. U.S.A.* **73**, 381–385.

Hass, P. E., Hotchkiss, A., Mohler, M., and Aggarwal, B. B. (1985). *J. Biol. Chem.* **260**, 12214–12218.

Helson, L., Green, S., Carswell, E., and Old, J. (1975). *Nature (London)* **258**, 731–732.

Hoffman, M. K., Oettgen, H. F., Old, L. J., Mittler, R. S., and Hammering, U. (1978). *J. Reticuloendothel. Soc.* **23**, 307–319.

Kull, F. C., and Cuatrecasas, P. (1984). *Proc. Natl. Acad. Sci. U.S.A.* **81**, 7932–7936.

Kull, F. C., Jr., Jacobs, S., and Cuatrecasas, P. (1985). *Proc. Natl. Acad. Sci. U.S.A.* **82**, 5756–5760.

Lee, S. H., Aggarwal, B. B., Rinderknecht, E., Assisi, F., and Chiu, H. J. (1984). *J. Immunol.* **133**, 1083.

Mannel, D. N., Moore, R. N., and Mergenhagen, S. E. (1980). *Infect. Immun.* **30**, 523–530.

Matthews, N. (1981). *Immunology* **44**, 135–142.

Matthews, N., and Watkins, J. F. (1978). *Br. J. Cancer* **38**, 302–309.

Nedwin, G. E., Naylor, S. L., Sakaguchi, A. Y., Smith, D., Jarrett-Nedwin, J., Pennica, D., Goeddel, D. V., and Gray, P. W. (1985). *Nucleic Acids Res.*, in press.

Pennica, D., Nedwin, G. E., Hayflick, J. S., Seeburg, P. H., Derynck, R., Palladino, M. A., Kohr, W. J., Aggarwal, B. B., and Goeddel, D. V. (1984). *Nature (London)* **312**, 724–729.

Pennica, D., Hayflick, J. S., Bringman, T. S., Palladino, M. A., and Goeddel, D. V. (1985). *Proc. Natl. Acad. Sci. U.S.A.* **82**, 6060–6064.

Picken, R. N., Mazaitis, A. J., Maas, W. K., Rey, M., and Heyneker, H. (1983). *Infect. Immun.* **42**, 269–275.

Proudfoot, N. J., and Brownlee, G. G.(1976). *Nature (London)* **263**, 211–214.

Ruff, M. R., and Gifford, G. E. (1981a). *Infect. Immun.* **31**, 380–385.

Ruff, M. R., and Gifford, G. E. (1981b). *In* "Lymphokines" (E. Pick, ed.), Vol. 2, pp. 235–275. Academic Press, New York.

Shalaby, M. R., Aggarwal, B. B., Rinderknecht, E., Svedersky, L. P., Finkle, B. S., and Palladino, M. A. (1985). *J. Immunol.* **135**, 2069–2073.

Shirai, T., Yamaguchi, H., Ito, H., Todd, C. W., and Wallace, R. B. (1985). *Nature (London)* **313**, 803–806.

Sugarman, B. J., Aggarwal, B. B., Hass, P. E., Figari, I. S., Palladino, M. A., and Shepard, H. M. (1985). *Science,* in press.

Torti, F. M., Dieckmann, B., Beutler, B., Cerami, A., and Ringold, G. M. (1985). *Science* **229**, 867–869.

Urban, J. L., Shepard, H. M., Sugarman, B. J., and Schreiber, H. (1985). Submitted to *Nature.*

Williamson, B. D., Carswell, E. A., Rubin, B. Y., Prendergast, J. S., and Old, L. D. (1983). *Proc. Natl. Acad. Sci. U.S.A.* **80**, 5397–5401.

Isolation and Expression of the Genes Coding for Mouse and Human Tumor Necrosis Factor (TNF) and Biological Properties of Recombinant TNF

JAN TAVERNIER, LUCIE FRANSEN,[1] ANNE MARMENOUT,[1]
JOSE VAN DER HEYDEN, RITA MUELLER,[2] MARIE-ROSE RUYSSCHAERT,[1]
ADRI VAN VLIET,[3] RITA BAUDEN, AND WALTER FIERS[4]

Biogent, 9000 Ghent, Belgium

I. Introduction

The activation of macrophages results, in addition to other phenomena such as enhanced phagocytosis and intracellular killing, in the release of soluble factors, the so-called monokines. Some of these monokines were found to mediate direct cytotoxic reactions. One such factor, tumor necrosis factor (TNF), is defined as a cytokine found in the sera of Mammalia which have been primed first by an injection of viable *Mycobacterium bovis*, strain Bacillus Calmette-Guerin (BCG), or some other immunostimulatory agent (e.g., *Corynebacterium parvum*, Zymosan) and followed 2–3 weeks later by an endotoxin challenge. When serum of such animals is passively transferred, it causes the hemorrhagic necrosis (and in some cases the complete regression) of certain transplanted tumors in mice (Carswell *et al.*, 1975). Serum from mice treated solely with BCG or endotoxin does not manifest such properties. TNF activity can also be detected in supernatants of stimulated peripheral blood leukocytes enriched for the monocyte fraction and is as such sometimes referred to as "monocyte cytotoxin" (Matthews, 1982; Hammerstrom, 1982; Stone-Wolff *et al.*, 1984), or it may be found in appropriately stimulated macrophage-related tumor cells as PU5-1.8 (Männel *et al.*, 1980). One report also mentions the production of a TNF activity by B lymphoblastoid cells transformed by Epstein–Barr virus and stimulated by a phorbol ester, but this activity most probably represents lymphotoxin (Williamson *et al.*, 1983).

Biologically, TNF in many respects resembles lymphotoxin (LT, currently also called TNF-β), a lymphokine secreted by stimulated lympho-

---

[1]Present address: Innogenetics N. V., 9710 Ghent, Belgium.

[2]Present address: Centro de Investigacion y de Estudios Avancados del I. P. N., Unidad Traquato, Iraquato, G.T.O. 36500, Mexico.

[3]Present address: P.G.S., 9000 Gent, Belgium.

[4]Present address: Laboratory of Molecular Biology, State University of Ghent, 9000 Ghent, Belgium.

cytes (Granger and Kolb, 1968). Indeed, LT manifests a comparable selective killing of a variety of tumor cells without marked species specificity. Also, the mechanism of action, the induction of RNA synthesis in target cells, the synergism with interferons, as well as the enhanced sensitivity of the target cells when pretreated with metabolic drugs such as actinomycin D are similar for both cytokines. Both factors can, however, be distinguished by their serological and biochemical properties. A role for these biological mediators in the natural immune surveillance and in the natural defense against malarial parasites has been suggested (Playfair et al., 1984).

Beside the induction of tumor necrosis in recipient animals, partially purified TNF also exhibits a pronounced cytotoxicity for a variety of tumor target cells in vitro (Carswell et al., 1975; Helson et al., 1975; Ostrove and Gifford, 1979) but not for normal nontransformed cell lines. This selective killing in vivo and in vitro occurs without any apparent species specificity. Partially purified TNF from rabbit serum has a molecular weights of around 35,000 (gel filtration) and 18,000 (SDS–PAGE). Its isoelectric point (IEP) is 5.1 (Matthews et al., 1980; Ruff and Gifford, 1980). Mouse TNF appears in higher molecular weight forms of around 250,000 and 150,000, and a lower molecular weight form of 50,000, with an IEP of 4.8 (Kull and Cuatrecasas, 1981). For a more detailed review on TNF induction, characterization, and action, we refer the reader to Ruff and Gifford (1981).

Several groups have recently established the molecular cloning of the genes coding for human TNF (Pennica et al., 1984; Shirai et al., 1985; Wang et al., 1985; Marmenout et al., 1985) and mouse TNF (Fransen et al., 1985). Here, we briefly review the research by our group. It comprises the isolation and expression of the mouse and human TNF genes, the purification of both TNF proteins, and initial results on the biological characterization.

II. Isolation of the Gene Coding for Mouse TNF

A. Induction and Detection of Mouse TNF-mRNA

Mouse TNF production was induced in vitro in the macrophage-related cell line PU5-1.8 by LPS treatment essentially as described by Männel et al. (1980). The secetion of TNF-activity was monitored by a cytotoxicity assay on L-929 cells in the presence of actinomycin D at 39.5°C (at this temperature the sensitivity is about 2.5 times higher than at 37°C) (Ruff and Gifford, 1981). In this assay, one TNF unit/ml represents the reciprocal of the dilution of TNF required to reduce cell sur-

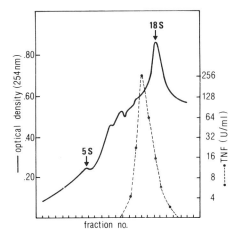

FIG. 1. Detection of mouse TNF mRNA. Poly(A)$^+$ RNA (250 μg) from LPS-stimulated PU5-1.8 cells was fractionated on a sucrose density gradient. The TNF activity was measured after translation in *Xenopus laevis* oocytes by a cytotoxicity assay on L-929 cells. The 5 S and 18 S ribosomal RNAs are indicated with arrows. (From Fransen *et al.*, 1985.)

vival by 50% within 18 hr. Cells were induced under optimal induction conditions (5 μg LPS/3.5 × 10^6 cells/ml in RPMI 1640 for 4 hr; this usually yielded 4–6 × 10^3 U/ml TNF), and cytoplasmic RNA was extracted using the NP-40 lysis protocol. Enrichment for TNF mRNA was by sequential oligo(dT) cellulose chromatography and 5–20% sucrose gradient fractionation. A typical profile of TNF activity found upon injection of the different mRNA fractions in *Xenopus laevis* oocytes is shown in Fig. 1. The TNF activity peaks at 17 S. Starting from 8 μg 17 S mRNA, approximately 30,000 clones were obtained following standard cDNA-cloning procedures (using GC-tailing in the *Pst*I restriction site of pAT153).

B. ISOLATION OF THE MOUSE TNF cDNA GENE

The screening of the cDNA library was accomplished by three different techniques: plus-minus hybridization, filter hybridization using chemically synthesized probes derived from protein sequencing data, and a hybridization–translation assay.

Two rounds of stringent plus-minus hybridization were performed directly on replicas of the cDNA colonies. The plus probe was a [^{32}P]cDNA synthesized from the sucrose-gradient fraction of mouse poly(A)$^+$ RNA showing the highest TNF biological activity after oocyte injection; the minus probe was cDNA synthesized from an equivalent fraction obtained from uninduced cultures. Out of 5000 colonies, 55

TNF FRAGMENT 3

MetLysLeuThrAspAsnGlnLeuValValProAlaAspGlyLeuTyrLeuIleTyr

TNF 3-1

ATGAAACTMACMGACAACCAACTMGTMGTMCCMGCMG
                          CAKGGKCGKCTGCCKGAKATGGAKTAKATGTTAA

                                TNF 3-4

TNF FRAGMENT 4

MetAlaTrpTyrGluProIleTyrLeuGlyGlyValPheGlnLeuGluLysGlyAspArgLeu

TNF 4-1

TGGTACGAACCMATMTACCTMGGCGGCGTCTTC

                          GCAGAAGGTTGAKCTTTTTCCKCTGTCATTAA

                              TNF 4-4

M = A ,C   K = A , T

FIG. 2. Design of oligonucleotide probes. The partial amino acid sequences of two CNBr-fragments of highly purified rabbit TNF are shown. Two overlapping oligonucleotide probes per amino acid sequence were chemically synthesized, taking into account the degeneracy of the genetic code, and the preferred choice for certain codons in eukaryotes. Both probes were radioactively labeled by a filling-in polymerization using Klenow enzyme in the presence of all four [α-^{32}P]deoxynucleoside triphosphates. (From Fransen *et al.*, 1985.)

FIG. 3. Map and nucleotide sequence of the mouse TNF cDNA gene. The diagram at the top represents the structure of the mouse TNF mRNA. The respective lengths in nucleotides of the different regions (corresponding to the incomplete 5' untranslated region, the presequence, the mature protein, and the 3' untranslated region) are indicated. Underneath, the areas present in the different cDNA clones p-mTNF-1, -2, and -3 are shown; wavy lines correspond to the homopolymer tails added during the cloning procedure. A map indicating the principal unique restriction cleavage sites as deduced by a computer search is also presented. Below, the complete nucleotide sequence and the deduced amino acid sequence (in 1-letter codes) corresponding to mouse pre-TNF is shown. A continuous-reading frame is present between nucleotides 157 and 864. The start and stop codons are fully boxed. The sequence flanking the start codon closely resembles the consensus sequence CCAUGG for eukaryotic initiation sites as proposed by Kozak (1984). The presequence, deduced by analogy with the human TNF structure, is underlined. Also indicated are the putative N-glycosylation signal and the two cysteine residues believed to be involved in an intrasubunit disulfide bridge. Two possible AATAAA glycosylation signals are indicated in dashed boxes.

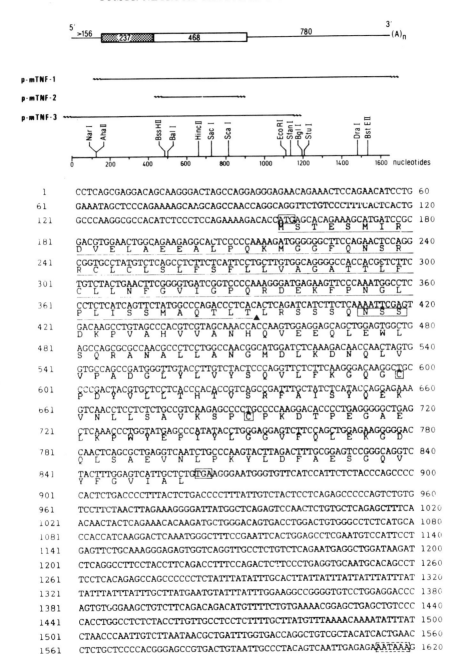

clones were thus selected. Plasmid DNA was individually extracted and repooled in 11 groups of 5 clones. To avoid background hybridization signals on the plasmid DNA, the inserts were separated from the plasmids by *Pst*I cleavage and subsequent agarose gel electrophoresis before transfer and fixation on a nitrocellulose filter. As a probe, two sets of partially overlapping, degenerate deoxyoligonucleotides derived from partial amino acid sequence data of highly purified rabbit TNF were chemically synthesized and radioactively labeled by a filling-in polymerization (Fig. 2). Upon hybridization under low stringency conditions, one positive clone was detected which is further designated as p-mTNF-1. Using an internal 252-bp *Rsa*I restriction fragment of this clone, two additional mouse TNF cDNA clones could be isolated from the 55 preselected colonies. Confirmation that the isolated cDNA clones were TNF-specific was initially obtained by demonstrating their ability to specifically hybridize to TNF mRNA in a hybridization–elution assay. the nucleotide structure and the derived amino acid sequence coding for mouse TNF is shown in Fig. 3. For more details on the isolation of the mouse TNF cDNA gene, refer to Fransen *et al.* (1985).

III. Isolation of the cDNA and Chromosomal DNA Genes Coding for Human TNF

The strategy for cDNA cloning of the human TNF gene completely parallels the procedure described above. As a source for human TNF mRNA, the U-937 cell line was chosen (Sundstrom and Nilsson, 1976). This histiocytic lymphoma cell line with monocyte characteristics was induced under serum-free conditions in the presence of bovine insulin (0.1 U/ml) by a combination of retinoic acid and the phorbol ester TPA. To achieve a reproducible induction, a conditioned medium from giant tumor cells containing colony stimulating factor (CSF) (Gibco) was added.

Human TNF-mRNA sedimented at 16 S and the appropriate poly(A)+ RNA fractions were converted into double-stranded cDNA as described. Upon insertion in the *Pst*I site of pAT153 using the GC-tailing technique, approximately 60,000 cDNA clones were obtained starting from 8 µg poly(A)+ RNA. In a colony hybridization experiment under low stringency conditions using a 297-bp internal *Pvu*II restriction fragment derived from the mouse TNF-cDNA clone, 26 out of 25,000 clones tested scored positive.

Analogously, a human genomic DNA library in λ Charon 4A (Lawn *et al.*, 1978) was screened as described in Tavernier *et al.* (1981). Out of several weakly hybridizing signals, one positive phage was selected using a probe derived from the human TNF cDNA clone. A more detailed description of the cloning procedure is given by Marmenout *et al.* (1985). The complete structure of the human TNF chromosomal gene is presented in Fig. 4.

IV. Structure of the Mouse and Human TNF Genes and Proteins

The nucleotide and amino acid sequences of mouse and human TNF genes and proteins are shown in Fig. 3 and Fig. 4, respectively.

Human and mouse TNF are both characterized by an unusually long presequence. As the N-terminus of mature human TNF produced by the U-937 cell line is Val-Arg-Ser-Ser-Ser- . . . , a region of 79 amino acids is cleaved off during the maturation process. Comparable results were obtained for TNF produced by PMA-stimulated human premonocytic HL-60 cells by the Genentech and Cetus groups (Aggarwal *et al.*, 1985; Wang *et al.*, 1985). On the basis of analogy with the NH_2-terminus of rabbit TNF, however, Shirai *et al.* (1985) argue that mature human TNF might be two amino acids shorter. Indicative of the biological importance of the presequence is the very high degree of conservation between the human and the mouse presequences (86%) at the amino acid level, which is even higher than that found for the mature proteins (79%). Several hypotheses regarding its biological role can be made. One possibility is that TNF is released only by damaged cells. This is, however, rather unlikely considering the efficient secretion obtained in *X. laevis* oocytes after injection with TNF mRNA or in transfected COS and CHO cells (see Section V). Second, alternative secretion pathways might exist in macrophages. Indeed, IL-1α and IL-1β, two other macrophage-released cytokines, also contain atypically long presequences (March *et al.*, 1985), and the existence of a membrane-associated IL-1 form in macrophages has been documented (Kurt-Jones *et al.*, 1985), while the lymphocyte analogue for TNF, lymphotoxin (also renamed as TNF-β), contains a standard signal peptide (Gray *et al.*, 1984).

It is also interesting to note that the TNF presequence contains a 20-amino acid-long hydrophobic region flanked by hydrophilic residues, and as such might also serve as an anchor signal (Fig. 5). The NH_2-terminal region is hydrophilic and contains several changed residues, both basic and acidic, and might represent a cytoplasmic domain. In that case, TNF might be released by clipping off the membrane-bound form. The presence of TNF on the membranes of induced macrophages has, however, not been demonstrated so far. Finally, it should be mentioned that two basic dipeptides (Lys-Lys, position 19, and Arg-Arg, position 28) are present and might be cleavage positions for the release of possibly biologically active peptides from the pre-TNF molecule.

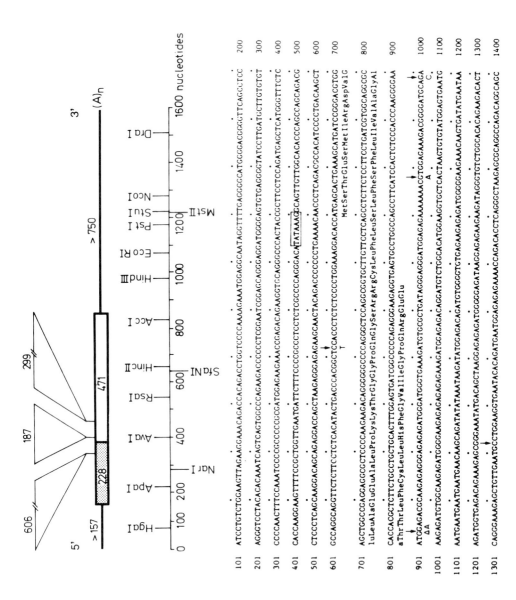

```
1401 CAGCTGTTCCTCCTTTAAGGGTGACTCCTCGATGTTAACCATTCTCCTTTCTCCCAACAGTTCCCAGCGACCTCTCTCTAATCAGCCTCTGGCCCAG        1500
                                                                  PheProArgAspLeuSerLeuIleSerProLeuAlaGln

1501 GCAGTCAGTAAGTGTCTCCAAACCTCTTTCCTAATTCTGGCTTTGGCTTGGGTAGCGTTAGTACCGGTATGGAACCA-TGGCGAAATTTAAAGTTT      1600
     AlaValA

1601 TGGTCTTGGGGAGGAGGATGGATGGCAGCGTGAAACTAGGGGGCTATTTTCTAGGAAGTTTAAGGGTCTCAGCTTTTTCTTTTCTCTCTCCTTCAGGATCAT      1700
                                                                                                     rgSerS

1701 CTTCTCGAACCCAGCAGTGACAAGCCTGTAGCCATGTTGAGGTAAGAGGTCTGAGGATGTGTCTTGGAACTTGGCAGGGCTAGGGATTGGGGATTCGAAGC      1800
     erSerArgThrProSerAspLysProValAlaHisValValA

1801 CCGGCTGATGGTAGGCAGGACAATGTGAGAAGGACTCGCTGAGCTCAAGGAAGGGTGAGGAACAGCACACGCCTTACTGGGATACTCAGA      1900

1901 ACGTCATGGCCAGGTGGGATGCTGGCATGCAGAACAGAGGAGCAGGAACCCGATGCTCGGGTGGCCAGAGCT-GAGGGCCAGGATGTGGAGAGTGAACCGA      2000

2001 CATGGCCACACTGACTCTCCTCCCTCCCTCCAGCAAACCCTCAAGCTGAGGGCAGCTCAGTGCTGAACCCCGGGGCCAATGCCCTCC      2100
                                                                              laAsnProGlnAlaGlyLeuGlnLeuGlnTrpLeuAsnArgArgAlaAsnAlaLeuLeuL

2101 TGGCCAATGGCGTGGAGCTGAGAGATAACCAGCTGCGTCGTCGTCCATCAGAGGGCCTGTACCTCATCTACTCCCAGGTCT-TTCAAGCGCCAAGGCTGCCC      2200
     euAlaAsnGlyValGluLeuArgAspAsnGlnLeuValValProSerGluGlyLeuTyrLeuIleTyrSerGlnValLeuPheLysGlyGlnGlyCysPr

2201 CTCCACCCATGTCTCCTCACCCACACCACATGCCATGCCCTCTCCTACCACACCAAGGTCAACCTCCTCTCCATCAAGAGCCCTCCCAGAGG      2300
     oSerThrHisValLeuLeuThrHisThrIleSerArgIleAlaValSerTyrGlnThrLysValAsnLeuLeuSerAlaIleLysSerProCysGlnArg

2301 GAGACCCCAGGAGGGCTGAGGCCAAGCCCTGGTATGAGCCCATCTATCTGGGAGGGGTCTTCAGCTGGAGAAGGGTGACCGACTCAGCCGTGAGATCA      2400
     GluThrProGluGlyAlaGluAlaLysProTrpTyrGluProIleTyrLeuGlyGlyVal:PheGlnLeuGluLysGlyAspArgLeuSerAlaGluIleA

2401 ATCGGCCGACTATCTGCGACTTTGCCGAGTCTGGCCAGGTCACTTTGGGATCATTGCCCTGTGAGGAGGAGCAACATCCAACCTTCCCAAAACGCCCTCCC      2500
     snArgProAspTyrLeuAspPheAlaGluSerGlyGlnValTyrPheGlyIleIleAlaLeuEnd

2501 CTGCCCCAATCCCTTTATTACCCCCTCCTTCAGCACCCTCAACCCTCTCTGCCTCAAAACAGAATTGGGGGTCTTAGGGTCGGAACCCAAGCTTAGAAC      2600

2601 TTTAAGCAACAAGACCACCACTTCGAAACCTGGGATTCAGGAATTGTCCCCGACCACTAGCAATTC  2686
```

FIG. 4. Map and nucleotide sequence of the human TNF chromosomal gene. A diagram at the top represents the structure of the human TNF chromosomal gene. The respective lengths in nucleotides of the different regions (corresponding to the 5' untranslated region, the presequence, the mature protein, and the 3' untranslated region) are indicated. Three introns are represented by triangles. A map of most unique restriction sites selected from a computer search is given below. Bottom, the complete nucleotide sequence and the deduced amino acid sequence (in 3-letter notation) corresponding to human pre-TNF is shown. A typical Goldberg–Hogness TATA sequence is boxed. The 3 introns divide the pre-TNF polypeptide into a large prepeptide (62 amino acids), 2 short exons (15 amino acids each), and most of the mature protein (139 amino acids). All introns are bound by consensus splice site sequences (Mount, 1982). No nucleotide substitutions were found between the exons of the genomic clone, the sequence of the cDNA clone p-hTNF-1, and the genomic sequence published by Shirai *et al.* (1985). However, 5 bp differences are found in the introns and 5' untranslated region (substitutions are indicated by arrows, and the alternative nucleotide is given underneath; deletions in our or their sequence are indicated by △ or ▽, respectively).

189

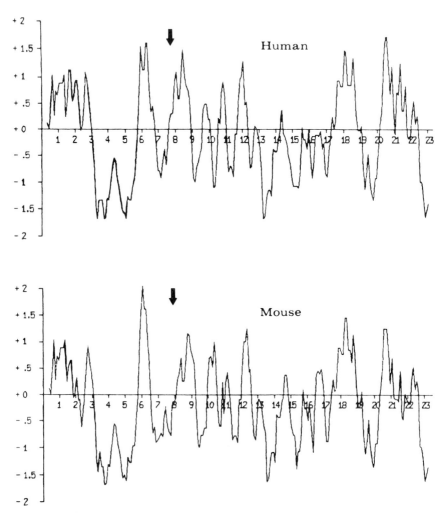

FIG. 5. Hydrophilicity plot of human and mouse TNF. Computer generated plots were determined according to the method of Hopp and Woods (1981). The arrows indicate the start of the mature proteins. The vertical axis represents hydrophilicity value; the horizontal axis represents amino acids $\times 10^{-1}$. (From Marmenout *et al.*, 1985.

Mature human and mouse TNF contain 157 and 156 amino acids, corresponding to calculated molecular weights of 17,356 and 17,202, respectively. This is in close agreement with the estimated 17 kDa value for natural human TNF as analyzed on denaturing SDS–PAGE gels. Whereas no glycosylation signal of the Asn-X-Ser/Thr type can be found n the human TNF sequence, one potential N-glycosylation signal is present at position 7 of the mature mouse TNF polypeptide. This is in agreement with published data regarding the glycosylated nature of mouse TNF (Green *et al.*, 1982). Two conserved cysteine residues, located at positions 69 and 101 in mature human TNF, might be involved in an intrasubunit disulfide bridge. The two regions at each side of the cysteine residues (48–64 and 119–133, mature human TNF numbering) are most conserved between human and mouse TNF and human lymphotoxin (Gray *et al.*, 1984) (Fig. 6), suggesting the functional importance of these domains. The overall homology between human TNF and lymphotoxin is 28%, or 43% when conservative changes are included. The two domains mentioned above, however, are both about 50% ho-

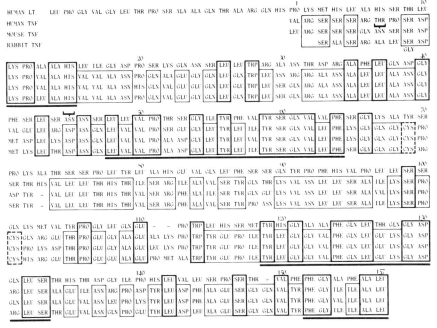

FIG. 6. Primary structure of tumor necrosis factors. Numbering above refers to the mature human TNF protein. Dashes indicate deletions required for optimal alignment. Bold and fine boxes indicate complete homologies between TNFs and LT, and between TNFs, respectively. The most conserved regions are underlined. Dashed boxes represent cysteine residues; potential N-glycosylation sites of mouse TNF and human LT are also indicated (⊔). The human LT sequence is from Gray *et al.* (1984), and the rabbit TNF sequence is from R. B. Wallace and H. Itoh (UK Patent Application GB 2 158 829 A) and our own unpublished results.

mologous. Both TNF and lymphotoxin also have a conserved region between residues 8 and 17 and have a conserved amino-terminus. The region between the two cysteines in TNF is not conserved when compared to LT. A possible explanation, as suggested by Pennica *et al.* (1984), is that this might be due to the absence of the cysteine residues in LT, so that in the latter protein a completely different primary structure is needed to obtain a comparable folding.

V. Expression and Characterization of Recombinant TNF

Expression of recombinant human TNF has been obtained both in prokaryotic (*E. coli*) and eukaryotic systems (COS-I cells, CHO cells).

The coding region for mature human TNF was engineered to allow high level expression upon derepression of the P_L transcriptional unit. Up to 870,000 U/ml of culture were detected after 4 hr induction while no significant activity could be found in control experiments (Marmenout *et al.*, 1985). More recently, *E. coli* strains producing even higher amounts were developed. The recombinant TNF was purified to >99% purity (J. Tavernier, unpublished results). This *E. coli*-derived TNF has a specific activity of about 2×10^7 U/mg protein, which is very similar to natural, U-937-derived TNF. Antiserum raised against purified U-937 TNF also neutralizes the recombinant TNF, indicating serological homology. Both proteins comigrate as a 17 kDa band on SDS–PAGE or as a 35 kDa protein on a gel filtration column, suggesting a noncovalent dimeric conformation (Fig. 7).

Using the strong SV40 late promoter, as present in the pSV529 vector (Gheysen and Fiers, 1982), expression of the complete TNF cDNA gene was obtained in monkey COS-1 cells. Upon transfection, up to 8000 U/ml TNF were secreted into the medium.

Expression in CHO cells was obtained upon cotransformation of CHO DHFR cells with pAdD26SV(A)-3 (Kaufman and Sharp, 1982) and a modified pSV2 vector (Mulligan and Berg, 1980) containing the human TNF cDNA gene under transcriptional control of the SV40 early promoter. Transformed cells were selected on the basis of their acquired DHFR+-phenotype, essentially as described by Scahill *et al.* (1983). The best producing lines were subjected to methotrexate amplification. Stable CHO lines, amplified to 20 nM methotrexate resistance and producing up to 10,000 U/ml, were thus selected (our unpublished results). This level of secretion is comparable to the TNF activity obtained after optimal induction of U-937 cells.

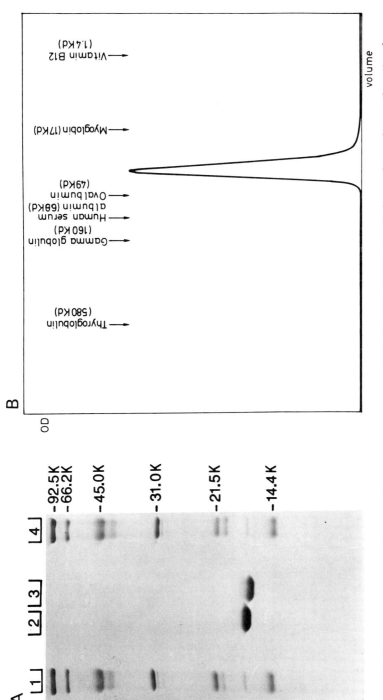

FIG. 7. Characterization of purified recombinant human and mouse TNF. (A) SDS–PAGE of purified recombinant human (lane 2) and mouse (lane 3) TNF. Lanes 1 and 4 represent marker proteins. (B) Gel filtration (TSK G3000 SW) profile of purified recombinant human TNF. Chromatography was carried out in PBS at a flow rate of 1 ml/min. The elution positions of the molecular weight markers are indicated by arrows. The derived molecular weight of recombinant human TNF is ~35,000. Recombinant mouse TNF migrates somewhat faster with a molecular weight of ~40,000.

VI. Biological Studies

A. DETECTION OF HIGH-AFFINITY RECEPTORS

The mechanism of action of TNF is still unknown. One first approach is to investigate the mode of interaction of TNF with its target cells. The availability of highly purified recombinant TNF in sufficient quantities allows one to search for specific, high-affinity receptors on the surface of different cells. Results of such a study are briefly discussed below (Baglioni *et al.*, 1985).

Recombinant human TNF was ^{125}I-labeled without significant loss of biological activity, as judged by the L-929 cytotoxicity assay. Both at 4 and at 37°C, specific binding was detected on the human TNF-sensitive HeLa-S2 cell line grown in suspension. Scatchard analysis of data from competition experiments indicated the presence of a single class of high-affinity receptors with a dissociation constant $K_d \sim 2 \times 10^{-10}\ M$ (Fig. 8). The number of binding sites was estimated to be about 6000. A large fraction of the bound TNF was shown to be internalized, presumably by receptor-mediated endocytosis, and subsequently degraded to acid-soluble products, most probably within the lysosomes. At present, it is unknown whether the internalization of TNF is a prerequisite for its biological action or whether the receptor binding provokes a membrane trigger

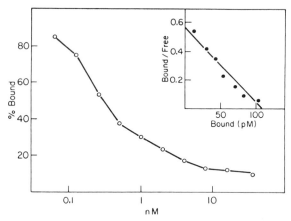

FIG. 8. Specific binding of ^{125}I-labeled TNF to Hela S2 cells. Suspension cultures (10^6 cells, 0.1 ml) of HeLa cells were incubated for 5 hr at 4°C with 0.02 nM ^{125}I-labeled TNF and increasing amounts of unlabeled TNF (abscissa). Without added competitor, 2670 cpm were bound. The cpm bound in the presence of competitor are given as a percentage of this value (ordinate). A Scatchard analysis of the binding data is shown in the inset. (From Baglioni *et al.*, 1985.)

signal. The inhibition of TNF activity by chloroquine, however, argues for a lysosomal involvement.

Analysis of ^{125}I-labeled TNF binding on the human Jurkat, Daudi, and Raji lymphoblastoid cell lines suggests a correlation between the presence of specific cell-surface TNF receptors and TNF sensitivity. It was found that only very little specific binding occurred to the Daudi and Raji cells, which are both insensitive to the cytotoxic effect of human TNF, while the TNF-sensitive Jurkat cells carry about 1100 receptors per cell. A screening for the presence of TNF receptors (and of receptors for other lymphokines such as IFN-γ) on tumor cells might be helpful for outlining a strategy for cancer therapy in individual cases.

It is also interesting to mention the likely identity between TNF and cachectin (Beutler *et al.*, 1985b). Indeed, a complete homology between the N-terminal residues of mouse cachectin and mouse TNF sequence was found. Cachectin causes a systemic suppression of lipoprotein lipase (LPL) activity, leading to a hypertriglyceridemic state (Rouzer and Cerami, 1980). A receptor-binding study using purified cachectin revealed the presence of high-affinity receptors on nontransformed tissues such as 3T3-L1 adipocytes, the C2 muscle cell line, and mouse liver membrane preparations. No cachectin receptors were found on erythrocytes or lymphocytes (Beutler *et al.*, 1985a). It was hypothesized that TNF (cachectin) might be involved in metabolic processes leading to a mobilization of host energy reserves upon invasion. These results indicate that the biological role of TNF might be a pleiotropic one, as is the case for the interferons, and thus might not be restricted to the immunological repertoire of an organism. The relationship with the selective tumoricidal activity of TNF is at present unclear.

B. *In Vitro* KILLING AND SYNERGISM WITH IFN-γ

The *in vitro* action of purified recombinant TNF on a set of well-characterized human malignant and nonmalignant cell lines, and the synergistic effect of IFN-γ on the TNF-induced cytotoxicity was investigated (Fransen *et al.*, 1986). Whereas all nontransformed cell lines tested (fibroblast cell lines FS-4 and E_1SM, and a lung cell line WI-38) were found to be insensitive, most transformed cell lines were to a higher or lesser degree sensitive to TNF action. A strong synergistic effect with IFN-γ was found in the case of different cervix, breast, colon, and ovary carcinoma cell lines, some of which were not sensitive, or were very weakly sensitive, to TNF alone. In some cases, this synergism was already evident with as little as 10 IU/ml IFN-γ. No difference was found between glycosylated IFN-γ produced by CHO cells and nonglycosylated, *E. coli*-derived IFN-γ. On the other hand, no synergism was detected in the case of the Jurkat A and C, the CEM, and the Raji lymphoblastoid cell lines, some of which are known not to carry membrane receptors for IFN-γ (Baglioni *et al.*, 1982).

This synergy was also seen between recombinant human TNF and murine IFN-γ in mouse cancer cell lines which were insensitive to the action of human TNF alone. Furthermore, studies on the species specificity of TNF indicate that both human and mouse TNF have similar effects, although human TNF generally exerts a more specific activity on human cells than does mouse TNF, and vice versa.

A different type of synergism was found with the metabolic drug actinomycin D. It has been shown that actinomycin D strongly enhances the sensitivity of many target cells to the cytotoxic effect of TNF (Ruff and Gifford, 1981). However, in this case, the selective killing is partially lost; some normal diploid cell lines (E_1SM, WI-38) become sensitive.

The mechanisms of synergy with IFN-γ or actinomycin D are at present unknown. Perhaps, the metabolic blocker actinomycin D might increase the sensitivity of the target cell by interference with a protective or repair mechanism, while IFN-γ might act by inducing an enhanced expression of TNF receptors.

VII. Concluding Remarks

The availability of the TNF gene and pure protein by recombinant DNA technology now allows a detailed analysis of the wide spectra of biological properties of this cytokine. A first major question regards the molecular basis of the discrimination between malignant and nonmaligant cells. Since TNF can act on many normal cells (e.g., cachectin activity), the dramatic selective cytotoxic effect of TNF seems not to be simply dependent on the presence or absence of its receptor (although its absence might explain one mechanism of TNF resistance). A detailed analysis of the effects of TNF after the receptor recognition event, on genetic and metabolic processes within the target cell might help to clarify this specific action on malignant cells, and perhaps the synergism found with IFN-γ and with metabolic drugs such as actinomycin D. Another major aspect regards the *in vivo* role of TNF. The role of this monokine is presumably not restricted to the immunological repertoire of an organism, but might be pleiotropic. A more profound understanding of its biological function and mechanism of action may help us to optimize the use of TNF in therapy.

ACKNOWLEDGMENTS

Part of this work was done in collaboration with Drs. E. Kawashima, A. Shaw (BIO-GEN, S. A.), R. Tizard (BIOGEN, Inc.), and C. Baglioni and S. McCandless (State

University of New York, Albany). We are grateful to Mr. B. van Oosterhout, Mrs. M. C. Vermeire and Mr. W. Drijvers for editing and artistic help. Biogent is a research laboratory of BIOGEN, S. A.

REFERENCES

Aggarwal, B. B., Henzel, W. J., Moffat, B., Kohr, W. J., and Harkins, R. N. (1985). *J. Biol. Chem.* **260**, 2345–2354.

Baglioni, C., Branca, A. A., D'Alessandro, S. B., Hossenlop, D., and Chadha, K. C. (1982). *Virology* **122**, 202–210.

Baglioni, C., McCandless, S., Tavernier, J., and Fiers, W. (1985). *J. Biol. Chem.* **260**, 13395–13397.

Beutler, B., Mahoney, J., Le Trang, N., Pekala, P., and Cerami, A. (1985a). *J. Exp. Med.* **161**, 984–995.

Beutler, B., Greenwald, D., Hulmes, J. D., Chang, M., Pan, Y.-C. E., Mathison, J., Ulevitch, R., and Cerami, A. (1985b). *Nature (London)* **316**, 552–554.

Carswell, E. A., Old, L. J., Kassel, R. L., Green, S., Fiore, N., and Williamson, B. (1975). *Proc. Natl. Acad. Sci. U.S.A.* **9**, 3666–3679.

Fransen, L., Mueller, R., Marmenout, A., Tavernier, J., Van der Heyden, J., Kawashima, E., Chollet, A., Tizard, R., Van Heuverswyn, H., Van Vliet, A., Ruysschaert, M. R., and Fiers, W. (1985). *Nucleic Acids Res.* **13**, 4417–4429.

Fransen, L., Van der Heyden, J., Ruysschaert, M. R., and Fiers, W. (1986). *Eur. J. Cancer Clin. Oncol.* **22**, 419–426.

Gheysen, D., and Fiers, W. (1982). *J. Mol. Appl. Genet.* **1**, 385–394.

Granger, G. A., and Kolb, W. P. (1968). *J. Immunol.* **101**, 111–116.

Gray, P. W., Aggarwal, B. B., Benton, C. V., Bringman, T. S., Henzel, W. J., Jarret, J. A., Leung, D. W., Moffat, B., Ng P., Svedersky, L. P., Palladino, M. A., and Nedwin G. E. (1984). *Nature (London)* **312**, 721–724.

Green, S., Dobrjansky, A., and Chiasson, M. A. (1982). *J. Natl. Cancer Inst.* **68**, 997–1004.

Hammerstrom, J. (1982). *Scand. J. Immunol.* **15**, 311–318.

Helson, L., Green, S., Carswell, E. A., and Old, L. J. (1975). *Nature (London)* **258**, 731–732.

Hopp, P., and Woods, K. R. (1981). *Proc. Natl. Acad. Sci. U.S.A.* **79**, 3824–3828.

Kaufman, R., and Sharp, P. (1982). *Mol. Cell. Biol.* **2**, 1304–1319.

Kull, F. C., and Cuatrecasas, P. (1981). *J. Immunol.* **126**, 1279–1283.

Kurt-Jones, E. A., Beller, D. I., Mizel, S. B., and Unanue, E. R. (1985). *Proc. Natl. Acad. Sci. U.S.A.* **82**, 1204–1208.

Lawn, R. M., Fritsch, E. F., Parker, R. C., Blake, G., and Maniatis, T. (1978). *Cell* **15**, 1157–1174.

Männel, D. N., Moore, R. N., and Mergenhagen, S. E. (1980). *Infect. Immun.* **30**, 523–530.

March, C. J., Mosley, B., Larsen, A., Cerretti, D. P., Braedt, G., Price, V., Gillis, S., Henney, C. S., Kronheim, S. R., Grabstein, K., Corlon, P. J., Hopp, T. P., and Cosman, D. (1985). *Nature (London)* **315**, 641–647.

Marmenout, A., Fransen, L., Tavernier, J., Van der Heyden, J., Tizard, R., Kawashima, E., Mueller, R., Ruysschaert, R., Van Vliet, A., and Fiers, W. (1985). *Eur. J. Biochem.*, **152**, 515–522.

Matthews, N., Ryley, H. C., and Neale, M. L. (1980). *Br. J. Cancer* **42**, 416–422.

Matthews, N. (1982). *Br. J. Cancer* **45**, 615–617.

Mount, S. M. (1982). *Nucleic Acids Res.* **10**, 459–472.

Mulligan, R., and Berg, P. (1980). *Science* **209**, 1422–1427.

Ostrove, J. M., and Gifford, G. E. (1979). *Proc. Soc. Exp. Biol. Med.* **160**, 354–358.

Pennica, D., Nedwin, G. E., Hayflick, J. S., Seeburg, P. H., Derynck, R., Palladino, M. A., Kohr, W. J., Aggarwal, B. B., and Goeddel, D. V. (1984). *Nature (London)* **312**, 724–729.

Playfair, J. H. L., Taverne, J., and Matthews, N. (1984). *Immunol. Today* **5**, 165–166.

Rouzer, C. A., and Cerami, A. (1980). *Mol. Biochem. Parasitol.* **2**, 31–38.

Ruff, M. R., and Gifford, R. E. (1980). *J. Immunol.* **125**, 1671–1677.

Ruff, M. R., and Gifford, R. E. (1981). *In* "Lymphokines" (E. Pick, ed.), Vol. 2, pp. 235–275. Academic Press, New York.

Scahill, S. J., Devos, R., Van der Heyden, J., and Fiers, W., (1983). *Proc. Natl. Acad. Sci. U.S.A.* **80**, 4654–4658.

Shirai, T., Yamaguchi, H., Ito, H., Todd, C. W., and Wallace, R. B. (1985). *Nature (London)* **313**, 803–806.

Stone-Wolff, D. S., Yip, Y. K., Kelker, H., Le, J., Henriksen-Destefano, D., Rubin, B. Y., Rinderknecht, E., Aggarwal, B. B., and Vilcek, J. (1984). *J. Exp. Med.* **159**, 828–843.

Sundstrom, C., and Nilsson, K. (1976). *Int. J. Cancer* **17**, 565–577.

Tavernier, J., Derynck, R., and Fiers, W. (1981). *Nucleic Acids Res.* **9**, 461–471.

Wang, A. M., Creasey, A. A., Ladner, M. B., Lin, L. S., Strickler, J., Van Arsdell, J. N., Yamamoto, R., and Mark, D. F. (1985). *Science* **228**, 149–154.

Williamson, B. D., Carswell, E. A., Rubin, B. Y., Prendergast, J. S., and Old, L. J. (1983). *Proc. Natl. Acad. Sci. U.S.A.* **80**, 5397–5401.

Molecular Characterization of Human Lymphotoxin

PATRICK W. GRAY

Department of Molecular Biology, Genentech, Inc., South San Francisco, California 94080

I. Introduction

Lymphotoxin (LT) is produced by mitogen-activated lymphocytes and was initially identified as a biological activity with anticellular effect on several tumor cell lines (Granger and Kolb, 1968; Ruddle and Waksman, 1968; Rosenau, 1968). Some neoplastic cell lines are directly lysed by LT, while others are growth inhibited. Primary cell cultures and some tumor cell lines are not growth inhibited by LT. This specificity for tumor cells led to *in vivo* studies which suggest that crude preparations containing LT have an antitumor effect (Papermaster *et al.*, 1980; Evans, 1982; Ransom *et al.*, 1982; Khan *et al.*, 1982).

Early attempts at purification of LT proved difficult because of the small amount and apparent heterogeneity of material secreted from activated lymphocyte cultures. Reported molecular weights of LT ranged from 10,000 to greater than 200,000 (Granger *et al.*, 1978). Aggarwal *et al.* (1984) reported the first convincing purification of LT to homogeneity and demonstrated that a 20,000-MW band observed by SDS–polyacrylamide gel electrophoresis retained biological activity. This form of LT was purified from the human lymphoblastoid cell line RPMI 1788 and had an apparent size of 60,000–70,000 MW when measured by molecular sieve chromatography. The 20,000-MW form appears to be derived from a 25,000-MW form of LT, which was subsequently characterized by Aggarwal *et al.* (1985a). Natural LT is thus susceptible to aggregation and degradation phenomena, which probably are responsible for the previously described heterogeneity. Additional complexity was caused by the presence of other cytotoxic factors, such as tumor necrosis factor. While the 1788-derived LT appeared to be less heterogeneous than that reported previously, antibodies raised against it neutralized all of the cytolytic activity produced by nonadherent lymphocytes (Stone-Wolff *et al.*, 1984). These results suggest that LT is the predominant cytotoxic lymphokine produced by the nonadherent fraction of peripheral blood mononuclear cells.

II. Isolation of LT cDNA

LT activity is measured by observation of cytolysis of a susceptible tumor cell line. The murine fibroblast line L-929 (Kramer and Granger,

199

1972) is particularly sensitive to lysis by LT in a rapid assay; actinomycin D-treated cells are exposed to LT for 18 hr and then stained with crystal violet. Only viable cells absorb the dye, and much of the assay is amenable to automation.

LT was isolated from stimulated RPMI 1788 cultures by adsorbtion to controlled pore glass followed by DEAE-cellulose chromatography, lentil-lectin Sepharose chromatography, and preparative native polyacrylamide gel electrophoresis (Aggarwal *et al.*, 1984, 1985a). The resulting homogeneous LT was subjected to microsequence analysis by the Edman degradation technique, and 155 residues of LT were determined. A small number of carboxy-terminal residues were not determined because of the limited availability of material and hydrophobic nature of this region.

A synthetic gene was constructed which encoded the 155 residues determined by sequencing, preceded by an ATG translational initiation codon (Gray *et al.*, 1984). The design of this synthetic gene presumed that the unknown carboxy-terminal residues would be unnecessary for biological activity; this has been observed for some other proteins such as interferon-α (IFN-α) (Levy *et al.*, 1981) and interferon-gamma (IFN-γ) (Burton *et al.*, 1985). The LT synthetic gene was constructed in three segments from synthetic oligonucleotides 16–20 bases in length (Gray *et al.*, 1984; Nedwin *et al.*, 1985a). The three segments were individually cloned, sequenced, and then ligated together with an expression plasmid containing a *trp* promoter. *Escherichia coli* cultures containing this expression plasmid were grown, but extracts were inactive when assayed for cytolysis of L-929 cells. This suggested that the carboxy-terminal residues which were not identified by protein sequencing (and consequently left out of the synthetic gene) were necessary for LT activity.

The three segments of the synthetic LT gene were used as probes to identify a natural LT cDNA sequence (Gray *et al.*, 1984). A culture of human peripheral blood lymphocytes was stimulated with mitogens and utilized for the isolation of messenger RNA. Complementary DNA was prepared from the mRNA and cloned in the vector λgt10. This library was screened with the synthetic radiolabeled LT gene segments under conditions of low stringency (Gray and Goeddel, 1983). Several phages hybridized to all three segments, and the longest cDNA insert was sequenced.

The lymphotoxin cDNA sequence is presented in Fig. 1. The LT cDNA structure is typical of other characterized cDNAs. The 5′ untranslated region is 170 base pairs long (Nedwin *et al.*, 1985b). The 3′ untranslated region is 626 base pairs in length and contains the consensus polyadenylation addition sequence AATAAA just upstream of the poly(A) tail.

```
  1 AGGGGCTCCGCACAGCAGGTGAGGCTCTCCTGCCCCATCTCCTTGGGCTGCCCGTGCTTCGTGCTTTGGACTACCGCCCAGCAGTGTCCTGCCCTCTGCC

                                                                        -30
                                                          met thr pro pro glu arg leu
101 TGGGCCTCGGTCCTCCTGCACCTGCTGCCTGGATCCCCGGCCTGCCTGGGCCTGGGCCTTGGTTCTCCCC ATG ACA CCA CCT GAA CGT CTC

          -20                                                        -10
    phe leu pro arg val cys gly thr thr leu his leu leu leu leu gly leu leu leu val leu leu pro gly ala
192 TTC CTC CCA AGG GTG TGT GGC ACC ACC CTA CAC CTC CTC CTT CTG GGG CTG CTG CTG GTT CTG CTG CCT GGG GCC

      -1  1                                  10                               20
    gln gly Leu Pro Gly Val Gly Leu Thr Pro Ser Ala Ala Gln Thr Ala Arg Gln His Pro Lys Met His Leu Ala
267 CAG GGG CTC CCT GGT GTT GGC CTC ACA CCT TCA GCT GCC CAG ACT GCC CGT CAG CAC CCC AAG ATG CAT CTT GCC

              30                               40
    His Ser Thr Leu Lys Pro Ala Ala His Leu Ile Gly Asp Pro Ser Lys Gln Asn Ser Leu Leu Trp Arg Ala Asn
342 CAC AGC ACC CTC AAA CCT GCT GCT CAC CTC ATT GGA GAC CCC AGC AAG CAG AAC TCA CTG CTC TGG AGA GCA AAC

      50                               60                               70
    Thr Asp Arg Ala Phe Leu Gln Asp Gly Phe Ser Leu Ser Asn Asn Ser Leu Leu Val Pro Thr Ser Gly Ile Tyr
417 ACG GAC CGI GCC TTC CTC CAG GAT CGT TTC TCC TTG AGC AAC AAT TCT CTC CTG GTC CCC ACC AGT GGC ATC TAC

              80                               90
    Phe Val Tyr Ser Gln Val Val Phe Ser Gly Lys Ala Tyr Ser Pro Lys Ala Thr Ser Ser Pro Leu Tyr Leu Ala
492 TTC GTC TAC TCC CAG GTG GTC TTC TCT GGG AAA GCC TAC TCT CCC AAG GCC ACC TCC TCC CCA CTC TAC CTG GCC

      100                              110                              120
    His Glu Val Gln Leu Phe Ser Ser Gln Tyr Pro Phe His Val Pro Leu Leu Ser Ser Gln Lys Met Val Tyr Pro
567 CAT GAG GTC CAG CTC TTC TCC TCC CAG TAC CCC TTC CAT GTG CCT CTC CTC AGC TCC CAG AAG ATG GTG TAT CCA

              130                              140
    Gly Leu Gln Glu Pro Trp Leu His Ser Met Tyr His Gly Ala Ala Phe Gln Leu Thr Gln Gly Asp Gln Leu Ser
642 GGG CTG CAG GAA CCC TGG CTG CAC TCG ATG TAC CAC GGG GCT GCG TTC CAG CTC ACC CAG GGA GAC CAG CTA TCC

      150                              160                        170 171
    Thr His Thr Asp Gly Ile Pro His Leu Val Leu Ser Pro Ser Thr Val Phe Phe Gly Ala Phe Ala Leu
717 ACC CAC ACA GAT GGC ATC CCC CAC CTA GTC CTC AGC CCT AGT ACT GTC TTC TTT GGA GCC TTC GCT CTG TAG   AA

791 CTTGGAAAAATCCAGAAAGAAAAAATAATTGATTTCAAGACCTTCTCCCCATTCTGCCTCCATTCTGACCATTTCAGGGGTCGTCACCACCTCTCCTTTG

891 GCCATTCCAACAGCTCAAGTCTTCCCTGATCAAGTCACCGGAGCTTTCAAAGAAGGAATTCTAGGCATCCCAGGGGACCCACACTCCCTGAACCATCCCT

991 GATGTCTGTCTGGCTGAGGATTTCAAGCCTGCCTAGGAATTCCCAGCCCAAAGCTGTTGGTCTTGTCCACCAGCTAGGTGGGGCCTAGATCCACACACAG

1091 AGGAAGAGCAGGCACATGGAGGAGCTTGGGGGATGACTAGAGGCAGGGAGGGGACTATTTATGAAGGCAAAAAAATTAAATTATTTATTTATGGAGGATG

1191 GAGAGAGGGAATAATAGAAGAACATCCAAGGAGAAACAGAGACAGGCCCAAGAGATGAAGAGTGAGAGGGCATGCGCACAAGGCTGACCAAGAGAGAAAG

1291 AAGTAGGCATGAGGGATCACAGGGCCCCAGAAGGCAGGGAAAGGCTCTGAAAGCCAGCTGCCGACCAGAGCCCCACACGGAGGCATCTGCACCCTCGATG

1391 AAGCCCAATAAACCTCTTTTCTCTGAAAAAAAAAAAAA
```

FIG. 1. Sequence of human LT cDNA. The sequence begins at the proposed start of the mRNA (Nedwin *et al.*, 1985b). Consequently, this sequence contains 100 extra residues at the 5' end which were not identified by cDNA cloning (Gray *et al.*, 1984).

The longest open-reading frame predicts a sequence which is completely homologous with the determined LT protein sequence. This is preceded by a sequence of 34 residues which has characteristics of a signal sequence (Kreil, 1981). The encoded carboxy-terminal region of the cDNA predicted an additional 16 residues not identified by protein sequencing. Using restriction endonuclease sites common to both sequences, DNA encoding these 16 residues was spliced into the previously constructed expression plasmid. Cultures containing the resulting hybrid synthetic gene/natural cDNA plasmid produced cytolytic activity when assayed on L-929 cells. This activity could be inhibited by both polyclonal and monoclonal sera prepared against natural LT, but preimmune serum did not affect the recombinant LT (Gray *et al.*, 1984).

III. LT Protein Structure

The expression of LT in *E. coli* made possible the preparation and isolation of recombinant LT which would be useful for understanding its activities and physicochemical characteristics. A murine monoclonal antibody derived to natural LT was isolated (C. V. Benton and T. S. Bringman, unpublished) and utilized for immunoaffinity purification (Gray *et al.*, 1984). Essentially homogeneous recombinant LT can be isolated from *E. coli* cultures by ammonium sulfate precipitation followed by chromatography on the monoclonal antibody-conjugated column.

Recombinant LT derived from *E. coli* is not glycosylated and consequently exhibits a lower molecular weight (18,600 compared with 25,000) than natural LT. Other biochemical parameters of recombinant LT are very similar to natural LT. Both preparations tend to aggregate under nondenaturing conditions and chromatograph on molecular sieving columns as multimers. Both natural and recombinant LT have similar thermolability profiles, with a $T_{1/2}$ of 75°C as presented in Fig. 2. Both preparations are insensitive to proteases such as trypsin, chymotrypsin, *Staphylococcus aureus* V8 protease, lysine C peptidase, and thermolysin (Aggarwal, 1985).

The carboxy-terminal region of LT is probably buried in the interior of the molecule, since LT is resistant to carboxypeptidase treatment. The amino-terminus of natural LT is relatively more hydrophilic and susceptible to proteolysis. Two forms of LT have been isolated from RPMI 1788 cells which differ in their amino-termini (Aggarwal *et al.*, 1985a); the smaller form (20,000 Da) lacks 23 residues compared with the larger form (25,000 Da). Both of these forms of LT have similar specific activities and both sizes have been engineered for expression in *E. coli* (Nedwin *et al.*, 1985a).

The cytolysis of murine L-929 cells by LT appears to be mediated by a specific cell surface receptor (Hass *et al.*, 1985). Human LT from both natural and recombinant sources was radiolabeled with [3H]propionyl succinimidate at lysine residues. This labeled LT was fully active in cell lysis and bound with high affinity ($K_d = 6.7 \times 10^{-11} M$) to a single class

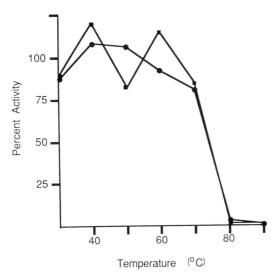

FIG. 2. Thermolability of LT. Both recombinant (■) and natural (●) LT preparations were purified to near homogeneity. Samples were incubated in triplicate for 1 hr at the indicated temperature (Nedwin *et al.*, 1985a).

of receptors. L-929 cells contained an average of 3200 binding sites per cell. Binding was specific and could be competitively inhibited with unlabeled LT or with antibodies specific for LT. The amount of LT bound to cells was directly proportional to the amount of observed cell lysis.

The primary sequence of LT is unique and exhibits no significant homology with other sequences reported in the Dayhoff data base (Aggarwal, 1985). However, significant homology is observed with tumor necrosis factor (TNF), which was cloned (Pennica *et al.*, 1984) and purified to homogeneity (Aggarwal *et al.*, 1985b) about the same time as LT. The mature forms of LT and TNF share 35% protein homology, as presented in Fig. 3. In addition, numerous conservative amino acid changes can be observed in this alignment. This striking homology suggests that LT and TNF have similar structures, which is supported by comparisons of hydrophobicity plots, as shown in Fig. 4. Although the signal sequences are not homologous, the secreted forms of LT and TNF each have a relatively hydrophilic amino-terminal region and a significant hydrophobic carboxy-terminus. This similarity is reflected in the biological activities of LT and TNF, as described below. Notable distinctions of protein structure of LT and TNF include glycosylation (LT only) and disulfide bonds (TNF only).

```
TNF                                                                              val arg ser    3
LT    leu pro gly val gly leu thr pro ser ala ala gln thr ala arg gln his pro lys met          20

TNF   ser ser arg thr pro ser asp |lys pro|val|ala his|val val ala asn|pro|gln ala glu         23
LT    his leu ala his ser thr leu |lys pro|ala|ala his|leu ile gly asp|pro|ser lys gln         40

TNF   gly gln|leu|gln|trp|leu asn arg arg ala asn|ala|leu|leu|ala asn|gly|val glu|leu|          43
LT    asn ser|leu|leu|trp|arg ala asn thr asp arg|ala|phe|leu|gln asp|gly|phe ser|leu|          60

TNF   arg asp|asn|gln|leu|val|val pro|ser glu|gly|leu|tyr|leu ile|tyr ser gln val|leu           63
LT    ser asn|asn|ser|leu|leu|val pro|thr ser|gly|ile|tyr|phe val|tyr ser gln val|val           80

TNF  |phe|lys|gly|gln gly cys pro --- --- --- ---|ser|thr his val leu|leu|thr|his|thr           79
LT   |phe|ser|gly|lys ala tyr ser pro lys ala thr|ser|ser pro leu tyr|leu|ala|his|glu          100

TNF   ile ser arg ile ala val ser|tyr|gln thr lys|val|asn|leu leu ser|ala ile|lys|ser          99
LT    val gln leu phe ser ser gln|tyr|pro phe his|val|pro|leu leu ser|ser gln|lys|met          120

TNF   pro cys gln arg glu thr|pro|glu gly ala|glu|ala lys|pro trp|tyr glu pro ile|tyr|         119
LT    val tyr --- --- --- ---|pro|gly leu gln|glu|--- ---|pro trp|leu his ser met|tyr|         134

TNF   leu|gly|gly val|phe|gln leu|glu lys|gly asp|arg|leu ser|ala glu ile asn arg pro          139
LT    his|gly|ala ala|phe|gln leu|thr gln|gly asp|gln|leu ser|thr his thr asp gly ile          154

TNF   asp tyr|leu|asp phe ala glu|ser|gly gln|val|tyr|phe gly|ile ile|ala leu|                 157
LT    pro his|leu|val leu ser pro|ser|thr ---|val|phe|phe gly|ala phe|ala leu|                 171
```

FIG. 3. Homology of the primary sequences of mature LT (Gray *et al.*, 1984) and TNF (Pennica *et al.*, 1984).

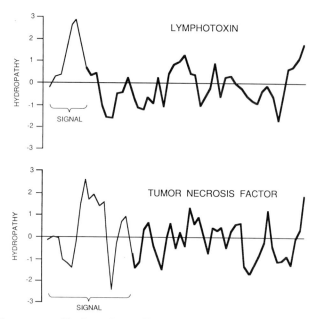

FIG. 4. Comparison of hydropathy profiles of LT (top) and TNF (bottom) by the method of Kyte and Doolittle (1982), using a width of 10 residues and a jump of 4 residues. See text for discussion.

IV. LT Gene Structure

The human LT gene was isolated from a human genomic-λ library using the LT synthetic gene segments as probes (Nedwin *et al.*, 1985b). The gene contains three intervening sequences and is about three kilobase pairs in length, as shown in Fig. 5. The first intron (287 bp) interrupts the 5′ untranslated region, while the second (86 bp) and third (247 bp) introns interrupt the signal and mature sequences, respectively. The primary transcript is processed into a 16 S messenger RNA, as shown by Northern hybridization (Gray *et al.*, 1984). The LT transcript is preceded by a characteristic "TATA" box (TATAAA) 28 base pairs upstream from the putative cap site (Nedwin *et al.*, 1985b).

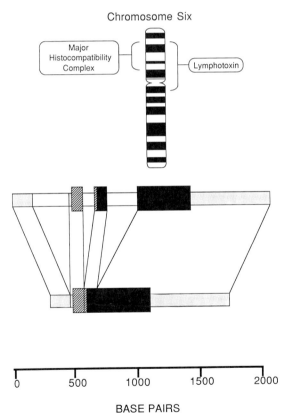

FIG. 5. Gene structure of human LT. Chromosomal localization is presented on top. The primary transcript (middle) contains three introns (open boxes) which are excised to produce the mRNA (bottom). Mature coding sequences are presented as filled boxes, the signal sequence is a hatched box, and 5′ and 3′ untranslated regions are stippled.

The LT gene structure is similar to that of the TNF gene (Nedwin *et al.*, 1985b) which also contains three introns. These genes are encoded by human chromosome 6 near the loci for the major histocompatibility complex. As shown by Pennica and Goeddel (this volume), only 1200 bp separate the two genes. Only the last exon of each gene is significantly homologous (56%) at the DNA level. Since the last exon of each gene codes for more than 80% of each secreted protein, the resultant mature proteins are quite homologous, as shown in Fig. 3.

The regulation of the LT and TNF genes is quite distinct. TNF is produced by macrophages 2–24 hr after induction, while LT is secreted by lymphocytes 8–72 hr following stimulation (Nedwin *et al.*, 1985a). Consistent with their independent regulation, little homology is observed in the promoter regions of the LT and TNF genes (Nedwin *et al.*, 1985b).

V. Biological Activity of LT

LT was initially characterized by its cytotoxic activity. It causes rapid lysis of some tumor lines, exhibits antiproliferative activity on others, and does not affect still others (Williamson *et al.*, 1983; Gray *et al.*, 1984). LT does not inhibit growth of normal cell lines and primary cell cultures.

LT exhibits an antitumor effect *in vivo*. In the classic tumor necrosis assay (Carswell *et al.*, 1975), LT causes hemorrhagic necrosis of methylcholanthrene-induced sarcoma in susceptible mice (Gray *et al.*, 1984). This is a rapid effect which is observed 24 hr following intratumoral injection.

LT appears to be an important regulatory molecule of the immune system. It can stimulate granulocytes in an antibody-dependent cellular cytotoxicity assay (Kondo *et al.*, 1981; Shalaby *et al.*, 1985). LT also stimulates osteoclasts to resorb bone tissue *in vitro* (Bertolini *et al.*, 1986).

LT and IFN-γ have a potent synergistic effect in antiproliferative assays *in vitro* (Stone-Wolff *et al.*, 1984; Lee *et al.*, 1984). This synergy may be a result of an increase in LT receptor number which is induced by IFN-γ (Aggarwal *et al.*, 1986). The potent antitumor activity found in natural preparations of lymphokines may be a result of synergistic activity of small amounts of both LT and IFN-γ (Stone-Wolff *et al.*, 1984).

TNF exhibits all of the biological activities which have so far been examined for LT. This may be a result of their recognition by the same receptor (Aggarwal *et al.*, 1986). LT and TNF may work in concert with each other by having similar bioactivities but independent modes of regulation. Other cytotoxic agents derived from hematopoietic cells have been described. Natural killer cells produce an anticellular factor which has been partially purified (Wright and Bonavida, 1981; Farram and Targan, 1983). Cytotoxic T lymphocytes produce cytolysin, a granule-encapsulated protein which causes lysis of both normal and neoplastic cells (Henkart *et al.*, 1984). Antibodies and DNA probes specific for LT and TNF will be useful in understanding the relationship of these cytotoxic factors to LT and TNF.

The cloning of LT cDNA was instrumental in characterizing LT and in understanding the heterogeneity of cytotoxic molecules. The availability of recombinant LT will aid the biological analysis of this lymphokine and help to define its role in the immune system and in controlling neoplasia.

REFERENCES

Aggarwal, B. B. (1985). *In* "Methods in Enzymology" (G. Di Sabato, J. J. Langone, and H. Van Vunakis, eds.), Vol. 116, pp. 441–448. Academic Press, New York.

Aggarwal, B. B., Moffat, B., and Harkins, R. N. (1984). *J. Biol. Chem.* **259**, 686–691.

Aggarwal, B. B., Henzel, W. J., Moffat, B., Kohr, W. J., and Harkins, R. N. (1985a). *J. Biol. Chem.* **260**, 2334–2344.

Aggarwal, B. B., Kohr, W. J., Hass, P. E., Moffat, B., Spencer, S. A., Henzel, W. J., Bringman, T. S., Nedwin, G. E., Goeddel, D. V., and Harkins, R. N. (1985b). *J. Biol. Chem.* **260**, 2345–2354.

Aggarwal, B. B., Eessalu, T. E., and Hass, P. E. (1986). *Nature (London)*, **318**, 665–667.

Bertolini, D. R., Nedwin, G. E., Bringman, T. S., Smith, D. D., and Mundy, G. R. (1986). *Nature (London)*, **319**, 516–518.

Burton, L. E., Gray, P. W., Goeddel, D. V., and Rinderknecht, E. (1985). *In* "The Biology of the Interferon System 1984" (H. Kirchner and H. Schellekens, eds.), pp. 403–409. Elsevier, Amsterdam.

Carswell, E. A., Old, L. J., Kassel, R. L., Green, S., Fiore, N., and Williamson, B. (1975). *Proc. Natl. Acad. Sci. U.S.A.* **72**, 3666–3670.

Evans, C. H. (1982). *Cancer Immunol. Immunother.* **12**, 181–190.

Farram, E., and Targan, S. R. (1983). *J. Immunol.* **130**, 1252–1256.

Granger, G. A., and Kolb, W.P. (1968). *J. Immunol.* **101**, 111–120.

Granger, G. A., Yamamoto, R. S., Fair, D. S., and Hiserodt, J. C. (1978). *Cell. Immunol.* **38**, 388–402.

Gray, P. W., and Goeddel, D. V. (1983). *Proc. Natl. Acad. Sci. U.S.A.* **80**, 5842–5846.

Gray, P., Aggarwal, B. B., Benton, C. V., Bringman, T. S., Henzel, W. J., Jarrett, J. A., Leung, D. W., Moffat, B., Ng, P., Svedersky, L. P., Palladino, M. A., and Nedwin, G. E. (1984). *Nature (London)* **312**, 721–724.

Hass, P. E., Hotchkiss, A., Mohler, M., and Aggarwal, B. B. (1985). *J. Biol. Chem.* **260**, 12214–12218.

Henkart, P. A., Millard, P. J., Reynolds, C. W., and Henkart, M. P. (1984). *J. Exp. Med.* **160**, 75–93.

Khan, A., Hill, N. O., Ridgway, H., and Webb, K. (1982). *In* "Human Lymphokines" (A. Khan and N. O. Hill, eds.), pp. 621–632. Academic Press, New York.

Kondo, L. L., Rosenau, W., and Wara, D. W. (1981). *J. Immunol.* **126**, 1131–1133.

Kramer, J. J., and Granger, G. A. (1972). *Cell. Immunol.* **3**, 88–100.

Kreil, G. (1981). *Annu. Rev. Biochem.* **50**, 317–348.

Kyte, J., and Doolittle, R. F. (1982). *J. Mol. Biol.* **157**, 105–132.

208 PATRICK W. GRAY

Lee, S. H., Aggarwal, B. B., Rinderknecht, E., Assisi, F., and Chiu, H. (1984). *J. Immunol.* **133**, 1083–1086.

Levy, W. P., Rubinstein, M., Shively, S., Del Valle, U., Lai, C.-Y., Moschera, J., Brink, L., Gerber, L., Stein, S., and Pestka, S. (1981). *Proc. Natl. Acad. Sci. U.S.A.* **78**, 6186–6190.

Nedwin, G. E., Jarrett-Nedwin, J. A., Leung, D. W., and Gray, P. W. (1985a). *In* "Cellular and Molecular Biology of Lymphokines" (C. Sorg and A. Schimpl, eds.), pp. 675–684. Academic Press, Orlando.

Nedwin, G. E., Naylor, S. L., Sakaguchi, A. Y., Smith, D., Jarrett-Nedwin, J., Pennica, D., Goeddel, D. V., and Gray, P. W. (1985b). *Nucleic Acids Res.* **13**, 6361–6373.

Nedwin, G. E., Svedersky, L. P., Bringman, T. S., Palladino, M. A., and Goeddel, D. V. (1985c). *J. Immunol.* **135**, 2492–2497.

Papermaster, B. W., Gilliland, C. D., McEntire, J. E., Smith, M. E., and Buchok, S. J. (1980). *Cancer* **45**, 1248–1253.

Pennica, D., Nedwin, G. E., Hayflick, J. S., Seeburg, P. H., Derynck, R., Palladino, M. A., Kohr, W. J., Aggarwal, B. B., and Goeddel, D. V. (1984). *Nature (London)* **312**, 724–729.

Ransom, J. H., Evans, C. H., and DiPaolo, J. A. (1982). *J. Natl. Cancer Inst.* **69**, 741–744.

Rosenau, W. (1968). *Fed. Proc., Fed. Am. Soc. Exp. Biol.* **27**, 34–38.

Ruddle, N. H., and Waksman, B. H. (1968). *J. Exp. Med.* **128**, 1267–1279.

Shalaby, M. R., Aggarwal, B. B., Rinderknecht, E., Svedersky, L. P., Finkle, B. S., and Palladino, M. A. (1985). *J. Immunol.* **135**, 2069–2073.

Stone-Wolff, D. S., Yip, Y. K., Kelker, H. C., Le, J., Henriksen, D., De Stefano, D., Rubin, B. Y., Rinderknecht, E., Aggarwal, B. B., and Vilcek, J. (1984). *J. Exp. Med.* **159**, 828–843.

Williams, T. W., and Bellanti, J. A. (1983). *J. Immunol.* **130**, 518–520.

Williamson, B. D., Carswell, E. A., Rubin, B. Y., Prendergast, J. S., and Old, L. J. (1983). *Proc. Natl. Acad. Sci. U.S.A.* **80**, 5397–5401.

Wright, S. C., and Bonavida, B. (1981). *J. Immunol.* **126**, 1516–1521.

Expression of Hemopoietic Growth Factor Genes in Murine T Lymphocytes

ANNE KELSO* AND NICHOLAS GOUGH†

*Cancer Research Unit, The Walter and Eliza Hall Institute of Medical Research and †Ludwig Institute for Cancer Research, Melbourne Tumour Biology Branch, Royal Melbourne Hospital, Parkville, Victoria 3050, Australia

I. Introduction

A. THE MURINE HEMOPOIETIC GROWTH FACTORS

Hemopoiesis is the process by which a small population of multipotential stem cells continuously gives rise to a large number of mature blood cells, representing eight distinct cellular lineages (for review, see Metcalf, 1984a, 1985a). In normal health the circulating levels of mature cells are tightly regulated, yet the system allows fluctuations to meet emergency situations, such as blood loss, infection, or reduced oxygen tension. There are undoubtedly many control mechanisms operating within this system, many of which are poorly understood. However, the ability to grow colonies of mature hemopoietic cells from progenitor cells in semisolid culture systems (Bradley and Metcalf, 1966; Pluznik and Sachs, 1966; Metcalf, 1984b) has proven invaluable in understanding the hierarchical structure of the progenitor cell populations and for identifying the molecules which control their growth and differentiation.

In the mouse, six distinct factors that stimulate the formation of hemopoietic cell colonies in soft agar cultures have been identified and characterized in some detail (Table I). Multi-CSF[1], which due to its wide spectrum of activities has a large number of synonyms, stimulates the growth and differentiation of multipotential stem cells and of progenitor cells committed to all of the nonlymphoid lineages including neutrophilic and eosinophilic granulocytes, macrophages, erythrocytes, megakaryocytes, and mast cells. The other factors have more restricted activities. GM-CSF stimulates the formation of granulocyte, macrophage,

[1]Abbreviations: cDNA, complementary DNA; CHX, cycloheximide; Con A, concanavalin A; CM, conditioned medium; CSF, colony stimulating factor; EO-CSF, eosinophil colony stimulating factor; G-CSF, granulocyte colony stimulating factor; GM-CSF, granulocyte–macrophage colony stimulating factor; IFN-γ, interferon-γ; IL-2, interleukin 2; IL-3, interleukin 3; kbp, kilobase pairs; MLC, mixed leukocyte culture; M-CSF, macrophage colony stimulating factor; mRNA, messenger ribonucleic acid; Multi-CSF, multi-lineage colony stimulating factor; rIL-2, recombinant interleukin 2.

209

TABLE I

MURINE HEMOPOIETIC GROWTH FACTORS

Name	Synonyms	Mature cells produced in vitro	Cellular sources in vitro	Molecular weight
Multi-CSF[a]	Interleukin 3 Burst-promoting activity Hemopoietic cell growth factor Mast cell growth factor P cell stimulating factor Hemopoietin 2 CSF-2α	Granulocytes Macrophages Eosinophils Erythrocytes Megakaryocytes Mast cells	T lymphocytes WEHI-3B myelomonocytic leukemia	19,000–29,000
GM-CSF[b]	MGI-1G CSF-2	Granulocytes Macrophages Eosinophils	T lymphocytes WEHI 274 monocytic leukemia Fibroblasts Krebs II ascites cells	23,000
M-CSF[c]	MGI-1M CSF-1	Macrophages (Granulocytes)	Fibroblast lines	70,000

G-CSF[d]	Granulocytes (Macrophages)	MGI-2 Differentiation factor	Monocytes/macrophages RIII-T3 mammary tumor Krebs II ascites cells	25,000
EO-CSF[e]	Eosinophils	Eosinophil differentiation factor Human-active EO-CSF	T lymphocytes	46,000
Erythropoietin[f]	Erythrocytes		[g]	40,000–45,000

[a] Johnson and Metcalf (1977); Burgess et al. (1980); Clark-Lewis and Schrader (1981); Nabel et al. (1981b); Yung et al. (1981); Iscove et al. (1982); Bazill et al. (1983); Ihle et al. (1983); Bartelmez et al. (1985); Cutler et al. (1985); Clark-Lewis et al. (1985a); Kelso and Metcalf, 1985a; Watson et al. (1985).

[b] Stanley et al. (1975); Burgess et al. (1977, 1981, 1986); Burgess and Metcalf (1980a); Metcalf et al. (1980) Clark-Lewis and Schrader (1982b); Koury and Pragnell (1982); Sachs (1982); Koury et al. (1983); Kelso et al. (1986); Metcalf and Nicola (1985).

[c] Worton et al. (1969); Austin et al. (1971); Stanley and Heard (1977); Johnson and Burgess (1978); Cronkite et al. (1982); Lanotte et al. (1982); Sachs (1982); Ben-Avram et al. (1985); Burgess et al. (1985).

[d] Burgess and Metcalf (1980b); Lotem et al. (1980); Sachs (1982); Nicola et al. (1983); Johnson et al. (1985); Metcalf and Nicola (1985).

[e] Metcalf et al. (1983); Kelso and Metcalf (1985b); Sanderson et al. (1985); Warren and Sanderson (1985); C. G. Begley, personal communication.

[f] Cutler et al. (1985b).

[g] Murine erythropoietin has been partially purified from anemic mouse serum (Cutler et al., 1985b). In the adult animal, the kidney appears to be the major source of erythropoietin. However, extrarenal sites of synthesis of erythropoietin exist, in particular the Kupffer cells of the fetal liver. A number of human renal tumors produce erythropoietin (see Metcalf, 1984a, for review).

and mixed granulocyte–macrophage colonies and, at higher concentrations, is also an effective stimulus for eosinophil colony formation. G-CSF preferentially stimulates the formation of granulocytic colonies, but at high concentrations also stimulates some granulocyte–macrophage and macrophage colonies. Conversely, M-CSF is almost exclusively a stimulus for macrophage colonies. A murine eosinophil differentiation activity has recently been described (Sanderson *et al.*, 1985) which is almost certainly the same as the human-active EO-CSF previously described by Metcalf *et al.* (1983). This factor has recently been shown to be capable of stimulating the formation of both murine and human eosinophilic colonies in soft agar cultures and is thus a true EO-CSF (C. G. Begley, personal communication). Erythropoietin acts within the erythroid lineage, stimulating the proliferation of relatively mature erythroid precursors. In addition to stimulating proliferation and differentiation of progenitor cells, all of these factors except erythropoietin have also been shown to affect the functional activities of mature end cells (Handman and Burgess, 1979; Hamilton *et al.*, 1980; Lopez *et al.*, 1983, 1986; D. Metcalf, personal communication).

The cell types that synthesize these hemopoietic growth factors *in vivo* and *in vitro* have generally been difficult to identify, in part because extracts and conditioned media from all organs and tissues contain some colony stimulating activity (Sheridan and Stanley, 1971; Nicola *et al.*, 1979; Nicola and Metcalf, 1981). Based largely on studies with cultured cell lines, tumors, and hybridomas, a minimal list of CSF-producing cells can be compiled (Table I). The ability of monocytes and macrophages, fibroblasts and lymphocytes to synthesize one or more CSFs may account for the ubiquity of these factors in freshly excised tissues, but it is clear that definitive identification of the producing cells *in vivo* must await application of techniques for detecting CSF mRNA and protein *in situ*.

All of the hemopoietic growth factors listed in Table I have been extensively purified, and their biochemical distinction, both from each other and from a number of other growth factors and cytokines, is well established. Partial amino acid sequence data have been obtained for all but EO-CSF (Ihle *et al.*, 1983; Clark-Lewis *et al.*, 1984; Ben-Avram *et al.*, 1985; Burgess *et al.*, 1985; Sparrow *et al.*, 1985; Watson *et al.*, 1985; N. A. Nicola *et al.*, personal communication). Molecular clones of cDNA and genomic sequences encoding murine GM-CSF and Multi-CSF have been obtained (Fung *et al.*, 1984; Gough *et al.*, 1984, 1985a; Yokota *et al.*, 1984; Campbell *et al.*, 1985; Miyatake *et al.*, 1985; Stanley *et al.*, 1985), and clonally pure factor produced (Yokota *et al.*, 1984; Delamarter *et al.*, 1985; Dunn *et al.*, 1985; Gough *et al.*, 1985a,b; Greenberger *et al.*, 1985; Hapel *et al.*, 1985; Rennick *et al.*, 1985). All of the biological activities previously ascribed to highly purified preparations of these factors are displayed in the recombinant material, demonstrating that all of these activities are indeed intrinsic to a single gene product and thus proving, in the case of Multi-CSF, that all of the differently named and identified factors are identical.

Because of the availability of cDNA clones encoding Multi-CSF and GM-CSF, and of cloned T lymphocyte lines which synthesize CSFs, the following discussion will be concerned mainly with the regulation of expression of Multi-CSF and GM-CSF in T lymphocytes. However, it is important to note that T lymphocytes are by no means the only cells capable of synthesizing these CSFs and hence that the activation of CSF production by T cells represents just one way in which the proliferation and maturation of hemopoietic cells may be regulated *in vivo*.

B. PRODUCTION OF HEMOPOIETIC GROWTH
   FACTORS BY T LYMPHOCYTES

When normal spleen cells are cultured *in vitro* with certain lectins, such as concanavalin A (Con A) or pokeweed mitogen, various soluble factors become detectable in the culture medium within a few hours. These include interleukin 2 (IL-2 or T cell growth factor), interferon-γ (IFN-γ), factor(s) affecting the growth and differentiation of B lymphocytes, and at least three distinct CSFs: GM-CSF, Multi-CSF and EO-CSF. A comparable but delayed production is observed when spleen cells are stimulated with antigen. Although complex cellular interactions are probably required to induce the production of these factors, in most cases the evidence is compelling that the factor-synthesizing cells are T lymphocytes.

In the case of the CSFs, the observation was first made by Parker and Metcalf (1974) that the presence of T lymphocytes was obligatory for production of CSF by lectin or alloantigen-stimulated spleen cells. It was subsequently shown by several groups that certain T cell lymphomas and hybridomas could secrete CSFs in the absence of any accessory cells, but stimulation with lectins or phorbol myristate acetate was usually necessary to activate CSF production (Ralph *et al.*, 1978; Howard *et al.*, 1979; Schrader *et al.*, 1980; Hilfiker *et al.*, 1981; Watson, 1983; Warren and Sanderson, 1985). However, the most direct evidence that normal T lymphocytes could produce CSF came from experiments with IL-2-dependent T cell lines and clones. These lines, whose proliferation is usually dependent on the continued presence of both IL-2 and antigen-presenting accessory cells, can sometimes be maintained for months or even years with retention of their original antigen specificity, surface antigen expression, and functional properties (Fathman and Fitch, 1982). They therefore represent powerful tools for the clonal analysis of various aspects of T lymphocyte function and phenotype. Numerous groups have reported the production of CSFs in cultures of such established T cell clones (Schreier and Iscove, 1980; Ely *et al.*, 1981; Nabel *et al.*, 1981a,b; Kelso *et al.*, 1982; Prystowsky *et al.*, 1982; Staber *et al.*, 1982; Guerne *et al.*, 1984; Kelso and Glasebrook, 1984; Fazekas de St. Groth *et al.*, 1986; Kelso and Metcalf, 1985a,b; Sanderson and Strath, 1985) or in limiting dilution cultures of T cells (Kelso and MacDonald, 1982; Staber *et al.*, 1982; Krammer *et al.*, 1983; Miller and Stutman, 1983; Hefneider *et al.*, 1984). With one exception (Nabel *et al.*, 1981a), significant CSF production by T cell clones depended on stimulation with the relevant antigen or a lectin such as Con A.

In addition to demonstrating that T lymphocytes can produce CSF, studies with both transformed and "normal" monoclonal T cell lines have shown that single clones are frequently able to produce more than one soluble factor. For example, A. L. Glasebrook's clone L2 and our own clone LB3 have been found to secrete at least four molecularly distinct activities: IL-2, IFN-γ, GM-CSF, and Multi-CSF (IL-3) (Prystowsky *et al.*, 1982; Kelso *et al.*, 1984; Kelso and Metcalf, 1985a). The coordinate production of several factors by many cloned lines has led to speculation that T cell lymphokines comprise a family of genes under common regulatory control (Staber *et al.*, 1982; Krammer *et al.*, 1983; Watson, 1983).

In this article, we present the results of molecular genetic and biological experiments relating to the control of expression of Multi-CSF and GM-CSF in IL-2-dependent T lymphocyte clones. Evidence is presented for the differential regulation of the genes encoding these growth factors, based on clonal variation in their expression, and marked differences in their activation by different stimuli. These results are reviewed in the context of recent advances in our knowledge of the structure and organization of the genes encoding Multi-CSF and GM-CSF.

II. Results

A. GM-CSF AND MULTI-CSF ARE NOT ENCODED BY A MULTIGENE FAMILY

Since GM-CSF and Multi-CSF (as well as G-CSF and M-CSF) are a set of growth factors displaying a range of overlapping activities, and since considerable biochemical heterogeneity has been observed for each of these factors, it has been speculated that these factors represent a multigene or supergene family within which there may be multiple related genes for each factor (Nicola *et al.*, 1979; Lotem *et al.*, 1980; Clark-Lewis and Schrader, 1981, 1982a; Sachs, 1982; Staber *et al.*, 1982; Watson, 1983; Sachs and Lotem, 1984; Clark-Lewis *et al.*, 1985; Cutler *et al.*, 1985a). Such a view is compounded by the gross biochemical similarities of three of the factors (GM-, Multi-, and G-CSF), all being glycoproteins of around 25,000 Da. The molecular cloning of cDNAs and genes encoding GM-CSF and Multi-CSF has revealed, however, that the situation is in fact far simpler.

The amino acid sequences of GM-CSF and Multi-CSF have been determined by partial amino acid sequence analysis of purified proteins (Ihle *et al.*, 1983; Clark-Lewis *et al.*, 1984; Sparrow *et al.*, 1985; Watson *et al.*, 1985) and by deduction from the nucleotide sequence of cloned cDNAs (Fung *et al.*, 1984; Gough *et al.*, 1984, 1985a; Yokota *et al.*, 1984). Despite the fact that these two factors display identical biological activities within the granulocyte–macrophage lineages, the primary sequences of these two factors show no statistically significant similarities. Furthermore, certain secondary and tertiary structural features of the two molecules predicted from their primary amino acid sequences (in particular the distribution of regions adopting α-helix or β-sheet and regions of hydrophobicity and hydrophilicity) display no similarities. Thus, it appears that these two factors are encoded by genes that have arisen independently of each other, rather than by divergent evolution from a common ancestral CSF gene, and thus they do not constitute members of a multigene family.

Although GM-CSF and Multi-CSF have no discernible structural relationship and hence are not members of the same multigene family, it is still conceivable that each factor represents an independent multigene family. In order to examine this possibility, the number of genes encoding GM-CSF-related and Multi-CSF-related factors has been assessed by Southern blotting. In the experiment shown in Fig. 1, high-molecular-weight genomic DNA from either BALB/c embryos or C57BL/6 livers was digested with *Eco*RI (tracks 1 and 2) or *Pst*I (tracks 3 and 4), subjected to electrophoresis through an agarose gel, transferred to nitrocellulose, and hybridized with a probe for the GM-CSF gene. In all cases only one fragment was detected: a 22 kbp *Eco*RI fragment and a 2.5 kbp *Pst*I fragment. Similar results have been obtained with several other restriction endonucleases, including *Bam*HI, *Hind*III (N. Gough, data not shown), *Sac*I (Lang *et al.*, 1985), *Kpn*I and *Bgl*I (E. Stanley, personal communication). If there is only one gene per hybridizing fragment, these data imply the existence of only one GM-CSF gene. Indeed, the GM-CSF gene has been cloned and its nucleotide sequence determined (Stanley *et al.*, 1985), confirming that the 2.5 kbp *Pst*I fragment does indeed contain only one GM-CSF gene. It is of course formally possible, although unlikely, that there are two (or more) GM-CSF genes flanked by identically located EcoRI, PstI, BamHI, HindIII, SacI, KpnI, and BglI sites, a situation which would give rise to the same Southern blot pattern as that in Fig. 1. The same pattern of hybridization is evident at all hybridization stringencies tested (from $0.2 \times$ SSC at 65°C to $6 \times$ SSC at 55°C), implying that there are no other genes in the murine genome having any close relationship to that of the GM-CSF gene (data not shown). The data in Fig. 1 (as well as in Fig. 9) also show that the number of GM-CSF genes and their general organization is the same in several mouse strains (BALB/c, C57, and AKR), as evidenced by a common 22 kbp EcoRI fragment and, in BALB/c and C57, a common 2.5 kbp PstI fragment.

Similarly, murine Multi-CSF has also been shown by Southern blotting to be encoded by a unique gene with no closely related genes in the murine genome (Campbell et al., 1985; Gough et al., 1985b; Miyatake et al., 1985). Thus, since there is only one GM-CSF and one Multi-CSF gene in the murine genome, the biochemically distinct GM- and Multi-CSFs produce by different sources must result from modifications that occur transcriptionally, translationally, or, most likely, posttranslationally.

Interestingly, both GM-CSF and Multi-CSF appear to be encoded on chromosome 11 in the mouse. For GM-CSF the result is essentially a negative one, since the current data derive from Southern blot analysis of mouse–Chinese hamster hybrid cell lines which have lost various mouse chromosomes (Gough et al., 1984). For example, the hybridization of a murine GM-CSF probe to mouse embryo DNA and DNA from 7 mouse–Chinese hamster hybrid cell lines is shown in Fig. 2. This experiment indicates that the 22-kbp EcoRI fragment bearing the murine GM-CSF gene (track 1) is absent from all of the hybrids (tracks 2–8). As chromosome 11 is the only mouse chromosome not retained in any of these lines (see Table 1 in Cory et al., 1983), a characteristic of mouse–Chinese hamster hybrids (Francke et al., 1977), it is likely that the GM-CSF gene is on this chromosome. Similar results have also been obtained for the murine Multi-CSF gene (Ihle and Kozak, 1984). The location of these two genes on the same chromosome raises the intriguing possibility that they are closely linked and perhaps under the influence of common regulatory elements.

Segments of chromosomal DNA encompassing both the GM-CSF and Multi-CSF genes have been cloned and the nucleotide sequence of each gene determined (Campbell et al., 1985; Miyatake et al., 1985; Stanley et al., 1985). The structure of these two genes and their corresponding

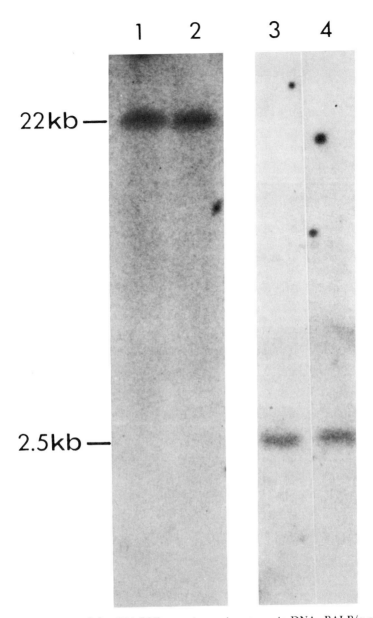

Fig. 1. Detection of the GM-CSF gene in murine genomic DNA. BALB/c embryo DNA (tracks 1 and 3) or C57BL/6 liver DNA (tracks 2 and 4) was digested with *Eco*RI (tracks 1 and 2) or *Pst*I (tracks 3 and 4), electrophoresed on a 0.8% agarose gel, and transferred to nitrocellulose (Southern, 1975). The filters were hybridized with a fragment spanning the entire cDNA insert of the cDNA clone pGM38 (Gough *et al.*, 1984) ^{32}P-labeled by nick translation (Rigby *et al.*, 1977). Hybridization was at 65°C in 2× SSC and washing at 65°C in 2× SSC.

1   2   3   4   5   6   7   8

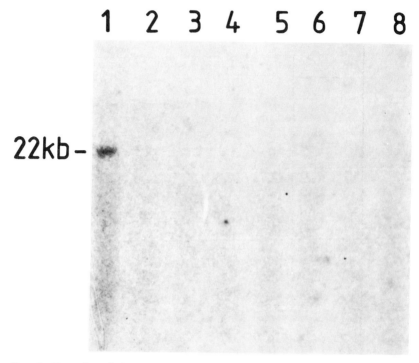

22kb-

FIG. 2. Detection of the murine GM-CSF gene in genomic DNA from a panel of mouse–Chinese hamster hybrid cell lines. In track 1, BALB/c mouse embryo DNA was electrophoresed, and in tracks 2–8, DNA from the hybrid clones I-18AHAT, I-18A-2a-8AG, EBS 58, EBS 11, EBS 4, I-13A-1a-8AG, and EAS 2 (Cory *et al.*, 1983). All DNAs were digested with *Eco*RI. The probe used for hybridization was the insert from the GM-CSF cDNA clone pGM38 (Gough *et al.*, 1984). The position of the 22-kbp *Eco*RI fragment bearing the GM-CSF gene (Gough *et al.*, 1984) is indicated.

mRNAs are illustrated in Fig. 3. In common with most other eukaryotic genes, the GM-CSF and Multi-CSF genes are segmented. That is, they are composed of segments ("exons") that are complementary to sequences present in the mature mRNA, but which are separated at the DNA level by "introns" or "intervening sequences," which are not retained in the corresponding mRNA (for a review, see Breathnach and Chambon, 1981). In Fig. 3, introns are depicted as lines and exons as blocks. During processing of the precursor RNA, the intervening sequences are removed to generate the mature mRNA species illustrated. For both genes, variant transcripts have been identified which include, at their 5′ ends, sequences encoded some distance from these loci (Stanley *et al.*, 1985; Gough *et al.*, 1985b; and see Gough and Burgess,

1987, for review). The significance of these alternative transcripts is not yet clear.

B. INDUCTION AND KINETICS OF CSF PRODUCTION IN T LYMPHOCYTE CLONES

We have established a number of stable long-term T cell clones in which to study the regulation of CSF production (Kelso and Metcalf, 1985a). These clones were obtained by single cell micromanipulation of T cell blasts activated in an allogeneic mixed lymphocyte culture (MLC), and maintained by regular restimulation with irradiated allogeneic spleen cells and a source of IL-2. Although clones could be generated with average plating efficiencies of approximately 20%, only a small percentage of these could be maintained for more than a few months. One clone, LB3, has now been in culture for 3.5 years and has retained the following properties: it expresses the surface antigen phenotype Thy-1$^+$ Lyt-2$^-$ L3T4$^+$, it is noncytolytic, its proliferation is IL-2 dependent, and it can be induced with Con A to secrete high titers of IL-2, IFN-γ, and CSFs (Kelso *et al.*, 1984; Kelso and Metcalf, 1985a). Because of its stability and high CSF production, it has been used for much of the work described below. However, most features of CSF production by this clone have also been observed in experiments with other clones of both the Lyt-2$^-$ L3T4$^+$ and the Lyt-2$^+$ L3T4$^-$ phenotypes.

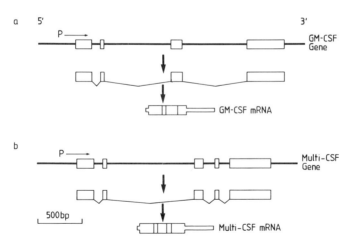

FIG. 3. Structures of the murine GM-CSF and Multi-CSF genes and mRNAs. Exons are depicted by boxes and intervening sequences by lines. P indicates the promoter adjacent to each of these genes (Campbell *et al.*, 1985; Miyatake *et al.*, 1985; Stanley *et al.*, 1985). Within the mature mRNAs, the untranslated regions are depicted by narrow boxes.

When clone LB3 was cultured with Con A, mRNA species encoding GM-CSF and Multi-CSF could be detected in cytoplasmic RNA from the cells (Fig. 4), and biologically active GM-CSF and Multi-CSF could be detected in the conditioned medium (CM). In the absence of Con A stimulation, neither the mRNAs nor the secreted proteins could be detected in significant quantities. Experiments in which GM-CSF and Multi-CSF probes were radioactively labeled to equivalent specific activity indicated that mRNA prepared 4–5 hr after stimulation of LB3 cells with Con A contained approximately 10-fold more GM-CSF than Multi-CSF transcripts. Similarly, preparative biochemical purification of CSFs from LB3 CM harvested 24–48 hr after Con A stimulation yielded 5–10 times more GM-CSF than Multi-CSF (R. L. Cutler, N. A. Nicola, L. Peterson, and A. W. Burgess, personal communication). Comparable results have been obtained with the independently derived clone D1, which is phenotypically similar to LB3. This clone can be induced by Con A to synthesize GM-CSF and Multi-CSF mRNA (Fig. 4) and to secrete these factors to about 10% of the level observed for LB3. There is thus a broad correlation between the relative quantities of GM-CSF and Multi-CSF detected at the mRNA and secreted protein levels of these two clones.

Two factor-dependent cell lines were used to quantitate CSF production by LB3 and other clones: FDC-P1, whose survival and proliferation are absolutely dependent on the presence of either GM-CSF or Multi-CSF (Dexter et al., 1980; Hapel et al., 1984; Metcalf, 1985b), and 32D cl 3, whose survival and proliferation are dependent exclusively on the presence of Multi-CSF (Greenberger et al., 1982; Metcalf, 1985b). Proliferation of FD and 32D cells was measured by [3H]thymidine incorporation in 100 μl microtiter cultures or by direct cell counting in 10 μl Terasaki microtest cultures after 2 days incubation of the target cells with CSF (Kelso et al., 1986). Two points should be noted about these assays. First, since there is no target cell population available that responds exclusively to GM-CSF, the presence of this factor in unfractionated CM has been deduced from the relative activities on FD and 32D cells. Second, assays of purified GM-CSF and Multi-CSF have revealed that FD cells and 32D cells exhibit very similar sensitivities to Multi-CSF, whereas FD cells are approximately 10 times more sensitive to Multi-CSF than GM-CSF in molar terms (D. Metcalf, personal communication).

The time course of CSF production by LB3 cells after Con A stimulation is shown in Fig. 5. CSF activities are presented as the reciprocal of the CM dilution which stimulated half-maximal proliferation of FD or 32D cells, standardized in both assays by comparison with a preparation

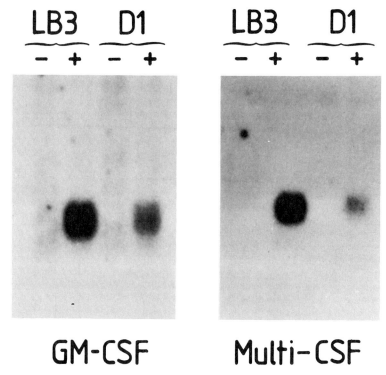

FIG. 4. GM-CSF and Multi-CSF transcripts in T lymphocyte clones LB3 and D1, with or without Con A stimulation. Polyadenylated cytoplasmic RNA prepared as described by Gough (1983) from unstimulated LB3 cells or from LB3 cells cultured at 10^6 cells/ml with 5 μg/ml Con A for 5 hr was fractionated on a 1% formaldehyde/agarose gel, transferred to nitrocellulose, and hybridized with either a GM-CSF probe (left panel) or a Multi-CSF probe (right panel). Both probes were ^{32}P-labeled by nick translation (Rigby *et al.*, 1977). Hybridization was in 2× SSC at 65°C and washing in 0.2× SSC at 65°C.

of purified Multi-CSF. As in many experiments with this and other clones (Kelso and Glasebrook, 1984; Kelso and Metcalf, 1985a), CSFs became detectable in the CM within 1–3 hr of stimulation and were secreted at an exponential rate for approximately 20 hr. Significant further production did not occur after 24 hr. Cessation of CSF production in such cultures is likely to be due, at least in part, to toxic effects of Con A on LB3 cells, but it is also observed with certain allogeneic tumor-reactive clones which transiently produce CSF when stimulated with the tumor cells under optimal conditions for clonal proliferation (unpublished observations).

A number of earlier experiments have suggested that LB3 and other

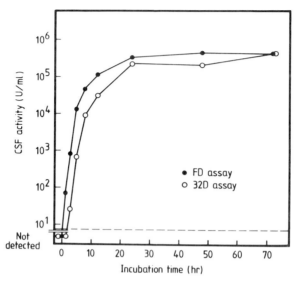

Fig. 5. Time course of CSF production by a Con A-stimulated T lymphocyte clone. LB3 cells were cultured at 10^6 cells/ml with 5 μg/ml Con A in 5% FCS. CM were harvested after the indicated incubation times and assayed for CSF on FD and 32D indicator cells. CSF titers were determined from dose–response curves standardized by comparison with a preparation of purified Multi-CSF (Cutler et al., 1985a).

clones release CSFs, IL-2, and IFN-γ with essentially identical kinetics (Kelso and Glasebrook, 1984; Kelso and Metcalf, 1985a; Fazekas de St. Groth et al., 1986). However, by using the FD and 32D assays, which are matched for sensitivity to Multi-CSF and differ only in their sensitivity to GM-CSF, it has become clear (Fig. 5) that GM-CSF production precedes Multi-CSF production by about 2 hr during the early stages of Con A stimulation of LB3 cells. At the 3-hr time point, for example, the ratio of the FD titer to the 32D titer is 30, which corresponds to a GM-CSF:Multi-CSF molar ratio of approximately 300. As in the incubation proceeds the FD:32D ratio progressively decreases, reaching a final value of approximately 1 by 24 hr, consistent with the observation that LB3 cells produce 5–10 times more GM-CSF than Multi-CSF.

C. CON A AND IL-2 INDUCE DIFFERENT PATTERNS
OF CSF PRODUCTION BY T CELL CLONES

The results described above indicate that Con A stimulation of LB3 cells induces transcription of the GM-CSF and Multi-CSF genes and secretion into the culture medium of biologically active GM-CSF and

Multi-CSF in the ratio of approximately 10:1. A somewhat different picture is seen when the same clone is cultured with IL-2 (Kelso *et al.*, 1986). As shown in Fig. 6, recombinant IL-2 (rIL-2) (kindly provided by Cetus Immune Corporation, Palo Alto, California) (Rosenberg *et al.*, 1983) induced a dose-dependent increase in CSF production above the low background level detected in CM of unstimulated cells. The dose–response curves for stimulation of CSF production, by this and other crude and purified sources of mouse and human IL-2, closely paralleled the dose–response curves for stimulation of LB3 cell proliferation, suggesting that IL-2 itself was the active moiety.

An interesting feature of the IL-2-induced CSF is that it stimulated FD cells at a concentration approximately 100-fold lower than was detectable in the 32D assay, indicating that it preferentially comprised GM-CSF. The FD:32D titer ratio of about 100 when IL-2 was the stimulus, or of 1–2 when Con A was the stimulus, was observed in all experiments over the full range of active concentrations of stimulus and over the full range of active LB3 cell concentrations. The possibility that IL-2 selectively inhibited either the induction of Multi-CSF synthesis or the activity of Multi-CSF in the 32D assay was discounted by experiments where inclusion of IL-2 failed to inhibit the production or detection of Multi-CSF from Con A-stimulated LB3 cells. In fact, experiments with certain other clones in which IL-2 also preferentially induced the

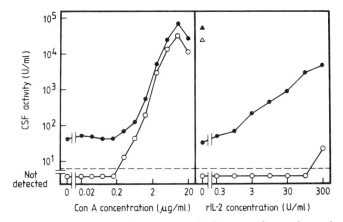

FIG. 6. Comparison of Con A and IL-2 as stimuli of CSF production by a T lymphocyte clone. LB3 cells were cultured at 5×10^5 cells/ml with the indicated concentrations of Con A or recombinant IL-2 (rIL-2) in 5% FCS. CM were harvested after 24 hr (left panel, experiment 1) or 48 hr (right panel, experiment 2) and assayed for CSF on FD and 32D indicator cells. The CSF titers induced by 5 μg/ml Con A in experiment 2 are indicated by the triangles. ●, FD assay; ○, 32D assay.

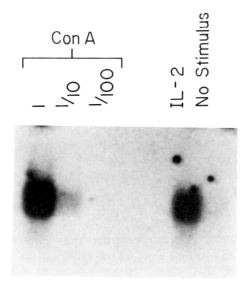

FIG. 7. GM-CSF transcripts in LB3 cells cultured with Con A or IL-2. Polyadenylated cytoplasmic RNA from LB3 cells cultured at 10^6 cells/ml for 4.5 hr with 5 μg/ml Con A, EL-4 supernatant (150 U/ml IL-2), or culture medium alone was probed for GM-CSF transcripts. RNA (5μg) was electrophoresed in tracks 1, 4, and 5, and 10-fold serial dilutions of Con A-stimulated LB3 RNA were electrophoresed in tracks 2 and 3.

production of GM-CSF revealed that combined stimulation with Con A (or allogeneic cells) and recombinant IL-2 synergistically enhanced production of both GM-CSF and Multi-CSF compared to either stimulus alone.

Hybridization of mRNA from IL-2-stimulated LB3 cells with a GM-CSF cDNA probe (Fig. 7) indicated that IL-2 induced the accumulation of GM-CSF transcripts to about one-third of the level induced by Con A. In most experiments, IL-2 stimulated secretion of GM-CSF to 1–10% of the level produced by Con A-stimulated cells. The quantitative discrepancy between the mRNA levels detected after 5 hr incubation and the cumulative protein production over 24 or 48 hr could reflect kinetic differences between Con A- and IL-2-induced transcription of the GM-CSF gene. Alternatively, they may indicate differences in the post-transcriptional regulation of CSF synthesis induced by the two stimuli. Experiments are in progress to discriminate between these possibilities.

D. CLONAL HETEROGENEITY IN CSF PRODUCTION BY T CELLS

In addition to looking at CSF production by certain well-characterized T lymphocyte clones like LB3, we have screened a large number of short-term clones for their ability to synthesize CSFs. In an earlier study of 55 clones (Kelso and Metcalf, 1985b), it was found that 80% could produce some CSF when stimulated with Con A. Of these, half secreted GM-CSF only. The other half secreted Multi-CSF and could be shown, in the 12 cases tested by biochemical fractionation, to have also produced GM-CSF. By screening the clone CM in agar cultures of human bone marrow, it was also shown that 13% of the clones tested produced detectable EO-CSF; all of the EO-CSF-producing clones synthesized Multi-CSF.

In recent experiments using improved conditions of cell density and stimulus (Con A and recombinant IL-2 together) and the most sensitive microassays for detection of CSFs, it was found that all of a group of 56 clones produced detectable CSF (Table II). Most of these produced Multi-CSF, which may or may not have been accompanied by GM-CSF, and a small group produced only GM-CSF. These results are consistent with a number of other studies showing heterogeneity in the combinations of lymphokines secreted by T cell clones (Prystowsky et al., 1982; Guerne et al., 1984; Kelso and Glasebrook, 1984). By contrast, a group of 48 subclones of the LB3 line and 12 subclones of the D1 line, tested in the same way as the clones from mixed leukocyte culture, all produced CSF active in both the FD and 32D assays, mirroring the activities of their parental lines.

Both the MLC clones and the subclones of LB3 and D1 varied in the

TABLE II

CSF PRODUCTION BY T LYMPHOCYTE CLONES AND SUBCLONES[a]

Source of clones	Number tested[b]	Positive clones (%)		
		FD$^+$32D$^+$	FD$^+$32D$^-$	FD$^-$32D$^-$
MLC	56	89	11	0
Clone LB3	48	100	0	0
Clone D1	12	100	0	0

[a] Clones were obtained by micromanipulation of single cells from 5-day C57BL/6 anti-DBA/2 mixed leukocyte cultures, or from cultures of the clones LB3 and D1, into microtiter wells containing irradiated DBA/2 spleen cells and a source of IL-2. After 9–12 days incubation, clones were expanded in a single passage with irradiated spleen cells and IL-2, then washed and cultured at 10^6 cells/ml with 5 μg/ml Con A and 100 U/ml recombinant IL-2 (or Con A alone in the case of D1) with 1% fetal calf serum for 24–48 hr. CM from these cultures were assayed for CSFs on FD and 32D indicator cells. Assay results were standardized by comparison with a purified preparation of Multi-CSF.

[b] Data are pooled from four experiments for MLC clones (average cloning efficiency, 17%) and one experiment each for LB3 (cloning efficiency, 64%) and D1 (84%).

total levels of CSF produced, but whereas the FD titers secreted by the LB3 subclones varied over a 100-fold range, those secreted by the MLC clones varied over a range of 10^7. In addition, CM from the MLC clones were very heterogeneous in their ratios of FD:32D titer, which ranged from one to several hundred, indicating that they varied markedly in the relative quantities of GM-CSF and Multi-CSF produced (Fig. 8). No correlation was noted between the FD:32D ratio and the total level of CSF production. By contrast, the FD:32D ratio in CM from the LB3 subclones all varied within a 10-fold range, suggesting that the relative quantities of GM-CSF and Multi-CSF produced in response to a given stimulus are a stable and heritable property of the line. Repeated testing of the 12 subclones of D1 over an 8-week period further indicated that the FD:32D ratio remained approximately constant among the clones in independent tests. Taken together with the observed variations between unrelated clones, the apparent stability of individual clones and their

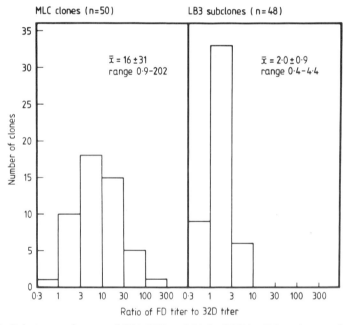

FIG. 8. Relative production of GM-CSF and Multi-CSF by T lymphocyte clones and subclones. The ratios of the CSF titers obtained in FD and 32D assays were calculated from the data described in Table II for the 50 MLC clones which secreted detectable Multi-CSF and all 48 subclones of clone LB3.

subclones suggests that one of the consequences of T lymphocyte maturation must be the acquisition of a stable, clonotypic pattern of lymphokine production.

E. GM-CSF AND MULTI-CSF GENES ARE NOT REARRANGED IN T LYMPHOCYTES

One means by which a stable pattern of growth factor production might be imposed upon a clone of T lymphocytes could involve rearrangement of the genes encoding the relevant factors. This is an intriguing possibility since several products of mature lymphoid cells are encoded by genes that undergo rearrangements resulting in a clonotypic pattern of gene expression (for reviews see Tonegawa, 1983; Hood et al., 1985). We have therefore examined the context of the GM-CSF gene in a variety of T lymphocyte lines by Southern blotting. For example, Fig. 9 shows the hybridization pattern of EcoRI-digested DNA from several different T lymphocyte lines. The lines ST1, ST4, BAL9, and TIKAUT make no detectable GM- or Multi-CSF on stimulation with Con A, whereas YAC1, LB3, EL4, and BW5147 produce GM- and Multi-CSF to differing levels. These lines represent a variety of different states of T cell differentiation and display a range of different surface markers. In all cases the only hybridizing fragment evident is the 22 kbp-EcoRI fragment present in nonlymphoid DNA (BALB/c embryo, C57BL/6 liver, or AKR liver DNA), and thus in no case is there evidence for any rearrangements to the DNA within the 22 kbp spanning the GM-CSF gene. Similarly, the Multi-CSF gene has been shown to be in germ-line configuration in the T cell line C1.Ly1+2−/9, which produces this factor on stimulation with Con A, and in mouse spleen DNA (Miyatake et al., 1985); thus it can be concluded that DNA rearrangement is not a necessary prerequisite for production of these factors by T lymphocytes. There are, however, reports of DNA rearrangements adjacent to the Multi-CSF gene in the myelomonocytic leukemic cell line WEHI-3B(D−) (Miyatake et al., 1985; Ymer et al., 1985). This line, which is one of the few non-T lymphocyte sources of Multi-CSF, displays constitutive, rather than inducible, production of Multi-CSF. Ymer et al. (1985) have demonstrated that there has been a retroviral insertion just upstream of the promoter of the Multi-CSF gene in this line and that this insertion appears to be responsible for its unregulated expression. It has been speculated that such unregulated Multi-CSF expression might be a step in the genesis of a factor-independent myeloid leukemia (Ymer et al., 1985).

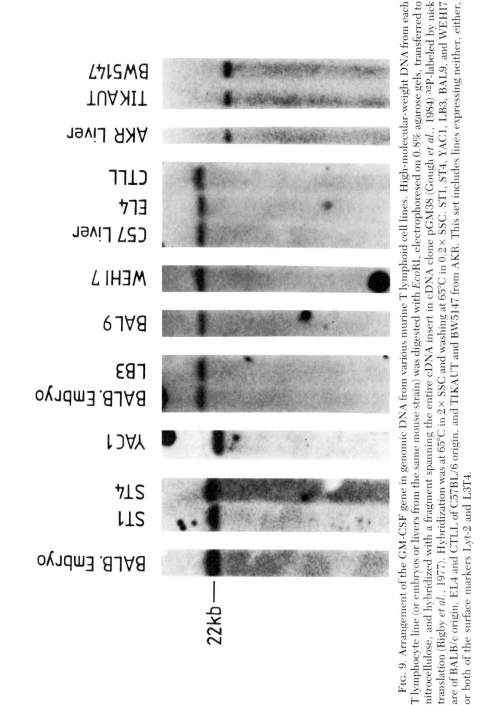

FIG. 9. Arrangement of the GM-CSF gene in genomic DNA from various murine T lymphoid cell lines. High-molecular-weight DNA from each T lymphocyte line (or embryos or livers from the same mouse strain) was digested with EcoRI, electrophoresed on 0.8% agarose gels, transferred to nitrocellulose, and hybridized with a fragment spanning the entire cDNA insert in cDNA clone pGM38 (Gough et al., 1984) [32P]-labeled by nick translation (Rigby et al., 1977). Hybridization was at 65°C in 2× SSC and washing at 65°C in 0.2× SSC. ST1, ST4, YAC1, LB3, BAL9, and WEHI7 are of BALB/c origin, EL4 and CTLL of C57BL/6 origin, and TIKAUT and BW5147 from AKR. This set includes lines expressing neither, either, or both of the surface markers Lyt-2 and L3T4.

F. Metabolic Requirements for Induction of GM-CSF and Multi-CSF in Cloned T Cells

Some of the metabolic requirements for CSF production by Con-A-stimulated LB3 cells were assessed by inclusion of inhibitors in the cultures either at the time of, or 2 hr before, Con A addition (Table III). No dependence on cellular proliferation could be demonstrated using the S phase inhibitors hydroxyurea or cytosine arabinoside. This is consistent with observations that Con A itself substantially inhibited clonal proliferation and that the rate and quantity of CSF production was equivalent when LB3 cells were in the exponential or plateau phases of growth (Kelso and Metcalf, 1985a). By contrast, experiments with the inhibitors actinomycin D and cycloheximide suggested that CSF production requires *de novo* synthesis of RNA and protein, as would be predicted from the accumulation of abundant GM-CSF and Multi-CSF transcripts in these cells after stimulation (Fig. 4).

Evidence that protein synthesis is required only for the synthesis of CSF itself, rather than for Con A induction of CSF gene expression, was obtained in the experiment shown in Fig. 10. Messenger RNA prepared from LB3 cells stimulated with Con A in the presence of cycloheximide

TABLE III

Effect of Metabolic Inhibitors on CSF Production
by Con A-Stimulated LB3 Cells[a]

Clone	Stimulus	Inhibitor	Time of inhibitor addition	CSF activity on FD cells (U/ml)
LB3	No stimulus	—	—	15
LB3	Con A	—	0 hr	15,384
		Hydroxyurea		14,761
		Actinomycin D		799
		Cycloheximide		425
LB3	Con A	—		10,811
		Hydroxyurea	−2 hr	8,698
		Actinomycin D		254
		Cycloheximide		15

[a] LB3 cells were cultured at 5×10^5 cells/ml in culture medium alone or with the following inhibitors: hydroxyurea (300 μg/ml), actinomycin D (5 μg/ml), cycloheximide (10 μg/ml). Con A (5 μg/ml) was added either immediately or after 2 hr incubation. Conditioned media were harvested 24 hr after addition of Con A, passed through Sephadex G-25M PD-10 columns to remove inhibitors, and then assayed in agar cultures of FD indicator cells. No inhibition of CSF activity was observed in control CM, which were mixed with the inhibitors and passed through PD-10 columns to test the efficacy of inhibitor removal, with the exception of actinomycin D, where inhibition was observed at the highest doses of CM assayed.

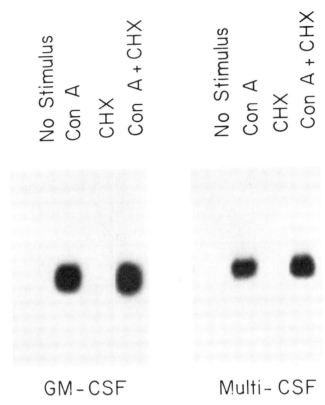

FIG. 10. Effect of cycloheximide on Con A induction of GM-CSF and Multi-CSF gene expression. Polyadenylated cytoplasmic RNA from unstimulated LB3 cells or from LB3 cells cultured at 10^6 cells/ml with either 5 μg/ml Con A or 10 μg/ml cycloheximide, or both, was probed for GM-CSF transcripts (left panel) or Multi-CSF transcripts (right panel). Cells were cultured for 4.5 hr with cycloheximide or Con A, or for 2 hr with cycloheximide, and a further 4.5 hr with cycloheximide plus Con A.

hybridized strongly with the GM-CSF probe (left panel) or Multi-CSF probe (right panel) despite the fact that cycloheximide reduced production of biologically active CSF from the cells by 99%. This experiment also showed that cycloheximide on its own did not induce GM-CSF or Multi-CSF transcription (third track in each panel), implying that these genes are not regulated by a labile repressor protein whose synthesis would be inhibited by cycloheximide.

III. Discussion

The development of monoclonal T lymphocyte lines and specific assays for their products has provided many insights into the mechanisms controlling production of hemopoietic growth factors and other lymphokines at the cellular level. With the advent of molecular cloning, it is anticipated that a detailed understanding of the regulation of the genes encoding these factors at the molecular level will soon emerge. In this article we have attempted to draw together recent results from our laboratories concerning the organization of the GM-CSF and Multi-CSF genes and their expression in cloned T lymphocyte lines. In light of these results, the following paragraphs discuss some of the issues which a model for CSF gene regulation should accommodate.

The observation that some monoclonal T cell populations can be induced to secrete several different lymphokines concomitantly suggests that expression of these factors may be coordinately regulated. This is supported by findings that clones producing high titers of one lymphokine tend to produce high titers of others (Guerne *et al.*, 1984; Kelso and Glasebrook, 1984; Kelso and Metcalf, 1985b) and that production of two different factors remains associated in subclones of a lymphoma which generates nonproducing variants at a high frequency (Watson, 1983). These results support the idea that lectins or antigen induce the synthesis of different lymphokines by a common pathway.

In several gene systems short DNA segments upstream of the transcriptional start site have been implicated, directly or circumstantially, in the induction or tissue-specific expression of the corresponding gene (Hen *et al.*, 1982; Pelham and Bienz, 1982; Hache *et al.*, 1983; Payvar *et al.*, 1983; Scheidereit *et al.*, 1983; Dudler and Travers, 1984; Falkner and Zachau, 1984; Fowlkes *et al.*, 1984; Parslow *et al.*, 1984; Searle *et al.*, 1984, 1985; Wu, 1984; Ryals *et al.*, 1985; Goodbourn *et al.*, 1985; Grosschedl and Baltimore, 1985; Mason *et al.*, 1985; Mattaj *et al.*, 1985; and see Davidson *et al.*, 1983, for review and further references). Therefore, Stanley *et al.* (1985) have searched the 5′ flanking regions of the GM-CSF, Multi-CSF (Campbell *et al.*, 1985; Miyatake *et al.*, 1985), IL-2 (Fujita *et al.*, 1983; Fuse *et al.*, 1984), and IFN-γ (Gray and Goeddel, 1982) genes for the presence of common nucleotide sequences which might play a role in lectin- or antigen-mediated activation of these genes and have noted a family of closely related decanucleotides which exist between 80 and 270 nucleotides upstream of the TATA box component of the promoter (Table IV). The elements identified adjacent to the GM-CSF, Multi-CSF, and IL-2 genes are in the same orientation as each other with respect to their corresponding gene, whereas the decanucleotide adjacent to the IFN-γ gene occurs in the opposite orientation. Whether the orientation of this element with respect to its adjacent gene would be critical for its proposed function is unclear since analogous elements in certain other gene systems have been shown to operate independently of orientation (Mattaj *et al.*, 1985). Thus, a candidate

TABLE IV

A FAMILY OF HOMOLOGOUS SEQUENCES WITHIN THE 5′ FLANKING REGIONS
OF VARIOUS HEMOPOIETIC GROWTH FACTOR GENES[a]

	Factor	Sequence	Location[b]	Relatedness[c]				
				I	II	III	IV	V
I	Murine GM-CSF	5′-GAGATTCCAC-3′	−78	—	10	8	8	7
II	Murine Multi-CSF(1)	5′-GAGATTCCAC-3′	−265	10	—	8	8	7
III	Murine Multi-CSF(2)	5′-GAGGTTCCAT-3′	−84	8	8	—	6	8
IV	Murine/human IL-2[d]	5′-GGGATTTCAC-3′	−175/−172	8	8	6	—	5
V	Human IFN-γ[e]	5′-GAGTTTCCTT-3′	−138	7	7	8	5	—

[a] This table is based on that of Stanley *et al.* (1985).

[b] The location corresponds to the distance between the 5′ nucleotide of the region of homology and the 5′ nucleotide of the TATA box element of the promoter.

[c] The number of matched positions between one element and another is given as a measure of the relatedness of one element to all other members of the family. The probability (P) of a random decanucleotide being matched at $m/10$ positions, where each nucleotide has an equal 1/4 chance of occurrence, is $\{10!/[(10-m)!m!]\}(1/4)^m(3/4)^{10-m}$. Thus, for a 5/10 match, $P \cong 0.05$; 6/10, $P \cong 0.01$; 7/10, $P \cong 0.003$; 8/10 $P \cong 0.004$ and 10/10, $P \cong 0.0000009$. The probability of chance occurrence of sequences with the observed degree of similarity to that of the GM-CSF decanucleotide within the region −78 to −265 of these genes is approximately 3×10^{-6} [calculated according to Davidson *et al.* (1983) with L = 187].

[d] In order to allow for the relatedness of the decanucleotides within the murine and human IL-2 genes that must exist purely as a result of the close similarity of the two genes, only one of these sequences is considered for statistical purposes.

[e] The decanucleotide adjacent to the IFN-γ gene occurs in the opposite orientation compared with the homologous elements of the other genes.

sequence has been identified which may play a role in the coordinate activation of these genes. However, this remains to be established experimentally.

Our analysis of the synthesis of GM-CSF and Multi-CSF by T cell clones, however, indicates that production of these factors is not obligatorily linked, but can in fact be dissociated at several levels: (1) the appearance of GM-CSF precedes that of Multi-CSF by about 2 hr in the CM of a Con A-stimulated clone; (2) in certain clones which secrete both GM-CSF and Multi-CSF when cultured with Con A or the relevant antigen, stimulation with IL-2 preferentially induces the production of GM-CSF; and (3) unrelated clones exhibit marked variation in total CSF production and in the relative amounts of GM-CSF and Multi-CSF produced, whereas sibling clones show much smaller variations in both parameters.

Thus, although a common element in the DNA adjacent to four different genes (GM-CSF, Multi-CSF, IL-2, IFN-γ) responsive to lectin- or antigen-mediated induction may be involved in transmitting the induction signal to those genes, the results presented here implicate additional factors which regulate the levels to which these genes are expressed. Obvious candidates are structural modifications to the DNA, such as methylation or chromatin structure, which might affect the level of expression of, or even silence, a particular gene. Whatever their nature, it is clear from the stable patterns of factor production by T cell clones that these additional levels of control must be heritable.

Yet another level at which CSF gene expression must be controlled is suggested by the observation that GM-CSF can be produced by a number of cell types that do not produce Multi-CSF (Table I). It is interesting to note that although GM-CSF production is inducible in some of these cell types, the inductive signals differ from those described for T lymphocytes. For example, whereas T cells can be stimulated to synthesise GM-CSF and Multi-CSF by IL-2 or by antigen (or lectins which mimic the action of antigen), GM-CSF (but not Multi-CSF) synthesis is induced in Krebs ascites cells by lipopolysaccharide (Metcalf and Nicola, 1985) and possibly in fibroblasts by diterpene esters (Koury *et al.*, 1983) and retroviruses (Koury and Pragnell, 1982). And so, while any model of CSF gene regulation must accommodate the linked production of GM- and Multi-CSF in T cells stimulated with antigen or lectins, it must also account for the ability of different signals to stimulate selectively GM-CSF expression in other cell types. Two alternative explanations could be considered for this latter problem. On the one hand, LPS and diterpene esters might induce GM-CSF transcription by the same intracellular pathways as antigen and lectins, but some feature of the Multi-CSF gene confers tissue specificity on its expression. On the other hand, the biochemical pathways mediating LPS induction of the GM-CSF gene might be different from those mediating antigen or lectin induction and involve genetic elements unique to the GM-CSF gene.

In summary, we believe that the cellular and molecular data now available point to the existence of at least three levels of control of GM-CSF and Multi-CSF expression: (1) common regulatory sequences that may be shared with genes for other T lymphocyte products (IFN-γ and IL-2), and that account for the coordinate induction of synthesis of all these factors in many T cell lines; (2) heritable features that may act pre- or posttranscriptionally and that account for the stable differences between T cell clones in the relative quantities of different factors produced; and (3) tissue-specific elements that account for the production of GM-CSF by a number of cell types which do not produce Multi-CSF.

With the present interest in the regulation of synthesis of the CSFs and other growth factors, it is anticipated that many of the mechanisms which control their expression at these different levels will soon be elucidated.

NOTE ADDED IN PROOF. It has recently been shown both by genetic analysis using an interspecies cross (*Mus musculus* × *Mus spretus*) and by Southern blot analysis of large DNA fragments separated by pulsed-field gradient gel electrophoresis that the murine GM-CSF and Multi-CSF genes are very tightly linked on chromosome 11, lying no more than 250 kbp apart (M. Bucan, D. Barlow, H. Lehrach, B. L. M. Hogan, and N. M. Gough, submitted for publication). These two CSF genes are tightly linked to the SPARC gene, which has been assigned by *in situ* chromosome hybridization to subband B1 on murine chromosome 11 [I. J. Mason, D. Murphy, M. Münke, U. Francke, R. W. Elliott, and B. L. M. Hogan, *EMBO J.*, **5**, 1831 (1986)].

ACKNOWLEDGMENTS

We are grateful to Don Metcalf and Tony Burgess for comments on the manuscript, Tony Kyne for help with statistics and computing, Dr. A. Raubitschek for providing recombinant IL-2, Annette Futter, Cathy Quilici, and Yvonne Wiluszynski for technical assistance, and Sue Blackford for preparation of the manuscript. A. K. is supported by the National Health and Medical Research Council (Canberra), the Carden Fellowship Fund of the Anti-Cancer Council of Victoria, and The National Cancer Institute (Bethesda) Grant CA-22556.

REFERENCES

Austin, P. E., McCulloch, E. A., and Till, J. E. (1971). *J. Cell Physiol.* **77**, 121–134.
Bartelmez, S. H., Sacca, R., and Stanley, E. R. (1985). *J. Cell. Physiol.* **122**, 362–369.
Bazill, G. W., Haynes, M., Garland, J., and Dexter, T. M. (1983). *Biochem. J.* **210**, 747–759.
Ben-Avram, C. M., Shively, J. E., Shadduck, R. K., Waheed, A., Rajavashisth, T., and Lusis, A. J. (1985). *Proc. Natl. Acad. Sci. U.S.A.* **82**, 4486–4489.
Bradley, T. R., and Metcalf, D. (1966). *Aust. J. Exp. Biol. Med. Sci.* **44**, 287–300.
Breathnach, R., and Chambon, P. (1981). *Annu. Rev. Biochem.* **50**, 349–383.
Burgess, A. W., and Metcalf, D. (1980a). *Blood* **56**, 947–958.
Burgess, A. W., and Metcalf, D. (1980b). *Int. J. Cancer* **26**, 647–654.
Burgess, A. W., Camakaris, J., and Metcalf, D. (1977). *J. Biol. Chem.* **252**, 1998–2003.
Burgess, A. W., Metcalf, D., Russell, S. H. M., and Nicola, N. A. (1980). *Biochem. J.* **185**, 301–314.
Burgess, A. W., Bartlett, P. F., Metcalf, D., Nicola, N. A., Clark-Lewis, I., and Schrader, J. W. (1981). *Exp. Hematol.* **9**, 893–903.
Burgess, A. W., Metcalf, D., Sparrow, L. G., and Nice, E. C. (1986). *Biochem. J.* **235**, 805–814.
Burgess, A. W., Metcalf, D., Kozka, I. J., Simpson, R. J., Vairo, G., Hamilton, J. A., and Nice, E. C. (1985). *J. Biol. Chem.* **260**, 16004–16011.

Campbell, H. D., Ymer, S., Fung, M.-C., and Young, I. G. (1985). *Eur. J. Biochem.* **150**, 297–304.

Clark-Lewis, I., and Schrader, J. W. (1981). *J. Immunol.* **127**, 1941–1947.

Clark-Lewis, I., and Schrader, J. (1982a). *J. Immunol.* **128**, 175–180.

Clark-Lewis, I., and Schrader, J. (1982b). *J. Immunol.* **128**, 168–174.

Clark-Lewis, I., Kent, S. B., and Schrader, J. W. (1984). *J. Biol. Chem.* **259**, 7448–7494.

Clark-Lewis, I., Thomas, W. R., and Schrader, J. W. (1985). *Exp. Hematol.* **13**, 304–311.

Cory, S., Gerondakis, S., and Adams, J. M. (1983). *EMBO J.* **2**, 213–216.

Cronkite, E. P., Harigaya, K., Garnett, H., Miller, M. E., Honikel, L., and Shadduck, R. K. (1982). *In* "Experimental Haematology Today 1982" (S. J. Baum, G. D. Ledney, and S. Thierfelder, eds.), pp. 11–18. Karger, Basel.

Cutler, R. L., Metcalf, D., Nicola, N. A., and Johnson, G. R. (1985a). *J. Biol. Chem.* **260**, 6579–6587.

Cutler, R. L., Johnson, G. R., and Nicola, N. A. (1985b). *Exp. Hematol.* **13**, 899–905.

Davidson, E. H., Jacobs, H. T., and Britten, R. J. (1983). *Nature (London)* **301**, 468–470.

Delamarter, J. F., Mermod, J.-J., Liang, C.-M., Elliason, J. F., and Thatcher, D. (1985). *EMBO J.* **4**, 2575–2581.

Dexter, T. M., Garland, J., Scott, D., Scolnick, E., and Metcalf, D. (1980). *J. Exp. Med.* **152**, 1036–1047.

Dudler, R., and Travers, A. A. (1984). *Cell* **38**, 391–398.

Dunn, A. R., Metcalf, D., Stanley, E., Grail, D., King, J., Nice, E. C., Burgess, A. W., and Gough, N. M. (1985). *In* "Cancer Cells 3: Growth Factors and Transformation" (J. Feramisco, B. Ozanne, and C. Stiles, eds.), pp. 227–234. Cold Spring Harbor Lab., Cold Spring Harbor, New York.

Ely, J. M., Prystowsky, M. B., Eisenberg, L., Quintans, J., Goldwasser, E., Glasebrook, A. L., and Fitch, F. W. (1981). *J. Immunol.* **127**, 2345–2349.

Falkner, F. G., and Zachau, H. G. (1984). *Nature (London)* **310**, 71–74.

Fathman, C. G., and Fitch, F. W., eds. (1982). "Isolation, Characterization and Utilization of T Lymphocyte Clones." Academic Press, New York.

Fazekas de St. Groth, B., Thomas, W. R., McKimm-Breschkin, J. L., Clark-Lewis, I., Schrader, J. W., and Miller, J. F. A. P. (1986). *Int. Arch. Allergy Appl. Immunol.* **79**, 169–177.

Fowlkes, D. M., Mullis, N. T., Comeau, C. M., and Crabree, G. R. (1984). *Proc. Natl. Acad. Sci. U.S.A.* **81**, 2313–2316.

Francke, U., Lalley, P. A., Moss, W., Ivy, J., and Minna, J. D. (1977). *Cytogenet. Cell Genet.* **19**, 57–84.

Fujita, T., Takaoka, C., Matsui, H., and Taniguchi, T. (1983). *Proc. Natl. Acad. Sci. U.S.A.* **80**, 7437–7441.

Fung, M. C., Hapel, A. J., Ymer, S., Cohen, D. R., Johnson, R. M., Campbell, H. D., and Young, I. G. (1984). *Nature (London)* **307**, 233–237.

Fuse, A., Fujita, T., Yasumitsu, H., Kashima, N., Hasegawa, K., and Taniguchi, T. (1984). *Nucleic Acids Res.* **12**, 9323–9331.

Goodbourn, S., Zinn, K., and Maniatis, T. (1985). *Cell* **41**, 509–520.

Gough, N. M. (1983). *J. Mol. Biol.* **165**, 683–699.

Gough, N. M., and Burgess, A. W. (1987). *In* "Growth and Maturation Factors" (G. Guroff, ed.). Wiley, New York, in press.

Gough, N. M., Gough, J., Metcalf, D., Kelso, A., Grail, D., Nicola, N. A., Burgess, A. W., and Dunn, A. R. (1984). *Nature (London)* **309**, 763–767.

Gough, N. M., Metcalf, D., Gough, J., Grail, D., and Dunn, A. R. (1985a). *EMBO J.* **4**, 645–653.

Gough, N. M., King, J., Metcalf, D., and Dunn, A. R. (1985b). Submitted.

Gray, P. W., and Goeddel, D. V. (1982). *Nature (London)* **298**, 859–863.

Greenberger, J. S., Hapel, A., Nabel, G., Eckner, R. J., Newberger, P.E., Ihle, J., Denburg, J., Moloney, W. C., Sakakeeny, M., and Humphries, K. (1982). In "Experimental Hematology Today 1982" (S. J. Baum, G. D. Ledney, and S. Thierfelder, eds.), pp. 195–209. Karger, Basel.

Greenberger, J. S., Humphries, R. K., Messner, H., Reid, D. M., and Sakakeeny, M. A. (1985). *Exp. Hematol.* **13**, 249–260.

Grosschedl, R., and Baltimore, D. (1985). *Cell* **41**, 885–897.

Guerne, P.-A., Piguet, P.-F., and Vassalli, P. (1984). *J. Immunol.* **132**, 1869–1871.

Hache, R. J. G., Wiskocil, R., Vasa, M., Roy, R. N., Lau, P. C. K., and Deeley, R. G. (1983). *J. Biol. Chem.* **258**, 4556–4564.

Hamilton, J. A., Stanley, E. R., Burgess, A. W., and Shadduck, R. K. (1980). *J. Cell. Physiol.* **103**, 435–445.

Handman, E., and Burgess, A. W. (1979). *J. Immunol.* **122**, 1134–1137.

Hapel, A. J., Warren, H. S., and Hume, D. A. (1984). *Blood* **64**, 786–790.

Hapel, A. J., Fung, M. C., Johnson, R. M., Young, I. G., Johnson, G., and Metcalf, D. (1985). *Blood* **65**, 1453–1459.

Hefneider, S. H., Conlon, P. J., Dower, S. K., Henney, C. S., and Gillis, S. (1984). *J. Immunol.* **132**, 1863–1868.

Hen, R., Sassone-Corsi, P., Corden, J., Gaub, M. P., and Chambon, P. (1982). *Proc. Natl. Acad. Sci. U.S.A.* **79**, 7132–7136.

Hilfiker, M. L., Moore, R. N., and Farrar, J. J. (1981). *J. Immunol.* **127**, 1983–1987.

Hood, L., Kronenberg, M., and Hunkapiller, T. (1985). *Cell* **40**, 225–229.

Howard, M., Burgess, A., McPhee, D., and Metcalf, D. (1979). *Cell* **18**, 993–999.

Ihle, J. N., Keller, J., Oroszlan, S., Henderson, L. E., Copeland, T. D., Fitch, F., Prystowsky, M. B., Goldwasser, E., Schrader, J. W., Palaszynski, E., Dy, M., and Lebel, B. (1983). *J. Immunol.* **131**, 282–287.

Ihle, J. N., and Kozak, C. A. (1984). National Cancer Institute, Frederick Cancer Research Facility Annual Report.

Iscove, N. N., Roitsch, C. A., Williams, N., and Guilbert, L. J. (1982). *J. Cell. Physiol. Suppl.* **1**, 65–78.

Johnson, G. R., and Burgess, A. W. (1978). *J. Cell Biol.* **77**, 35–47.

Johnson, G. R., and Metcalf, D. (1977). *Proc. Natl. Acad. Sci. U.S.A.* **74**, 3879–3882.

Johnson, G. R., Whitehead, R., and Nicola, N. A. (1985). *Int. J. Cell Cloning* **3**, 91–105.

Kelso, A., and Glasebrook, A. L. (1984). *J. Immunol.* **132**, 2924–2931.

Kelso, A., and MacDonald, H. R. (1982). *J. Exp. Med.* **156**, 1366–1379.

Kelso, A., and Metcalf, D. (1985a). *Exp. Hematol.* **13**, 7–15.

Kelso, A., and Metcalf, D. (1985b). *J. Cell. Physiol.* **123**, 101–110.

Kelso, A., Glasebrook, A. L., Kanagawa, O., and Brunner, K. T. (1982). *J. Immunol.* **129**, 550–556.

Kelso, A., MacDonald, H. R., Smith, K. A., Cerottini, J.-C., and Brunner, K. T. (1984). *J. Immunol.* **132**, 2932–2938.

Kelso, A., Metcalf, D., and Gough, N. M. (1986). *J. Immunol.* **136**, 1718–1725.

Koury, M. J., and Pragnell, I. B. (1982). *Nature (London)* **299**, 638–640.

Koury, M. J., Balmain, A., and Pragnell, I. B. (1983). *EMBO J.* **2**, 1877–1882.

Krammar, P. H., Echtenacher, G., Gemsa, D., Hamann, U., Hultner, L., Kaltmann, B., Kees, U., Kubelka, C., and Marcucci, F. (1983). *Immunol. Rev.* **76**, 5–28.

Lang, R. A., Metcalf, D., Gough, N. M., Dunn, A. R., and Gonda, T. J. (1985). *Cell* **43**, 531–542.

Lanotte, M., Metcalf, D., and Dexter, T. M. (1982). *J. Cell. Physiol.* **112**, 123–127.

Lopez, A. F., Nicola, N. A., Burgess, A. W., Metcalf, D., Battye, F. L., Sewell, W. A., and Vadas, M. A. (1983). *J. Immunol.* **131**, 2983–2988.

Lopez, A. F., Begley, C. G., Williamson, D. J., Warren, D. J., Vadas, M. A. and Sanderson, C. J. (1986). *J. Exp. Med.* **163**, 1085–1099.

Lotem, J., Lipton, J. H., and Sachs, L. (1980). *Int. J. Cancer* **25**, 763–771.

Mason, J. O., Williams, G. T., and Neuberger, M. S. (1985). *Cell* **41**, 479–487.

Mattaj, I. W., Lienhard, S., Jiricny, J., and de Robertis, E. M. (1985). *Nature (London)* **316**, 163–167.

Metcalf, D. (1984a). "The Haemopoietic Colony Stimulating Factors." Elsevier, Amsterdam.

Metcalf, D. (1984b). "The Clonal Culture of Haemopoietic Cells." Elsevier, Amsterdam.

Metcalf, D. (1985a) *Science* **229**, 16–22.

Metcalf, D. (1985b). *In* "Experimental Approaches for the Study of Haemoglobin Switching" (G. Stomatoyannopoulos and A. Neinhuis, eds.), pp. 323–377. Academic Press, New York.

Metcalf, D., and Nicola, N. A. (1985). *Prog. Cancer Res. Ther.* **32**, 215–232.

Metcalf, D., Johnson, G. R., and Burgess, A. W. (1980). *Blood* **55**, 138–147.

Metcalf, D., Cutler, R. L., and Nicola, N. A. (1983). *Blood* **61**, 999–1005.

Miller, R. A., and Stutman, O. (1983). *J. Immunol.* **130**, 1749–1753.

Miyatake, S., Yokota, T., Lee, F., and Arai, K. (1985). *Proc. Natl. Acad. Sci. U.S.A.* **82**, 316–320.

Nabel, G., Greenberger, J. S., Sakakeeny, M. A., and Cantor, H. (1981a). *Proc. Natl. Acad. Sci. U.S.A.* **78**, 1157–1161.

Nabel, G., Galli, S.J., Dvorak, A. M., Dvorak, H. F., and Cantor, H. (1981b). *Nature (London)* **291**, 332–334.

Nicola, N. A., and Metcalf, D. (1981). *J. Cell Physiol.* **109**, 253–264.

Nicola, N. A., Burgess, A. W., and Metcalf, D. (1979). *J. Biol. Chem.* **254**, 5290–5299.

Nicola, N. A., Metcalf, D., Matsumoto, M., and Johnson, G. R. (1983). *J. Biol. Chem.* **258**, 9017–9021.

Parker, J. W., and Metcalf, D. (1974). *J. Immunol.* **112**, 502–510.

Parslow, T. G., Blair, D. L., Murphy, W. J., and Granner, D. K. (1984). *Proc. Natl. Acad. Sci. U.S.A.* **81**, 2650–2654.

Payvar, F., De Franco, D., Firestone, G. L., Edgar, B., Wrange, O., Okret, S., Gustafsson, J.-A., and Yamamoto, K. R. (1983). *Cell* **35**, 381–392.

Pelham, H. R. B., and Bienz, M. (1982). *EMBO J.* **1**, 1473–1477.

Pluznik, D. H., and Sachs, L. (1966). *Exp. Cell Res.* **43**, 553–563.

Prystowsky, M. B., Ely, J. M., Beller, D. I., Eisenberg, L., Goldman, J., Goldman, M., Goldwasser, E., Ihle, J., Quintans, J., Remold, H., Vogel, S. N., and Fitch, F. W. (1982). *J. Immunol.* **129**, 2337–2344.

Ralph, P., Broxmeyer, H. E., Moore, M. A. S., and Nakoinz, I. (1978). *Cancer Res.* **38**, 1414–1419.

Rennick, D. M., Lee, F. D., Yokota, T., Arai, K.-I., Cantor, H., and Nabel, G. J. (1985). *J. Immunol.* **134**, 910–914.

Rigby, P. W. J., Dieckmann, M., Rhodes, C., and Berg, P. (1977). *J. Mol. Biol.* **113**, 237–251.

Rosenberg, S. A., Grimm, E. A., McGrogan, M., Doyle, M., Kawasaki, E., Koths, K., and Mark, D. F. (1984). *Science* **223**, 1412–1415.

Ryals, J., Dierks, P., Ragg, H., and Weissmann, C. (1985). *Cell* **41**, 497–507.

Sachs, L. (1982). *J. Cell. Physiol. Suppl.* **1**, 151–164.

Sachs, L., and Lotem, J. (1984). *Nature (London)* **312,** 407.

Sanderson, C. J., and Strath, M. (1985). *Immunology* **54,** 275–279.

Sanderson, C. J., Warren, D. J., and Strath, M. (1985). *J. Exp. Med.* **162,** 60–74.

Scheidereit, C. Geisse, S., Westphal, H. M., and Beato, M. (1983). *Nature (London)* **304,** 749–752.

Schrader, J. W., Arnold, B., and Clark-Lewis, I. (1980). *Nature (London)* **283,** 197–199.

Schreier, M. H., and Iscove, N. N. (1980). *Nature (London)* **287,** 228–230.

Searle, P. F., Davison, B. L., Stuart, G. W., Wilkie, T. M., Norstedt, G., and Palmiter, R. D. (1984). *Mol. Cell. Biol.* **4,** 1221–1229.

Searle, P. F., Stuart, G. W., and Palmiter, R. D. (1985). *Mol. Cell. Biol.* **5,** 1480–1489.

Sheridan, J. W., and Stanley, E. R.(1971). *J. Cell. Physiol.* **78,** 451–460.

Southern, E. M. (1975). *J. Mol. Biol.* **98,** 503–517.

Sparrow, L. G., Metcalf, D., Hunkapiller, M. W., Hood, L. E., and Burgess, A. W. (1985). *Proc. Natl. Acad. Sci. U.S.A.* **82,** 292–296.

Staber, F. G., Hultner, L., Marcucci, F., and Krammer, P. H. (1982). *Nature (London)* **298,** 79–82.

Stanley, E., Metcalf, D., Sobieszczuk, P., Gough, N. M., and Dunn, A. R. (1985). *EMBO J.* **4,** 2569–2573.

Stanley, E. R., and Heard, P. M. (1977). *J. Biol. Chem.* **252,** 4305–4312.

Stanley, E. R., Hansen, G., Woodcock, J., and Metcalf, D. (1975). *Fed. Proc., Fed. Am. Soc. Exp. Biol.* **34,** 2272–2278.

Tonegawa, S. (1983). *Nature (London)* **302,** 575–581.

Warren, D. J., and Sanderson, C. J. (1985). *Immunology* **54,** 615–623.

Watson, J. D. (1983). J. Immunol. **131,** 293–297.

Watson, J. D., Prestidge, R. L., Booth, R. J., Urdal, D. L., Mochizuki, E. Y., Conlon, P. J., and Gillis, S. (1985). *In* "Mediators in Cell Growth and Differentiation" (R. J. Ford and A. L. Maizel, eds.), pp. 315–325. Raven, New York.

Worton, R. G., McCulloch, E. A., and Till, J. E. (1969). *J. Cell. Physiol.* **74,** 171–182.

Wu, C. (1984). *Nature (London)* **311,** 81–84.

Ymer, S., Tucker, W. Q. J., Sanderson, C. J., Hapel, A. J., Campbell, H. D., and Young, I. G. (1985). *Nature (London)* **317,** 255–258.

Yokota, T., Lee, F., Rennick, D., Hall, C., Arai, N., Mosmann, T., Nabel, G., Cantor, H., and Arai, K. (1984). *Proc. Natl. Acad. Sci. U.S.A.* **81,** 1070–1074.

Yung, Y. P., Eger, R., Tertian, G., and Moore, M. A. S. (1981). *J. Immunol.* **127,** 794–799.

Cloning and Expression of the Murine Interleukin 3 Gene

H. D. CAMPBELL, M.-C. FUNG, A. J. HAPEL*, AND I. G. YOUNG

*Medical Molecular Biology Unit and *Department of Medicine and Clinical Science, John Curtin School of Medical Research, The Australian National University, Canberra, A.C.T. 2601, Australia*

I. Introduction

Interleukin 3 (IL-3) is a hemopoietic growth factor distinguished from the other colony stimulating factors (CSFs) which regulate hemopoiesis (Nicola and Vadas, 1984) by the broad spectrum of biological activities it possesses. This multitargeted lymphokine has been studied under a variety of names, including burst-promoting activity, histamine-producing–cell-stimulating factor, P cell stimulating factor, CFUs-stimulating activity, mast cell growth factor, Thy-1-inducing factor, multicolony stimulating factor, hemopoietic growth factor, and multilineage hemopoietic growth factor. There is now a general consensus that a single polypeptide can account for all the activities measured in the various assays. This evidence derives both from the biological properties of purified IL-3 and experiments with recombinant IL-3 (see below).

IL-3 is believed to support the growth and differentiation of pluripotent stem cells leading to the production of all the different blood cell types. While there is substantial evidence for direct effects of IL-3 on myeloid cells, there is currently no unequivocal evidence for direct effects on cells committed to the T or B lymphocyte lineages. The biological properties of IL-3 have recently been reviewed by Iscove and Roitsch (1985).

The availability of highly sensitive assays for IL-3, together with IL-3-producing cell lines as a source of mRNA, has enabled the isolation of cDNA clones encoding this lymphokine. These clones have provided an important entry point to molecular studies of IL-3 and the regulation of its expression as well as yielding recombinant IL-3 for further studies of its biological properties.

II. Cloning of cDNA for Murine Interleukin 3

The cloning of cDNA coding for murine interleukin 3 was reported early in 1984 by Fung *et al.* The basic assay for IL-3 mRNA used in this work involved translation of mRNA in *Xenopus laevis* oocytes, followed by the measurement of IL-3 activity in the oocyte incubation medium using the IL-3-dependent cell line 32D cl-23 (Greenberger *et al.*, 1983;

239

Ihle *et al.*, 1982; Hapel *et al.*, 1984). Comparison of poly(A)+ mRNA from the constitutive IL-3 producer WEHI-3, and from the T cell lymphoma line EL-4 following phorbol myristate acetate stimulation, suggested that WEHI-3 was the better source of translatable IL-3 mRNA.

Poly(A)+ mRNA from WEHI-3 was then fractionated by sucrose density gradient centrifugation, resulting in a 10- to 20-fold purification of the IL-3 mRNA (~12 S). The purified IL-3 mRNA was used to synthesize cDNA (Land *et al.*, 1981), which was inserted at the *Pst*I site of the plasmid pAT153 by GC tailing (Michelson and Orkin, 1982).

The cDNA library of ~5000 clones prepared in this manner was screened by the "hybrid release translation" method (Parnes *et al.*, 1981). Briefly, this involved hybridization of WEHI-3 mRNA to linearized plasmid DNA which was bound to nitrocellulose. Groups of 10 clones were screened. The RNA was then eluted from the filters and assayed for IL-3 mRNA.

One positive pool of 10 clones was detected. Individual clones from this group were rescreened in the same manner, and a single positive clone was obtained. The cDNA insert in this clone was short (139 bp), and, based on its nucleotide sequence, a synthetic oligonucleotide 21-mer was synthesized and used as a hybridization probe to screen a second library enriched for cDNA fragments >500 bp. In this way a longer cDNA clone was obtained which contained the complete IL-3 coding region. Its nucleotide sequence (Sanger *et al.*, 1977, 1982), together with the deduced primary structure of murine IL-3, is shown in Fig. 1.

At about the same time Yokota *et al.* (1984) isolated a cDNA clone coding for a murine mast cell growth factor (MCGF) activity. A cloned T cell line known to produce MCGF after Con A stimulation (Nabel *et al.*, 1981) was used as the source of mRNA. An unfractionated cDNA library was screened by the hybrid release method using *Xenopus laevis* oocytes for translation, and activity was detected using a factor-dependent cloned mast cell line. From an initial positive pool of 672 clones, a single positive clone was obtained by a three-part strategy. This involved further hybrid release translation, narrowing the number of clones down from 672 to 48, hybridization analysis utilizing T cell and Con A stimulation-specific cDNA probes, narrowing the number down from 48 to 3, and finally, further hybrid release translation to identify a single positive clone. This clone was then used to isolate full-length cDNA clones by hybridization analysis of a size-fractionated cDNA library. A feature of this study was the use of the pcD cloning vector (Okayama and Berg, 1983), which allows expression of cDNA inserts following transfection into monkey COS cells. Thus, the fact that clones containing the com-

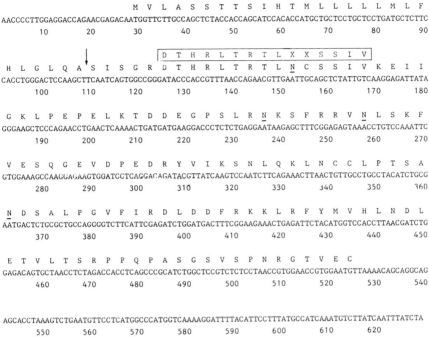

```
                        M  V  L  A  S  S  T  T  S  I  H  T  M  L  L  L  L  L  M  L  F
AACCCCTTGGAGGACCAGAACGAGACAATGGTTCTTGCCAGCTCTACCACCAGCATCCACACCATGCTGCTCCTGCTCCTGATGCTCTTC
      10        20        30        40        50        60        70        80        90

                    |                   D  T  H  R  L  T  R  T  L  X  X  S  S  I  V
                    ↓                  ┌──────────────────────────────────────────────┐
  H  L  G  L  Q  A  S  I  S  G  R  D  T  H  R  L  T  R  T  L  N  C  S  S  I  V  K  E  I  I
CACCTGGGACTCCAAGCTTCAATCAGTGGCCGGGATACCCACCGTTTAACCAGAACGTTGAATTGCAGCTCTATTGTCAAGGAGATTATA
        100       110       120       130       140       150       160       170       180

  G  K  L  P  E  P  E  L  K  T  D  D  E  G  P  S  L  R  N  K  S  F  R  R  V  N  L  S  K  F
GGGAAGCTCCCAGAACCTGAACTCAAAACTGATGATGAAGGACCCTCTCTGAGGAATAAGAGCTTTGGAGAGTAAACCTGTCCAAATTC
        190       200       210       220       230       240       250       260       270

  V  E  S  Q  G  E  V  D  P  E  D  R  Y  V  I  K  S  N  L  Q  K  L  N  C  C  L  P  T  S  A
GTGGAAAGCCAAGGAGAAGTGGATCCTCAGGACAGATACGTTATCAAGTCCAATCTTCAGAAACTTAACTGTTGCCTGCCTACATCTGCG
        280       290       300       310       320       330       340       350       360

  N  D  S  A  L  P  G  V  F  I  R  D  L  D  D  F  R  K  K  L  R  F  Y  M  V  H  L  N  D  L
AATGACTCTGCGCTGCCAGGGGTCTTCATTCGAGATCTGGATGACTTTCGGAAGAAACTGAGATTCTACATGGTCCACCTTAACGATCTG
        370       380       390       400       410       420       430       440       450

  E  T  V  L  T  S  R  P  P  Q  P  A  S  G  S  V  S  P  N  R  G  T  V  E  C
GAGACAGTGCTAACCTCTAGACCACCTCAGCCCGCATCTGGCTCCGTCTCTCCTAACCGTGGAACCGTGGAATGTTAAAACAGCAGGCAG
        460       470       480       490       500       510       520       530       540

AGCACCTAAAGTCTGAATGTTCCTCATGGCCCATGGTCAAAAGGATTTTACATTCCTTTATGCCATCAAATGTCTTATCAATTTATCTA
        550       560       570       580       590       600       610       620
```

FIG. 1. Nucleotide sequence of cDNA for murine IL-3 and predicted amino acid sequence of the protein. The sequence is that of a cDNA clone from WEHI-3B. The N-terminal sequence of Ihle *et al.* (1983) for purified IL-3 is boxed. The arrow represents the predicted cleavage point of the leader peptide (Von Heijne, 1983). Reports by Clark-Lewis *et al.* (1984) and Conlon *et al.* (1985) have indicated that cleavage of the leader peptide to yield mature IL-3 may occur one residue to the left of the arrow. Potential N-glycosylation sites are underlined.

plete MCGF coding sequence had been obtained was verified by direct expression of the clones to yield MCGF activity. The nucleotide sequence of the MCGF cDNA proved to be identical with that of the IL-3 cDNA except for a single nucleotide difference.

Some features of IL-3 have been elucidated from the nucleotide sequence of the cDNA and the predicted primary structure of the protein. Among these is the presence of a hydrophobic leader sequence of ~27 amino acids at the N-terminus of IL-3, based on the assumption that translation begins at the first methionine codon. It should be noted, however, that a clone starting at nucleotide 41 (Fig. 1) can still express high levels of IL-3 (Yokota *et al.*, 1984), indicating that alternative start sites are possible. The cleavage point of the putative leader sequence (Fung *et al.*, 1984) was originally predicted by empirical rules (Von

Heijne, 1983). This analysis suggested that mature IL-3 might start at serine (residue 28). The N-terminal sequence obtained by Ihle *et al.* (1983), by Edman degradation of purified IL-3, commences a further 5 residues on at aspartate, immediately after an arginine residue (Fig. 1), suggesting that, subsequent to signal peptide removal, a further proteolytic processing step may occur to yield mature IL-3. It is possible, however, that the N-terminal sequence of Ihle *et al.* (1983) was generated during purification by adventitious proteolysis. In this connection it is interesting that Clark-Lewis *et al.* (1984) and Conlon *et al.* (1985) have reported a different N-terminal sequence for purified IL-3 starting with alanine (residue 27), 6 residues ahead of the sequence of Ihle *et al.* (1983).

Another feature is the presence of the four potential N-glycosylation sites (Fig. 1). Glycosylation of the nearest of these to the N-terminus would explain the inability to identify asparagine at this position on Edman degradation (Ihle *et al.*, 1983). The exact nature and extent of glycosylation of IL-3 *in vivo*, and its functional role, if any, remain to be determined. IL-3 is believed to carry significant amounts of carbohydrate (Metcalf, 1985), including sialic acid, which contribute to its heterogeneity when examined, for example, by isoelectric focusing, and make it appear larger than predicted from its primary structure when run on SDS–gel electrophoresis (Weber *et al.*, 1972).

Also of significance for studies with purified IL-3 are the complete absence of tryptophan and the presence of only 2 tyrosine residues per molecule. This must be taken into account when using absorbance at 280 nm to quantitate IL-3. The calculated value for the molar absorption coefficient at 280 nm (Edelhoch, 1967) is 2560 or 2800/M/cm, depending on whether the four cysteine residues are free or in disulfide bridges, respectively.

Comparison of the predicted amino acid sequence of IL-3 with the sequences of GM-CSF (Gough *et al.*, 1984, 1985), IL-2 (Taniguchi *et al.*, 1983), and interferon-γ (Gray *et al.*, 1982) has not revealed any significant sequence homology, nor has any homology with any other known protein been detected.

III. Cloning of the Gene for Murine Interleukin 3

The cDNA clones for IL-3 have been used to show, via Southern hybridization analysis (Southern, 1975), that there is a single copy of the IL-3 gene in the mouse genome (Miyatake *et al.*, 1985; Campbell *et al.*, 1985). This was demonstrated for a range of mouse strains, including BALB/c and C57BL/6J from which the cell lines used by Fung *et al.*

(1984) for the cloning of IL-3 and Yokota *et al.* (1984) for the cloning of MCGF were derived, respectively. The single nucleotide difference (which results in a single amino acid difference) between the sequences of the murine IL-3 and MCGF clones therefore probably represents allelic variation between BALB/c and C57BL/6J mice. This comparison is restricted to the short (28 bp) 5′ untranslated portions and the coding regions of the respective cDNA clones. In the case of GM-CSF, a similar comparison of cDNA clones from BALB/c and C57BL/6J shows three nucleotide differences (but once again a single amino acid change) in the same regions, as well as a further five differences in the 3′ untranslated portion (Gough *et al.*, 1984, 1985).

In the Southern hybridization analyses, the IL-3 gene appeared to reside on a single, ~8.5-kb *Eco*RI fragment in genomic DNA from BALB/c mice. Campbell *et al.* (1985) cloned this *Eco*RI fragment from BALB/c liver DNA using the λgtWES.λB system (Leder *et al.*, 1977). The *Eco*RI digested chromosomal DNA was first enriched ~40-fold for the 8.5 kb fragment by agarose gel electrophoresis. The size-fractionated λ library obtained was screened by plaque hybridization (Benton and Davis, 1977) using a probe derived from the IL-3 cDNA, and clones containing the gene were isolated. The IL-3 gene was then localized to a 3.7-kb *Hinc*II/*Eco*RI fragment of the 8.5-kb clone by further hybridization analysis and chain termination sequencing of double-stranded plasmid DNA with specific oligonucleotide primers (Campbell *et al.*, 1985; H. D. Campbell, unpublished results).

The nucleotide sequence of 3490 bp encompassing the IL-3 gene was determined on both strands by the chain termination method (Sanger *et al.*, 1977, 1982; Deininger, 1983). The nucleotide sequence of this region is shown in Fig. 2. The chromosomal organization of the murine IL-3 gene, together with some features mentioned in the following discussion, is depicted in Fig. 3.

Miyatake *et al.* (1985) (see Otsuka *et al.*, this volume) have also cloned and sequenced the murine IL-3 gene using the MCGF cDNA as a probe. The gene was cloned from a BALB/c mouse sperm library in λ Charon 4A. A 3140 bp region covering the IL-3 gene was sequenced, 60% of it on both strands. Apart from four bases (222, 224, 434 and 1057, Fig. 2) present in the sequence of Campbell *et al.* (1985) which are absent from the sequence of Miyatake *et al.* (1985), there are no other differences.

Analysis of the nucleotide sequence of the IL-3 gene (Campbell *et al.*, 1985; Miyatake *et al.*, 1985) has revealed a number of features of interest. The coding sequence is interrupted by four introns, of 96, 993, 135, and 122 bp in order from the 5′ end of the gene. All of the introns interrupt the coding region between codons and are thus of class 0 (Sharp, 1980).

```
CTAGAGATACACTTAGCTCTGGCTACCACCAGACGACTAGCCACCATGGAAGTTTAACCATGTGCCAGAATGCCACCAAGTTCAAGTCTGCTCCAGTGACTCTGGTGACTACC
        10        20        30        40        50        60        70        80        90       100       110       120

TCTATCAGGTAGGGTGTACAGTCACCACATAGGCTGTACAGTTTCTGCAGGTCAAGTTTGTAGGATGGTAGGATGAGATTCCACTGCATAGAAAGCCAAGCTGCCTCAGAGCCAGCGCTA
       130       140       150       160       170       180       190       200       210       220       230       240

CTTCCTCCCACAACCTGTTTCCACTCCGTCCATCTCTATGACAAAGGAAGAAGAGATGCCTTTGAATAAGCAGTCTTTCTTCCCATGTGACAGTCTTTCTGATAATCTGACTACTAGAAATGTGATGAATAA
       250       260       270       280       290       300       310       320       330       340       350       360

GTTTGTGGTTTGCTATGGAGGTTCCATGTCAGATAAAGCTGCTTCTGATGCCTGCCTCCCCCGCCCGGCCCGCCCACCCCTCTGAATACATATAAGTGAGGCTCCT
       370       380       390       400       410       420       430       440       450       460       470       480

           M   V   L   A   S   S   T   T   S   I   H   T   M   L   L   L   L   M   L   F   H   L   G   L   L   Q   A
GTGGCTTCTTCAGGAACCCCTGGAGGACCAGAACGAGACAATGGTTCTTGCCAGCTTCACCACCAGCATCCACCACATGCTGCTCCTGCTGATGCTCTTCCACCTGGGACTCCAAGC
       490       500       510       520       530       540       550       560       570       580       590       600

 S   I   S   G   R   D   T   H   R   L   T   R   T   L   N   C   S   S   I   V   K   E   I   I   G   K   L   P ⌈intron 1 →
TTCAATCAGTGGCCGGGATACCCACCGTTTAACCAGACAGTTGAATTGCAGCTCTATTGTCAAGGAGATTATAGGAGAGTCCCAGTGAGTAACGCTGGTGAGGTTGGCTGTGGTCAGCGCC
       610       620       630       640       650       660       670       680       690       700       710       720

         ← intron 1⌉ E   P   E   L   K   T   D   D   E   G   P   S   L   R⌈intron 2 →
GGCTCAACAGGTGCCTCAGCCAGTGACGCCTCATGATTCTTCTTTCTTTCTTGTGTTCTCATGTCCTCACAGGAACCTGAACTCAAAACTGATGATGAAGGACCCTCTCTGAGCGTAAGAGCCCTGCTTTG
       730       740       750       760       770       780       790       800       810       820       830       840

GGATATTCTTGGGTTCCATCTATCTCCGCTCGGTGACTTCAGCCATCGCATGCCTTGCTCAGCCATCACTCCACGATGCCTTGCTCATTTTGCATCTATCTCAGTGGGTTATTAAGGAAATCATCAGATGACTC
       850       860       870       880       890       900       910       920       930       940       950       960

TCAAGCCTCAGTATATACCTCAGTGCAATAATGAAAGTTACCTTTTAGGATAATCAATGAAGACAGCTGTGGTGAACCGTGGGTGCTCTGGCTGCTGGCTCGCAGGCCTCTGGCTCCACTTTCAGTGG
       970       980       990      1000      1010      1020      1030      1040      1050      1060      1070      1080

GGATGCCATTGCCCCTGTGACTTTTGTGTCTTTTGCTTTTCTCCTCTGCCAAAACTGAAGTTGTGTTTCTACTTCCGCCAGCCCCAGACATTACTATTTGTAGTTATTTTCCTAGT
      1090      1100      1110      1120      1130      1140      1150      1160      1170      1180      1190      1200

TTGATACAATAGTTATGTCTTGTTTTTATTTGTTTGGACCTAACATGAAGTTCTTTGCAAGAGTCTATATTTCCCCTCCCTAGGAACATGTTGGAGCCTAGGAGCTTATACGGATTTTCT
      1210      1220      1230      1240      1250      1260      1270      1280      1290      1300      1310      1320

TCTAGGTATCCAGAAAATTCTTAATTAAATTAAAGCATTGGCCTGGGTTTTTGGCCATCTTGGTATTTTCCTTGCCTTTCTCTAGAGTCTTTGTCTGAGATATACACTAGCTTTTAGCCCCAGG
      1330      1340      1350      1360      1370      1380      1390      1400      1410      1420      1430      1440

TCAAGTACAGACAAATCTGCTTAGATCCTTCACACAGCTGCCAGGAGTTAAGACCTGGTGCTTGGAGAAAACAGGCCCTTGTCTGAGATATACACTAGCTTTTAGCCCCAGG
      1450      1460      1470      1480      1490      1500      1510      1520      1530      1540      1550      1560

ATAATGAAGGGACAGGAATAAGGCTGTTCAAAGAAATCTCAAATAGCAGGCACACTTCCCTAGCTCTGATCTCTCCAGCTCTCCAGTCTCCAGTCTCAAATCCCCAGCTCTTTTCCTTTCC
      1570      1580      1590      1600      1610      1620      1630      1640      1650      1660      1670      1680

AGTTCTCACCTCCCTGCTCTCACCTCTCTGGATCTCATCTCCTGGCTTGCTCTCAACTCCCCAAGCTCTTTCATTTCCAGTTCACCTCACCTCCCAGCTCTCACCTCCCAGCTCTCCAGTCTCCCAGCCTTTACATAAAGA
      1690      1700      1710      1720      1730      1740      1750      1760      1770      1780      1790      1800

     ← intron 2⌉ N   K   S   F   R   R   V   N   L   S   K   F   V   E   S   Q   G   E   V   D   P   E   D   R   Y   V   I   K   S   N   L   Q⌈intron 3
TTTCTTGCCCTCTTAGAATAGACGTTTCGGACGAGTAAAATCGTGGAAAGCCAAGGACAGATACGTTATCAAGTCCAATCTTCAGTGTGTGG
      1810   ⌊1820      1830      1840      1850      1860      1870      1880      1890      1900      1910      1920
```

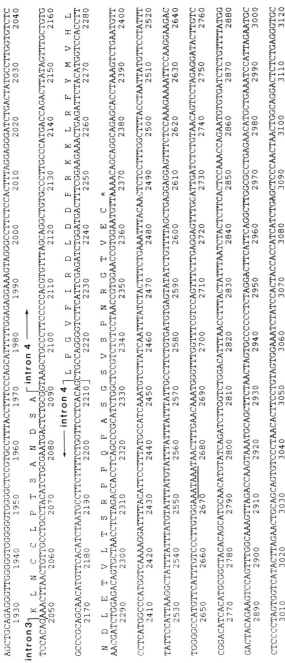

FIG. 2. Nucleotide sequence of the murine IL-3 gene and flanking regions. The sequence is that of the IL-3 gene isolated from BALB/c liver DNA by Campbell *et al.* (1985). The predicted amino acid sequence of IL-3 (Fig. 1) is aligned above the corresponding portions of the nucleotide sequence. Introns are indicated. The TATA box and AATAAA polyadenylation signal are underlined. The vertical arrow marks the start of transcription. (Reproduced from Campbell *et al.*, 1985, with permission of the *European Journal of Biochemistry.*)

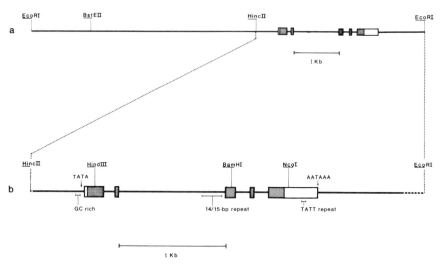

FIG. 3.   Organization of the murine IL-3 gene. a, The 8.5-kb *Eco*RI fragment containing the IL-3 gene from BALB/c DNA. b, The 3.7-kb *Hinc*II–*Eco*RI fragment containing
the IL-3 gene. Campbell *et al.* (1985) determined the nucleotide sequence of this fragment, excluding the dotted portions at the ends. The boxes on the lines indicate the
exons. Shaded portions of the boxes indicate IL-3 coding sequences and the unshaded
portions indicate the untranslated regions of the IL-3 mRNA. Unique *Hind*III, *Bam*HI
and *Nco*I sites in the 3.7-kb fragment are shown. The locations of the TATA box, AATAAA
polyadenylation signal, and the GC-rich region upstream of the TATA box are indicated.
Areas of tandem repeats, one based on a 14/15-bp repeating unit, the other on a TATT
unit, are also indicated.

The sequence of the exons is in exact agreement with the sequence of the
IL-3 cDNA from WEHI-3 (Fung *et al.*, 1984), establishing that the
unprocessed primary structure of IL-3 is identical in WEHI-3 and
BALB/c mice.

A conventional TATA box (Breathnach and Chambon, 1981; Nevins,
1983) is present 31 nucleotides upstream from the start of transcription,
as is typical of many eukaryotic promoters. Several potential CAAT box
sequences (Breathnach and Chambon, 1981) are present upstream from
the TATA box, the two closest being at nucleotides 381–389 and 392–400
(Fig. 2). These are separated from the TATA box by a very GC-rich
region (nucleotides 410–450, Fig. 2) in which 37 out of 41 bases are G or
C. This region exhibits marked strand asymmetry, with 29 Cs on the
coding strand, and is a candidate for an enhancer sequence (McKnight *et
al.*, 1984; McKnight and Kingsbury, 1982; Gidoni *et al.*, 1984; Khoury
and Gruss, 1983; Gruss, 1984). Experiments to test this are in progress.

A single AATAAA sequence, often referred to as a "polyadenylation signal" (Nevins, 1983; Proudfoot and Brownlee, 1976) is present in the 1123-bp-sequenced region beyond the translational termination codon. The exact site of endonucleolytic cleavage of the precursor mRNA to yield the 3' poly(A) attachment site (Montell *et al.*, 1983; Higgs *et al.*, 1983) is 12–14 bp downstream from the AATAAA sequence (Miyatake *et al.*, 1985).

The largest intron contains a tandem repeating sequence made up of ~12 copies of a 14- to 15-bp sequence. This repetitive element is located close to the 3' end of the intron. The consensus sequence for the repeats exhibits some homology with a human genomic repetitive DNA sequence isolated by hybridization with the BK virus enhancer sequence (Rosenthal *et al.*, 1983). This human sequence does exhibit some weak enhancer-like activity (Rosenthal *et al.*, 1983). The repeat in the IL-3 intron also shows some homology with a repeat within a human myoglobin gene intron (Weller *et al.*, 1984). We have also noticed that this IL-3 repeat shows some similarity to a highly conserved 21-bp repeat sequence present in the U3 region of the long terminal repeats (LTRs) of both HTLV-I and HTLV-II (Seiki *et al.*, 1983; Shimotohno *et al.*, 1984; Sodroski *et al.*, 1984). An alignment of these sequences is shown in Fig. 4. It has been suggested that these repeats in HTLV-I and -II may play a part in conferring lymphoid cell specificity on these retroviruses (Shimotohno *et al.*, 1984; Sodroski *et al.*, 1984). The possible enhancer activity of the IL-3 intron repeat is under examination.

Another tandem repetitive element is present in the IL-3 gene between the translational termination codon and the polyadenylation signal (Campbell *et al.*, 1985). This element appears to be based on a TATT repeat unit and resembles similarly located areas of the human IL-2 gene (Degrave *et al.*, 1983; Fujita *et al.*, 1983; Holbrook *et al.*, 1984), members of the human interferon-α gene family (Goeddel *et al.*, 1981), and the murine GM-CSF gene (Stanley *et al.*, 1985).

BKV homolog GGTTATCACCTCCCT
IL-3   AGCTCTCACCTCCCT
                            C
HTLV-I&II   GGCTCTGACGTCTCC

FIG. 4. Alignment of consensus sequences for various repeats. The alignment of the consensus sequence for the 14/15-bp tandem repeat in intron 2 of the IL-3 gene with part of a consensus sequence for the human BKV-like 21-bp tandem repeats (Rosenthal *et al.*, 1983) was noted by Campbell *et al.* (1985) and Miyatake *et al.* (1985). The alignment of the IL-3 repeat consensus with part of the consensus sequence for a conserved 21-bp repeat present in the U3 region of the LTRs of HTLV-I and -II (Seiki *et al.*, 1983; Shimotohno *et al.*, 1984; Sodroski *et al.*, 1984) is also shown.

A number of lymphokines are produced by T lymphocytes following stimulation with antigen or mitogen. For IL-3, IL-2 and interferon-γ, control of expression appears to be exerted at the transcriptional level since mRNA for these lymphokines can be detected in stimulated T lymphocytes but not in unstimulated ones (Yokota *et al.*, 1984; Taniguchi *et al.*, 1981, 1983). There is little highly significant homology between the 5' and 3' flanking regions of the IL-2 and interferon-γ genes (Gray and Goeddel, 1982; Degrave *et al.*, 1983; Fujita *et al.*, 1983). On comparison of the murine IL-3 gene with the human IL-2 and interferon-γ genes, it was found that all three genes contained the sequence TTTC-CAGTT (Campbell *et al.*, 1985). Two copies of this sequence are present in the tandem repeat in intron 2 of the IL-3 gene; in the IL-2 gene a single copy is also present in intron 2, whereas in the interferon-γ gene, a single copy is present 3' to the polyadenylation signal. It is possible that such a sequence could play a role in the coordinate expression of these genes by activated T lymphocytes. It is now feasible to test the role of the various sequence elements outlined here in the control of IL-3 gene expression.

IV. Expression of IL-3 from Recombinant DNA Constructs

A. EXPRESSION IN EUKARYOTIC CELLS

The expression of IL-3 from IL-3 cDNA clones in eukaryotic cells has provided an opportunity to examine the range of biological activities possessed by IL-3 without some of the problems associated with the use of purified factors from "normal" biological sources. Hapel *et al.* (1985) and Rennick *et al.* (1985) have studied the biological properties of recombinant IL-3 with broadly similar findings.

Hapel *et al.* (1985) recloned an IL-3 cDNA into pSV2*neo* (Southern and Berg, 1982) and transfected monkey COS-1 cells with the resulting construct. The chromatographic properties of the transiently expressed IL-3 on diethylaminoethyl Sephacel and phenyl Sepharose were the same as those of IL-3 produced by WEHI-3, and the expressed IL-3 was purified 10,000-fold in this way. The expressed material exhibited growth factor activity for IL-3-dependent cell lines and mast cells ("P" cells), the ability to induce 20αSDH in nu/nu splenic lymphocytes, as well as colony stimulating activity for granulocyle–macrophage, eosinophil, megakaryocyte, natural-killer-like, erythroid, and multipotential colony forming cells from murine fetal liver and adult bone marrow.

The broad range of biological activities exhibited by this expressed material includes all of those previously attributed to IL-3 and to a number of other factors/activities postulated to be identical with IL-3 on the basis of studies with highly purified material from WEHI-3- or spleen-conditioned medium (e.g., Ihle *et al.*, 1982, 1983), or with antibodies to such material (Bowlin *et al.*, 1984), and on the basis of other criteria. These other factors have included erythroid colony stimulating factor, burst-promoting activity, hemopoietic cell growth factor, P cell stimulating factor, multipotential colony stimulating factor, and MCGF.

In the complementary study by Rennick *et al.* (1985), a full-length IL-3 cDNA which had been cloned directly in a eukaryotic expression vector (Section II) was employed. In addition to some of the activities mentioned above, it was shown that the expressed factor exhibited Thy-1-inducing factor activity. The absence of T cell growth factor activity and B cell growth or differentiation factor activity was also reported.

As a control to correct for any background activities present, Hapel *et al.* (1985) used medium from COS cells transfected with empty vector, i.e., pSV2-*neo* (Southern and Berg, 1982), without any insert. Rennick *et al.* (1985) used medium from mock-transfected COS cells and, in some instances, medium from cells transfected with an incomplete IL-3 cDNA in the expression vector. The necessity for this type of control is illustrated by the finding (Hapel *et al.*, 1985) that control vector-transfected COS cell medium contained a low but detectable level of macrophage CSF; it was suggested that this may have been responsible for the increased percentage of macrophage colonies in bone marrow cultures stimulated by the expressed IL-3 relative to purified IL-3.

This type of problem can only be completely overcome when recombinant IL-3 is prepared in large amounts by high-level expression of the cDNA in bacteria, yeast, or in mammalian cells and subsequently purified to homogeneity. Expression in mammalian cells has the advantage for some applications that at least partially correct posttranslational processing (glycosylation, etc.) is expected to occur. Recently, with the availability of the complete amino acid sequence, IL-3 and some analogues have been prepared by solid phase peptide synthesis (Clark-Lewis *et al.*, 1986), providing an alternative approach to the study of the biological properties of IL-3.

B. EXPRESSION IN *ECHERICHIA COLI*

High-level expression of IL-3 in microorganisms such as *E. coli* provides recombinant IL-3 in large amounts which is free of contaminating eukaryotic proteins such as other growth factors.

Initial work from this laboratory (M.-C. Fung and I. G. Young, unpublished) established that biologically active IL-3 could be produced in

E. coli, indicating that glycosylation is not essential for activity. The most promising results were obtained using fusion constructs where the coding sequence for IL-3 was fused to the promoter, ribosome binding site, and a short portion of the N-terminal coding sequence of the *E. coli* β-galactosidase gene. These experiments have now been considerably extended in collaboration with Biotechnology Australia Pty. Ltd. (S. Clark *et al.*, unpublished) and highly purified recombinant IL-3 prepared in milligram quantities. The IL-3 expressed in *E. coli* has all of the biological activities described above for IL-3 expressed in monkey COS-1 cells. Bacterial expression of IL-3 has also been reported by Kindler *et al.* (1986).

The availability of relatively large amounts of recombinant IL-3 purified from *E. coli* has permitted us to produce several anti-IL-3 monoclonal antibodies. Lewis rats were immunized with several weekly injections of IL-3, and spleen cells were fused to EX-63 mouse myeloma cells three days after a final intravenous injection of 10^6 units. Serum from the sacrificed rats was shown to neutralize IL-3 activity measured on FDC-P1 cells and to inhibit proliferation of FDC-P1-IL3. Several antibody-producing hybridoma clones were identified by binding of antibody in culture supernatants to IL-3 coated plates, using an ELISA assay. Two types of antibody were found. One type, an IgM, bound strongly to both recombinant and "natural" IL-3, while another type, an IgG, bound preferentially to recombinant IL-3. The IgM antibody has proven useful in detecting IL-3 production in single cells by immunohistochemistry. This antibody is now being used as the basis of sensitive radioimmunoassays and enzyme-linked assays for IL-3 (P. Townsend and A. Hapel, unpublished).

C. RETROVIRAL EXPRESSION

Abnormal expression of a growth factor gene by a cell also expressing a functional receptor for that factor has been postulated as one possible mechanism by which a cell may become tumorigenic (Todaro and De Larco, 1978; Heldin and Westermark, 1984; Sporn and Roberts, 1985; Waterfield *et al.*, 1983; Doolittle *et al.*, 1983; Hunter, 1985). Constitutive synthesis of IL-3 by WEHI-3B cells may be related to the leukemic nature of this cell line by the operation of such an autocrine loop at some stage of the evolution of the tumor (Ymer *et al.*, 1985).

In order to more directly test this concept, we have been interested in the use of retroviral expression vectors. A recombinant retrovirus containing the murine IL-3 gene has been constructed using the "shuttle" vector fpGV-1 (Robins, *et al.*, 1986; Jhappan *et al.*, 1986). This vector was originally derived from HT-1 MSV and contains the bacterial ColE1 origin of replication, the SV40 origin of replication, and the neomycin resistance gene from transposon Tn5. The *Hinc*II-*Nco*I fragment of the murine IL-3 gene (Campbell *et al.*, 1985) was inserted into the M13-derived polylinker in the viral vector using *Eco*RI linkers. The clone fpGV-IL3 contains the IL-3 gene in the same transcriptional orientation as the viral genome.

In order to reconstitute infective virions, fpGV-IL3 was transfected into COS cells which had previously been infected with HIX virus. HIX is a recombinant helper virus which cannot transform cells but provides the necessary replicative functions in *trans*. The host range of HIX includes both murine and human cells. The supernatant from this transfection was used to infect NIH 3T3 cells which were subsequently selected in the presence of G418. These cells produced levels of IL-3 comparable to those produced by WEHI-3B (D⁻) cells.

The viral DNA from the G418-resistant, IL-3-producing NIH 3T3 cells was isolated by the shuttle method (Robins *et al.*, 1986) This procedure involves fusion of these cells to COS cells, Hirt extraction of low MW DNA, transformation of *E. coli*, and selection on kanamycin or neomycin. Analysis of these plasmid clones revealed that the *Eco*RI fragment carrying the IL-3 gene was ~1kb smaller than in the original clone, indicating that the IL-3 gene in fpGV-IL3 had been processed.

fpGV-IL3 was used to infect FDC-P1 cells, and the infected cells were selected in the presence of G418 and the absence of IL-3. A new cell line, FDC-P1-IL3, was derived in this way which proliferated independently of exogenous IL-3. The proliferation of FDC-P1-IL3 was blocked by anti-IL-3 antiserum, and this inhibition could be overcome by addition of GM-CSF. These data demonstrate that the independent growth of FDC-P1-IL3 requires secretion of IL-3, and that autocrine stimulation of cell growth has been achieved with these cells.

Culture supernatants from the FDC-P1-IL3 cell line were found to contain significant levels of IL-3 but did not contain detectable virus. The defective virus, however, could be rescued by superinfection with either HIX virus or the amphotropic virus 4070A. The failure of FDC-P1-IL3 to make infectious virus was an advantage in studies of the leukemic potential of this cell line since viral spread to host cells was precluded as a possible mechanism of leukemogenesis.

To test the leukemogenicity of the FDC-P1-IL3 cells, between 10⁶ and 10⁷ cells were injected intravenously into syngeneic (BALB/c) and allogeneic (NIH Swiss) mice. In BALB/c mice the FDC-P1-IL3 cells colonized the red pulp of spleen, the bone marrow, the liver, and the fatty tissues around the kidney, but not the lungs, lymph nodes, or thymus. In NIH Swiss inbred normal mice, FDC-P1-IL3 grew preferentially in lymph nodes, particularly mesenteric node, ovary, and mucosal surface (uterus, gut), while spleen enlargement was limited to a 2- to 3-fold increase in mononuclear cell number. Cells isolated from lymph nodes of NIH Swiss mice homed preferentially to lymph nodes in BALB/c mice. Cloned lines of such cells have now been shown to express elevated levels of receptor for IL-2 (R. Ceredig and A. Hapel, unpublished) compared to cloned lines derived from FDC-P1-IL3 passaged in BALB/c spleen. Addition of IL-2 to FDC-P1-IL3 or to FDC-P1 cells does not affect their rate of growth, suggesting that only low affinity receptors are present (Koyasu *et al.*, 1986). We are currently investigating the possibility that the low affinity receptor may play a role in homing or retention of leukemic cells in target organs, and that expression of particular receptors may influence metastasis in other tumor systems.

In contrast to FDC-P1 cells, normal bone marrow cells do not become leukemic when infected with the fpGV-IL3/HIX virus. Instead, such cells gave rise to continuous cultures containing predominantly P cells and a small proportion of granulocyte and uncommitted myeloid precursors. Such fpGV-IL3/HIX-infected cultures can be maintained for at least 11 months and can be passaged by splitting the culture every week. They provide a useful target for superinfection with other retroviral vectors containing *onc* genes.

V. Rearranged IL-3 Gene in WEHI-3B Leukemia

IL-3 is produced by T lymphocytes or T lymphomas only after stimulation with antigens, mitogens, or chemical activators such as phorbol esters. The myelomonocytic leukemia line WEHI-3B (Warner *et al.*, 1969; Metcalf and Nicola, 1982) also produces IL-3, but its production is constitutive (Metcalf *et al.*, 1969; Ralph *et al.*, 1976; Lee *et al.*, 1982) and the WEHI-3B cells do not appear to produce significant levels of any of the other lymphokines normally secreted by T lymphocytes after stimulation.

Southern transfer analysis of DNA from WEHI-3B has revealed genomic alteration in the vicinity of the IL-3 gene (Miyatake *et al.*, 1985; Campbell *et al.*, 1985; J. Ihle, personal communication). As well as the 8.5-kb *Eco*RI fragment which carries the IL-3 gene in BALB/c mice, from which WEHI-3B was originally derived, a second *Eco*RI fragment of 4 kb hybridizes with the IL-3 cDNA probe in WEHI-3B. It has been proposed by a number of workers that the genetic change leading to the constitutive synthesis of IL-3 may have been an important step in the development of the original leukemia from which the WEHI-3 cell line was derived (Iscove and Roitsch, 1985; Garland 1984;

Dexter and Allen, 1983; Schrader and Crapper, 1983). A differing view has also been expressed (Metcalf, 1985).

Recently, Ymer *et al.* (1985) have obtained and analyzed two groups of overlapping λ clones which span the altered IL-3 gene from WEHI-3 (4-kb *Eco*RI fragment) and the "normal" IL-3 gene from WEHI-3 (8.5-kb *Eco*RI fragment). It was found that the altered IL-3 gene contains a 5-kb insert 5' to the gene. This situation is shown in Fig. 5. The inserted element was identified as an intracisternal A particle (IAP) genome, as determined by nucleotide sequence analysis of the regions where the inserted element abuts the normal genomic sequence (see below).

IAPs (Finnegan, 1985) are a class of endogenous murine retrovirus-like particles found budding from the endoplasmic reticulum in mouse embryos and a variety of tumors (see Kuff and Fewell, 1985). There is no evidence that they are capable of functioning as infectious retroviruses. About 1000 IAP genomes are present in each copy of the haploid murine genome. These IAP genomes are analogous to the proviral forms of retroviruses (Varmus, 1982) and range in size up to 7 kb. IAP transcript levels are significantly elevated in some murine leukemias and other tumors (Augenlicht *et al.*, 1984).

Insertional mutations by IAP genomes have been reported for κ light chain genes (Kuff *et al.*, 1983), where inactivation of gene function occurred, and for the cellular oncogene c-*mos* (Canaani *et al.*, 1983), where the gene was activated (Horowitz *et al.*, 1984). Recently, an IAP genome

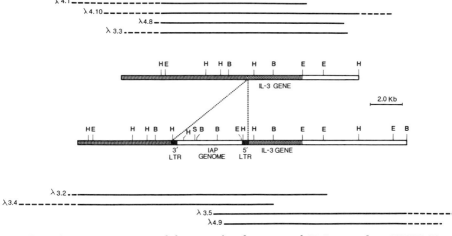

FIG. 5.   Restriction map of the normal and rearranged IL-3 genes from WEHI-3B. The inserted IAP genome and its LTRs are indicated. The λ clones from WEHI-3B, on which the map is based are shown. E, *Eco*RI; H, *Hind*III; B, *Bam*HI; S, *Sal*I.

has been found associated with one of the two renin genes of DBA/2 mice (Burt *et al.*, 1984), and there is some circumstantial evidence for gene activation in this case.

In WEHI-3, the IAP element is inserted in a head-to-head manner with respect to the IL-3 gene (Fig. 5), that is, the 5' LTR is close to the 5' end of the IL-3 gene. Its complete nucleotide sequence has now been obtained (Ymer *et al.*, 1986). The LTRs and adjacent sequences have features typical of retroviruses, and of IAPs in particular (Varmus, 1982; Ono and Ohishi, 1983; Chen and Barker, 1984), including transcriptional promoters, terminators, and polyadenylation signals. The IAP sequence immediately adjacent to the 5' LTR shows the expected phenylalanine tRNA primer binding site for (−) strand synthesis, and that adjacent to the 3' LTR shows the purine-rich (+) strand primer sequences. There is a 6-base (CACAAC) duplication of host sequence at the junctions of the insertion and the IL-3 gene as in other cases (Canaani *et al.*, 1983; Kuff *et al.*, 1983; Burt *et al.*, 1984).

The insertion is 215 bp upstream from the IL-3 gene's TATA box (Section III). The mechanism of activation of IL-3 expression by the IAP element is not yet clear. It appears that most IL-3 transcripts in WEHI-3B come from the IL-3 gene's normal promoter, since all three cDNA clones obtained from WEHI-3B (Fung *et al.*, 1984; H. D. Campbell, M.-C. Fung, and I. G. Young, unpublished results) have the same 5' end as full-length cDNA clones from a T cell line (Yokota *et al.*, 1984). One possibility is that the IAP genome provides an enhancer sequence which allows constitutive transcription from the normal IL-3 promoter. The LTRs (Chen and Barker, 1984) of IAP elements and other retroviruses contain sequences homologous to the SV40 core enhancer sequence, and in some cases the enhancer activity of LTR sequences has been demonstrated in expression systems (Christy *et al.*, 1985; Khoury and Gruss, 1983; Gruss, 1984). Alternatively, the IAP genome may abolish the effect of a *cis*-acting regulatory sequence by insertional inactivation or by moving it away from the IL-3 gene.

In order to directly examine the effect of the inserted IAP element on IL-3 gene expression, λ clone DNA containing copies of either the normal IL-3 gene from WEHI-3 or the rearranged IL-3 gene with the inserted IAP element was transfected into NIH 3T3 cells by the calcium phosphate precipitation technique (Graham and Bacchetti, 1983). Transient expression of IL-3 in supernatants from transfected cells was detected only when the IAP insertion was present and levels of IL-3 activity up to 22% of those produced by WEHI-3B cells were observed (Fig. 6; Ymer *et al.*, 1985). Similar results were obtained using monkey COS-1 cells.

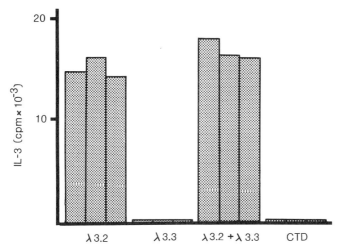

FIG. 6.   IL-3 production by NIH 3T3 cells following transfection with λ clones from WEHI-3B (Fig. 5). λ 3.2 contains a copy of the IL-3 gene with the IAP insertion, and λ 3.3 contains a copy of the IL-3 gene without the insertion. Clone DNA plus carrier calf thymus DNA (CTD) or CTD alone was used to transfect NIH 3T3 cells by the calcium phosphate method (Graham and Bacchetti, 1983). After 8 days, activity in the supernatants was assayed using 32D cl-23 cells (Ihle *et al.*, 1982; Hapel *et al.*, 1984). (Reproduced from Ymer *et al.*, 1985, with permission of *Nature.*)

These experiments provide direct evidence that the IAP insertion in the rearranged IL-3 gene in WEHI-3 is sufficient to bring about the unregulated expression of IL-3 from the altered gene and leave little doubt that the IAP insertion is responsible for the constitutive synthesis of IL-3 by WEHI-3. Further work is necessary to define the relationship, if any, between IL-3 gene activation and the development of the WEHI-3B leukemia.

VI. Conclusion

The cloning of cDNA for IL-3 (Fung *et al.*, 1984; Yokota *et al.*, 1984) has resulted in major advances in our knowledge of this lymphokine as discussed in the preceding sections. These advances have ranged from the primary structure of the IL-3 protein and the nucleotide sequence of the IL-3 gene and flanking regions to the delineation of the retroviral insertion which has brought about constitutive IL-3 synthesis by the leukemic cell line WEHI-3B. The control of IL-3 gene expression in both normal and malignant cells is a further area which is now under active investigation.

The construction of a retroviral expression vector carrying the IL-3 gene is allowing new approaches to be used to study the consequences of abnormal expression of the IL-3 gene in IL-3 dependent cells and in whole animals. There is increasing interest in the role of autostimulatory mechanisms in oncogenesis (Heldin and Westermark, 1984; Sporn and Roberts, 1985). A variety of circumstantial evidence supports the possible autocrine role of transforming growth factors (Todaro and De Larco, 1978; Derynck et al., 1984; Lee et al., 1985), and several oncogenes appear to be related to growth factors or their receptors (Waterfield et al., 1983; Doolittle et al., 1983; Downward et al., 1984; Sherr et al., 1985). Of interest in this regard is the IL-3 receptor which has not as yet been characterized in detail.

A potentially important application of IL-3 cDNA probes is in tissue hybridization. This technique has a number of applications and should provide a powerful approach for determining which cells produce IL-3 both normally and in various disease states.

Recombinant IL-3 protein, now available in large amounts as a result of expression studies in E. coli, should prove valuable in further biological studies of IL-3, in the generation of monoclonal antibodies against IL-3, and for studies of the IL-3 receptor. The next year or two should see further significant advances in our understanding of IL-3 and the biological processes in which it is involved.

While IL-3 has been extensively characterized in the mouse, little is known about IL-3 in other mammals. In hybridization studies of mammalian DNAs using the murine cDNA probe, we have failed to detect homologous sequences in most mammalian species other than rodents. This apparent low conservation of mammalian IL-3 genes contrasts with genes for other lymphokines. We have recently characterized the rat IL-3 gene and expressed this gene in monkey COS cells (Cohen et al., 1986). While the flanking regions, introns, and intron/exon junctions are highly conserved, there is relatively low conservation of sequence in the coding regions of the rat and mouse IL-3 genes. This is reflected in the amino acid homology which is only 54% for mature rat and mouse IL-3. Expression experiments have demonstrated that the rat IL-3 gene encodes a multilineage growth regulator which appears to have an analogous biological role to mouse IL-3. The low amino acid homology between rat and mouse IL-3 correlates with the demonstration that rat and mouse IL-3 show little cross reactivity. It appears that rat IL-3, together with its receptor, has evolved significantly away from the mouse IL-3 receptor system.

In terms of potential clinical applications, an important goal is the isolation of cDNA clones encoding human IL-3. To date, hybridization approaches using the murine IL-3 cDNA clones or oligonucleotide probes based on this sequence have not been successful. A number of laboratories are currently seeking to characterize the human equivalent of murine IL-3 and to isolate the gene concerned. The availability of cDNA clones for human IL-3 would provide a new window into the regulation of hemopoiesis in man.

ACKNOWLEDGMENTS

This work was supported in part by the Children's Leukaemia and Cancer Foundation.

REFERENCES

Augenlicht, L. M., Kobrin, D., Pavlovec, A., and Royston, M. E. (1984). *J. Biol. Chem.* **259**, 1842–1847.

Benton, W. D., and Davis, R. W. (1977). *Science* **196**, 180–182.

Bowlin, T. L., Scott, A. N., and Ihle, J. N. (1984). *J. Immunol.* **133**, 2001–2006.

Breathnach, R., and Chambon, P. (1981). *Annu. Rev. Biochem.* **50**, 349–383.

Burt, D. W., Reith, A. D., and Brammar, W. J. (1984). *Nucleic Acids Res.* **12**, 8579–8593.

Campbell, H. D., Ymer, S., Fung, M.-C., and Young, I. G. (1985). *Eur. J. Biochim.* **150**, 297–304.

Canaani, E., Dreazen, O., Klar, A., Rechavi, G., Ram, D., Cohen, J. B., and Givol, D. (1983). *Proc. Natl. Acad. Sci. U.S.A.* **80**, 7118–7122.

Chen, H. R., and Barker, N. C. (1984). *Nucleic Acids Res.* **12**, 1767–1778.

Christy, R. J., Brown, A. R., Gourlie, B. B., and Huang, R. C. C. (1985). *Nucleic Acids Res.* **13**, 289–302.

Clark-Lewis, I., Kent, S. B. H., and Schrader, J. W. (1984). *J. Biol. Chem.* **259**, 7488–7494.

Clark-Lewis, I., Aebersold, R., Ziltener, H., Schrader, J. W., Hood, L. E., and Kent, S. B. H. (1986). *Science*, **231**, 134–139.

Cohen, D. R., Hapel, A. J., and Young, I. G. (1986). *Nucleic Acids Res.* **14**, 3641–3658.

Conlon, P. J., Luk, K. H., Park, L. S., March, C. J., Hopp, T. P., and Urdal, D. L. (1985). *J. Immunol.* **135**, 328–332.

DeGrave, W., Tavernier, J., Duerinck, F., Plaetinck, G., Devos, R., and Fiers, W. (1983). *EMBO J.* **2**, 2349–2353.

Deininger, P. L. (1983). *Anal. Biochem.* **129**, 216–223.

Derynck, R., Roberts, A. B., Winkler, M. E., Chen, E. Y., and Goeddel, D. V. (1984). *Cell* **38**, 287–297.

Devos, R., Cheroutre, H., Taya, Y., Degrave, W., Van Heuverswyn, H., and Fiers, W. (1982). *Nucleic Acid Res.* **20**, 2487–2501.

Devos, R., Plaetinck, G., Cheroutre, H., Simons, G., Degrave, W., Tavernier, J., Remaut, E., and Fiers, W. (1983). *Nucleic Acids Res.* **11**, 4307–4323.

Dexter, T. M., and Allen, T. D. (1983). *J. Pathol.* **141**, 415–433.

Doolittle, R. F., Hunkapiller, M. W., Hood, L. E., Devare, S. G., Robbins, K. C., Aaronson, S. A., and Antoniades, H. N. (1983). *Science* **221**, 275–277.

Downward, J., Yarden, Y., Mayes, E., Scrace, G., Totty, N., Stockwell, P., Ullrich, A., Schlessinger, J., and Waterfield, M. D. (1984). *Nature (London)* **307**, 521–527.

Edelhoch, H. (1967). *Biochemistry* **6**, 1948–1954.

Finnegan, D. J. (1985). *Int. Rev. Cytol.* **93**, 281–326.

Fujita, T., Takaoka, C., Matsui, H., and Taniguchi, T. (1983). *Proc. Natl. Acad. Sci. U.S.A.* **80**, 7437–7441.

Fung, M. C., Hapel, A. J., Ymer, S., Cohen, D. R., Johnson, R. M., Campbell, H. D., and Young, I. G. (1984). *Nature (London)* **307**, 233–237.

Garland, J. M. (1984). *In* "Lymphokines" (E. Pick, ed.), Vol. 9, pp. 153–200. Academic Press, New York.

Gidoni, D., Dynan, W. S., and Tjian, R. (1984). *Nature (London)* **312**, 409–413.

Goeddel, D. V., Leung, D. W., Dull, T. J., Gross, M., Lawn, R. M., McCandliss, R., Seeburg, P. H., Ullrich, A., Yelverton, E., and Gray, P. W. (1981). *Nature (London)* **290**, 20–26.

Gottesman, S., Gottesman, M., Shaw, J. E., and Pearson, M. L. (1981). *Cell* **24**, 225–233.

Gough, N. M., Gough, J., Metcalf, D., Kelso, A., Grail, D., Nicola, N. A., Burgess, A. W., and Dunn, A. R. (1984). *Nature (London)* **309**, 7763–7767.

Gough, N. M., Metcalf, D., Gough, J., Grail, D., and Dunn, A. R. (1985). *EMBO J.* **4**, 645–653.

Graham, F. L., and Bacchetti, S. (1983). *In* "Techniques in the Life Sciences," Vol. B5. Elsevier, Amsterdam.

Gray, P. W., and Goeddel, D. V. (1982). *Nature (London)* **298**, 859–863.

Gray, P. W., Leung, D. W., Pennica, D., Yelverton, E., Najarian, R., Simonsen, C. C., Derynck, R., Sherwood, P. I., Wallace, D. M., Berger, S. L., Levinson, A. D., and Goeddel, D. V. (1982). *Nature (London)* **295**, 503–508.

Greenberger, K., Sakakeeny, A., Humphries, R. V., Eaves, C. S., and Eckner, R. J. (1983). *Proc. Natl. Acad. Sci. U.S.A.* **80**, 2931–2935.

Gruss, P. (1984). *DNA* **3**, 1–5.

Hapel, A. J., Warren, H. S., and Hume, D. A. (1984). *Blood* **64**, 786–790.

Hapel, A. J., Fung, M. C., Johnson, R. M., Young, I. G., Johnson, G., and Metcalf, D. (1985). *Blood* **65**, 1,453–1,459.

Heldin, C.-H., and Westermark, B. (1984). *Cell* **37**, 9–20.

Higgs, D. R., Goodbourn, S. E. Y., Lamb, J., Clegg, J. B., Weatherall, D. J., and Proudfoot, N. J. (1983). *Nature (London)* **306**, 398–400.

Holbrook, N. J., Smith, K. A., Fornace, A. J., Comeau, C. M., Wiskocil, R. C., and Crabtree, G. R. (1984). *Proc. Natl. Acad. Sci. U.S.A.* **81**, 1634–1638.

Horowitz, M., Luria, S., Rechavi, G., and Givol, D. (1984). *EMBO J.* **3**, 2937–2941.

Hunter, T. (1985). *Trends in Biochem. Sci.* **July**, 275–280.

Ihle, J. N., Keller, J., Greenberger, J. S., Henderson, L., Yetter, R. A., and Morse, H. C. (1982). *J. Immunol.* **129**, 1377–1383.

Ihle, J. N., Keller, J., Oroszlan, S., Henderson, L. E., Copeland, T. D., Fitch, F., Prystowsky, M. D., Goldwasser, E., Schrader, J. W., Palaszynski, E., Dy, M., and Lebel, B. (1983). *J. Immunol.* **131**, 282–287.

Iscove, N. N., and Roitsch, C. (1985). *In* "Cellular and Molecular Biology of Lymphokines" (C. Sorg and A. Schimpl, eds.). Academic Press, New York.

Jhappan, C., Vande Woude, G. F., and Robins, T. S. (1986). *J. Virol.*, in press.

Khoury, G., and Gruss, P. (1983). *Cell* **33**, 313–314.

Kindler, V., Thorens, B., De Kossodo, S., Allet, B., Eliason, J. F., Thatcher, D., Farber, N., and Vassalli, P. (1986). *Proc. Natl. Acad. Sci. U.S.A.* **83**, 1001–1005.

Koyasu, S., Yodoi, J., Nikaido, T., Tagaya, Y., Taniguchi, Y., Honjo, T., and Yahara, I. (1986). *J. Immunol.* **136**, 984–987.

Kuff, E. L., and Fewell, J. W. (1985). *Mol. Cell. Biol.* **5**, 474–483.

Kuff, E. L., Feenstra, A., Lueders, K., Smith, L., Hawley, R., Hozumi, N., and Shulman, M. (1983). *Proc. Natl. Acad. Sci. U.S.A.* **80**, 1992–1996.

Land, H., Grez, M., Hauser, H., Lindenmaier, W., and Schutz, G. (1981). *Nucleic Acids Res.* **9**, 2251–2266.

Langford, C. J., Klinz, F.-J., Donath, C., and Gallwitz, D. (1984). *Cell* **38**, 645–653.

Leder, P., Tiemeier, D., and Enquist, L. (1977). *Science* **196**, 175–177.

Lee, J. C., Hapel, A. J., and Ihle, J. N. (1982). *J. Immunol.* **128**, 2393–2398.

Lee, D. C., Rose, T. M., Webb, N. R., and Todaro, G. J. (1985). *Nature (London)* **313**, 489–491.

McKnight, S. L., and Kingsbury, R. (1982). *Science* **217**, 316–324.

McKnight, S. L., Kingsbury, R. C., Spence, A., and Smith, M. (1984). *Cell* **37**, 253–262.

Metcalf, D. (1985). *Science* **229**, 16–22.

Metcalf, D., and Nicola, N. A. (1982). *Int. J. Cancer* **30**, 773–780.

Metcalf, D., Moore, M. A. S., and Warner, N. L. (1969). *J. Natl. Cancer Inst.* **43**, 983–1001.

Michelson, A. M., and Orkin, S. H. (1982). *J. Biol. Chem.* **257**, 14773–14782.

Miyatake, S., Yokota, T., Lee, F., and Arai, K.-I. (1985). *Proc. Natl. Acad. Sci. U.S.A.* **82**, 316–320.

Montell, C., Fisher, E. F., Caruthers, M. H., and Berk, A. J. (1983). *Nature (London)* **305**, 600–605.

Nabel, G., Galli, S. J., Dvorak, A. M., Dvorak, H. F., and Cantor, H. (1981). *Nature (London)* **291**, 332–334.

Nevins, J. R. (1983). *Annu. Rev. Biochem.* **52**, 441–466.

Nicola, N. A., and Vadas, M. (1984). *Immunol. Today* **5**, 76–80.

Okayama, H., and Berg, P. (1983). *Mol. Cell Biol.* **3**, 280–289.

Ono, M., and Ohishi, H. (1983). *Nucleic Acids Res.* **11**, 7169–7179.

Parnes, J. R., Velen, B., Felsenfeld, A., Ramanathan, L., Ferrini, U., Appella, E., and Seidman, J. G. (1981). *Proc. Natl. Acad. Sci. U.S.A.* **78**, 2253–2257.

Proudfoot, N. J., and Brownlee, G. G. (1976). *Nature (London)* **263**, 211–214.

Ralph, P., Moore, M. A. S., and Nilsson, K. (1976). *J. Exp. Med.* **143**, 1528–1533.

Rennick, D. M., Lee, F. D., Yokota, T., Arai, K.-I., Cantor, H., and Nabel, G. J. (1985). *J. Immunol.* **134**, 910–914.

Robins, T. S., Vande Woude, G. F., Campbell, H. D., Young, I. G., and Hapel, A. J. Submitted .

Rosenthal, N., Kress, M., Gruss, P., and Khoury, G. (1983). *Science* **222**, 749–755.

Russell, D. R., and Bennett, G. N. (1982). *Gene* **20**, 231–243.

Sanger, F., Nicklen, S., and Coulson, A. R. (1977). *Proc. Natl. Acad. Sci. U.S.A.* **74**, 5463–5467.

Sanger, F., Coulson, A. R., Hong, G. F., Hill, D. F., and Petersen, G. B. (1982). *J. Mol. Biol.* **162**, 729–773.

Schrader, J. W., and Crapper, R. M. (1983). *Proc. Natl. Acad. Sci. U.S.A.* **80**, 6892–6896.

Seiki, M., Hattori, S., Hirayama, Y., and Yoshida, M. (1983). *Proc. Natl. Acad. Sci. U.S.A.* **80**, 3618–3622.

Sharp, P. A. (1980). *Cell* **23**, 643–646.

Sherr, C. J., Rettenmier, C. W., Sacca, R., Roussel, M. F., Look, A. T., and Stanley, E. R. (1985). *Cell*, **41**, 665–676.

Shimotohno, K., Golde, D. W., Miwa, M., Sugimura, T., and Chen, I. S. Y. (1984). *Proc. Natl. Acad. Sci. U.S.A.* **81**, 1079–1083.

Sodroski, J., Trus, M., Perkins, D., Patarca, R., Wong-Stahl, F., Gelmann, E., Gallo, R., and Haseltine, W. A. (1984). *Proc. Natl. Acad. Sci. U.S.A.* **81**, 4617–4621.

Southern, E. M. (1975). *J. Mol. Biol.* **98**, 503–517.

Southern, P. J., and Berg, P. (1982). *J. Mol. Appl. Genet.* **1**, 327–341.

Sporn, M. B., and Roberts, A. B. (1985). *Nature (London)* **313**, 745–747.

Stanley, E., Metcalf, D., Sobieszczuk, P., Gough, N. M., and Dunn, A. R. (1985). *EMBO J.* **4**, 2569–2573.

Taniguchi, T., Pang, R. H. L., Yip, Y. K., Henriksen, D., and Vilcek, J. (1981). *Proc. Natl. Acad. Sci. U.S.A.* **75**, 3469–3472.

Taniguchi, T., Matsui, H., Fujita, T., Takaoka, C., Kashima, N., Yoshimoto, R., and Hamuro, J. (1983). *Nature (London)* **302**, 305–310.

Todaro, G. J., and De Larco, J. E. (1978). *Cancer Res.* **38**, 4147–4153.

Varmus, H. E. (1982). *Science* **216**, 812–820.

Von Heijne, G. (1983). *Eur. J. Biochem.* **133**, 17–21.

Warner, N. L., Moore, M. A. S., and Metcalf, D. (1969). *J. Natl. Cancer Inst.* **43**, 963–982.

Waterfield, M. D., Scrace, G. T., Whittle, N., Stroobant, P., Johnsson, A., Wasteson, A., Westermark, B., Heldin, C.-H., Huang, J. S., and Deuel, T. F. (1983). *Nature (London)* **304**, 35–39.

Weber, K., Pringle, J. R., and Osborn, M. (1972). *In* "Methods in Enzymology" (C. H. W. Hirs and S. N. Timasheff, eds.), Vol. 26, pp. 3–27. Academic Press, New York.

Weller, P., Jeffreys, A. J., Wilson, V., and Blanchetot, A. (1984). *EMBO J.* **3**, 430–446.

Ymer, S., Tucker, W. Q. J., Sanderson, C. J., Hapel, A. J., Campbell, H. D., and Young, I. G. (1985). *Nature (London)*, **317**, 255–258.

Ymer, S., Tucker, W. Q. J., Campbell, H. D., and Young, I. G. (1986). *Nucleic Acids Res.* **14**, 5901–5918.

Yokota, T., Lee, F., Rennick, D., Hall, C., Arai, N., Mosmann, T., Nabel, G., Cantor, H., and Arai, K.-I. (1984). *Proc. Natl. Acad. Sci. U.S.A.* **81**, 1070–1074.

Organization of Chromosomal Genes for Interleukin 3 and Granulocyte–Macrophage Colony Stimulating Factor and Their Expression in Activated T cells

TAKESHI OTSUKA, SHOICHIRO MIYATAKE, TAKASHI YOKOTA,
JOAN CONAWAY, RON CONAWAY, NAOKO ARAI,
FRANK LEE, AND KEN-ICHI ARAI

DNAX Research Institute of Molecular and Cellular Biology, Palo Alto, California 94304

I. Signal Transduction during T Cell Activation and Expression of Lymphokines

Helper T cells activated by antigen or lectins such as concanavalin A produce several lymphokines. These secreted proteins affect the growth and differentiation of certain lymphopoietic and hematopoietic cells (Nabel *et al.*, 1981; Prytowsky *et al.*, 1982). Other proteins, such as the IL-2 receptor or nuclear oncogenes such as c-*myc* and p53 are also induced during T cell activation (Fig. 1). Although activation of protein kinase C and increased calcium influx (Nishizuka, 1984) have been suggested as early events in T cell activation (Weiss *et al.*, 1984; Kaibuchi *et al.*, 1985), the mechanism that regulates the coordinate induction of these genes is largely unknown.

To study the mechanism of lymphokine induction during T cell activation, we have chosen a molecular biology approach which includes (1) determination of the structure of chromosomal genes for several lymphokines, (2) characterization of regions required for regulated expression of lymphokine genes, and (3) identification of cellular components that interact with regulatory regions of lymphokine genes.

We have previously isolated a set of full-length lymphokine cDNA clones from activated mouse and human T cells using a pcD mammalian expression vector (Yokota *et al.*, 1984, 1985; Lee *et al.*, 1985). This paper describes results of our studies in the structure and expression of lymphokine genes with an emphasis on those encoding the hematopoietic growth factors, IL-3 (multi-CSF) and GM-CSF. Knowledge of the structure of these lymphokine genes and their regulatory regions will help to elucidate the molecular mechanisms linking antigen stimulation to the ultimate induction of lymphokine genes during T cell activation.

II. Structure of T Cell-Derived Lymphokine Genes

A. IL-3

The IL-3 gene isolated from a mouse sperm DNA library contains 5 exons and 4 introns (Fig. 2). The distance between the transcription

261

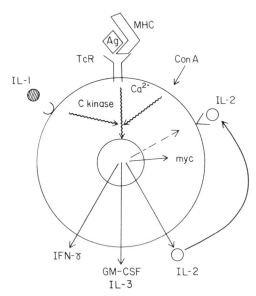

FIG. 1. Signal transduction during T cell activation. See text for discussion.

initiation site determined by S1 mapping and the nucleotide preceding the poly(A) stretch in the IL-3 cDNA clone is 2195 base pairs (bp). A "TATA"-like sequence is found 24 bp upstream from the transcription initiation site. This TATA box is preceded by a GC-rich region about 45-bp long which contains a C block in the sense strand.

One sequence which is conserved in the promoter region of many eukaryotic genes is the sequence GGCCAATCT, located ∼80 bp upstream of the cap site (Benoist *et al.*, 1980). We did not find a homologous sequence at ∼80 bp upstream of the cap site of the IL-3 gene. In

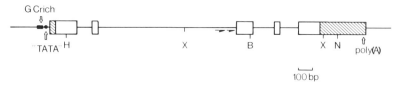

FIG. 2. Schematic representation of the mouse IL-3 gene. Open box, coding region of exons; hatched area, untranslated region; half arrows, the 73-bp duplicated sequence within the second introns; H, *Hind*III; X, *Xba*I; B, *Bam*HI; N, *Nco*I.

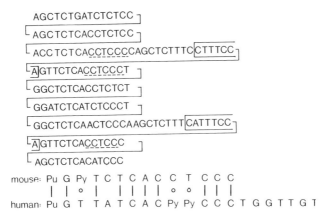

mouse: Pu G Py T C T C A C C T C C C
human: Pu G T T A T C A C Py Py C C C T G G T T G T

FIG. 3. Structure of repeated sequences in the mouse IL-3 gene. Above is the 14-bp and 73-bp repeat. A dashed line shows the GC-rich sequence that is found both in the SV40 GC-rich region upstream of the early promoter and in the BK virus enhancer sequence; a box defines the sequence that shares the homology with the complementary strand of the enhancer core sequence. Below is a comparison of consensus sequences of the 14-bp repeats in the mouse IL-3 gene and the 21-bp repeats in the human genome. Py, pyrimidine; Pu, purine.

the second intron of the IL-3 gene, there are 9 repeats of a closely related 14-bp sequence, interrupted by 2 segments of unique sequence. The region encompassing 8 of the repeats can be divided into two 73-bp direct repeats. Within each 73-bp repeat is a sequence homologous to the complementary strand of the enhancer core sequence (Weiher *et al.*, 1983) (Fig. 3). In addition, the IL-3 14-bp repeats share strong homology with a series of 20-bp repeats in the human genome having enhancer activity in several cell types (Rosenthal *et al.*, 1983). All of these sequences contain the sequence C-C-T-C-C-C which is similar to the sequence C-C-G-C-C-C found in the GC-rich region of the SV40 early promoter.

Southern blotting analysis performed with DNA isolated from spleen, cloned helper T cells, and the WEHI-3 cell line showed that there is only one copy of IL-3 gene in the mouse haploid genome (Miyatake *et al.*, 1985). Since one allele of the IL-3 gene is altered in WEHI-3 cells, we speculated that this rearrangement leads to the constitutive expression of IL-3 in WEHI-3 cells. Recently, Ymer *et al.* (1985) reported that this alteration is due to the insertion of a large terminal repeat derived from an intracisternal A particle genome into the 5' flanking region of the IL-3 gene.

B. GM-CSF

1. Structure of Mouse and Human GM-CSF Genes

There is a single copy gene encoding mouse GM-CSF (Gough *et al.*, 1984). Southern blotting analysis performed with chromosomal DNA isolated from HeLa cells, which are nonproducers, and Mo cells, which are constitutive producers of human GM-CSF, showed the same hybridization pattern indicating that each human haploid genome contains a single copy of the GM-CSF gene.

No detectable rearrangements were found in the GM-CSF gene in the Mo cell line. Therefore, constitutive production of lymphokines in Mo T cells may depend on a certain common activator rather than a gene rearrangement.

The mouse and human GM-CSF genes isolated from genomic λ phage libraries of mouse sperm and human placenta contain four exons and three introns (Fig. 4). The distance between the transcription initiation site determined by S1 mapping and the nucleotide preceding the poly(A) stretch in the human and mouse cDNA clones is 2376–2378 bp and 2371 bp, respectively.

As is the case for several other lymphokine genes (Gray and Goeddel, 1982, 1983; Fujita *et al.*, 1983; Fuse *et al.*, 1984; Miyatake *et al.*, 1985), each intron interrupts the reading frame precisely between codons. The

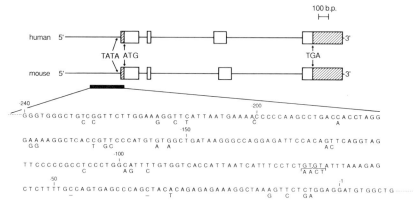

FIG. 4. Schematic representation of human and mouse GM-CSF genes. Open box, coding region of exons; hatched box, untranslated region; thin line, introns and the flanking region; thick bar, sequence of the highest homology in the 5' flanking region. The nucleotide sequence of this region of the human GM-CSF gene is shown at the bottom. Mouse nucleotides differing from the human sequence are shown underneath. Nucleotides missing in the mouse gene are indicated by bars. Nucleotides are numbered negatively upstream of the first base of the initiation codon.

consensus sequences for splicing junctions, G/GTAAG for the donor splice site and AG for the acceptor splice site, were found in all boundaries between introns and exons (Breathnach *et al.*, 1978).

"TATA"-like sequences are found 20–25 bp upstream from the transcription initiation sites of both genes. In the 5' flanking region of the mouse GM-CSF gene, 14 contiguous GT dinucleotides are found at about 1 kb upstream from the cap site. This sequence is found in the flanking region of many different mammalian genes and it is known to form a left-handed form of DNA (Wang *et al.*, 1979; Haniford *et al.*, 1983; Nordheim and Rich, 1983a,b). Such a sequence was reported to have an enhancer activity (Hamada *et al.*, 1984).

2. Comparison of Mouse and Human GM-CSF Genes

Both human and mouse GM-CSF genes are organized in a similar manner (Fig. 4). The sizes of exons 2, 3, and 4 (defined from the beginning of exon 4 to the stop codon TGA) are identical in both species and, therefore, each exon encodes exactly the same number of amino acid residues in both species. However, exon 1 of human GM-CSF gene is 9 bp longer than exon 1 of mouse GM-CSF. In addition, the length of each intron is nearly the same in both genes. The mouse GM-CSF gene contains four direct repeats in the second intron, but these repeated sequences are not found in the introns of the human GM-CSF gene. Nucleotide sequences of the mouse and human GM-CSF cDNA clones share ~70% homology and the amino acid sequences share ~50% homology (Lee *et al.*, 1985).

In general, intron sequences show more diversity than exon sequences. However, stretches which show >70% homology are clustered in each intron. The most highly conserved sequences (87% homology) were found in the region extending ~240 bp upstream of the initiator ATG codon (Fig. 4). Upstream sequences beyond this point show very little or no homology. The remarkable conservation of the overall structure and the nucleotide sequence of the human and mouse GM-CSF genes indicate that they evolved from a common ancestral gene. We conclude that the GM-CSF cDNA clone isolated from a Con A-stimulated human helper T cell clone encodes the human homologue of mouse GM-CSF.

C. COMPARISON OF 5' FLANKING REGIONS OF LYMPHOKINE GENES

Despite the lack of any convincing homology among four T cell-derived lymphokines (IL-2, IL-3, GM-CSF, and IFN-γ), some common features could be recognized (Fig. 5). All four genes have a relatively

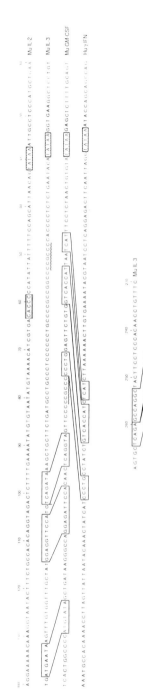

Fig. 5. The 5' flanking sequence of four different lymphokine genes (mouse IL-2, mouse IL-3, mouse GM-CSF, and human IFN-γ). Nucleotides are numbered negatively upstream of the transcription initiation site. Boxes with diagonal lines define a "TATA"-like sequence. The wavy line shows the GC-rich sequence that is found both in the SV40 GC-rich region upstream of the early promoter and in the herpes simplex virus gene promoter. A similar sequence found in mouse IL-2 is defined by a heavily shaded box. The open boxes show the regions which share homology between mouse IL-3 and mouse GM-CSF, and homology between mouse GM-CSF and human IFN-γ.

short second exon (40–70 bp), while the fourth exon is the longest. The first introns of IL-2, IL-3, and GM-CSF are of nearly the same size (90–100 bp). To find the potential consensus sequences which might be involved in regulated expression of lymphokine genes, the 5' flanking region sequences of these lymphokine genes were compared. Some sequence homologies were detected in some of the lymphokine genes.

In many mammalian genes the sequence GGGCGG, or the complementary sequence CCGCCC, appears in the 5' upstream region. This sequence element is known to be required for transcription of SV40 early genes and the herpes virus thymidine kinase gene, both *in vivo* and *in vitro* (Fromm and Berg, 1982; McKnight *et al.*, 1984). The transcription factor Spl specifically binds to this sequence element. (Dynan and Tijan, 1983). In the 5' upstream region of mouse IL-3 and mouse and human GM-CSF, this GC-rich sequence element is found about 50 bp and 80 bp from the cap site, respectively. A similar sequence, CACCC, is found about 60 bp upstream from the cap site of both mouse and human IL-2 genes. The requirement of this sequence for efficient transcription of the β-globin gene has been suggested by tranfection experiments (Dierks *et al.*, 1983), as well as by sequence analysis of DNA from β-thalassemia patients (Treisman *et al.*, 1983; Orkin *et al.*, 1982), but there is no such sequence in the 5' flanking region of the human IFN-γ gene.

There are some other sequence homologies in the 5' upstream region of mouse IL-3 and human and mouse GM-CSF. One is located about 90–130 bp from the cap site, and the other is located 240–260 bp from the cap site. An additional region of homology between mouse and human GM-CSF and human IFN-γ is located 50–70 and 80–100 bp upstream of transcription initiation sites of GM-CSF and IFN-γ genes, respectively. Whether or not these sequence elements are involved in the coordinate expression of the hematopoietic growth factor genes in T cells is under investigation.

III. Expression of Lymphokine Genes

A. INDUCTION OF LYMPHOKINE mRNAs

Induction for both human and mouse lymphokines at transcription level can be observed in activated T cells after Con A exposure. Approximately 10% of total T cell mRNA is induced after 10 hr. For example, Northern blot analysis with Con A-induced and uninduced mRNA prepared from the mouse helper T cell clone, LB2-1, showed that a mouse IL-3 cDNA probe hybridized to a single mRNA which was strongly inducible by Con A (Fig. 6). Similar results were also obtained for mouse

LB2-1

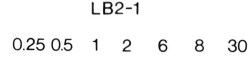

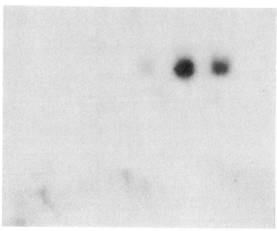

probe: Mu IL-3

FIG. 6. Northern blotting of a cloned mouse helper T cell line, LB2-1, using a mouse IL-3 specific cDNA probe. Numbers indicate the time (hr) after Con A treatment.

GM-CSF, IL-2, and IFN-γ. The transcripts of all these genes were detected within 2 hr after the addition of Con A, and the maximum level was observed for all these genes at about 5–8 hr. The frequency of mRNA specific for each gene is 0.1–1.0% of the total mRNA of activated helper T cells.

Human helper T cell clones showed strong induction of GM-CSF (Fig. 7), IL-2, and IFN-γ mRNAs after Con A exposure. GM-CSF mRNA induced in helper T-cells represents about 0.5–1.0% of the total mRNA; in contrast, Mo T cells produced low levels of GM-CSF mRNA constitutively.

B. EXPRESSION OF THE IL-3 GENE IN L CELLS

We have isolated stable transformants of L cells cotransfected with the IL-3 genomic clone (pλMGM12-4) DNA and pSV2neo. Of 12 clones, 11 showed relatively high IL-3 activity (Table I) (Miyatake et al., 1985). To examine the promoter function of the 5′ flanking region of the IL-3 gene, plasmid DNAs which carried the whole IL-3 gene and its flanking region (pλMGM12-4), or the 5′ flanking region fused with CAT (pSVIL3cat),

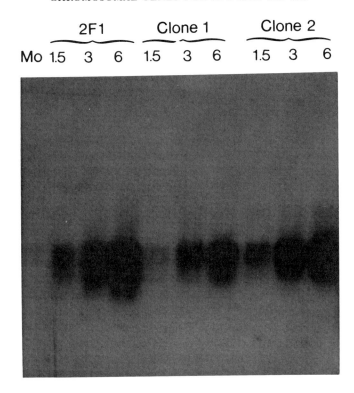

probe: Hu GM-CSF

FIG. 7. Northern blotting of cloned human T cells 2Fl, clone 2 and clone 3, and HTLV-transformed human T cell line Mo using a human GM-CSF specific cDNA probe. Numbers indicate the time (hr) after Con A treatment.

were transfected into L cells. Later (48 hr), the transient expression level was measured as IL-3 activity in supernatant or by CAT activity in cell extracts, respectively. In both cases, very little activity was detected, suggesting that the IL-3 promotor is not efficient in L cells. Why then do L cell stable transformants produce large quantities of IL-3? Southern blotting of chromosomal DNA from the highest producing stable transformant revealed that there were about one hundred integrated copies of the IL-3 gene. This suggests that the relatively high IL-3 production in these cells might be due to a copy number effect. Alternatively, two plasmids, pλMGM12-4 and pSV2neo, are ligated together in the integrated form, which may juxtapose SV40 promoter and enhancer sequences to the IL-3 gene, resulting in higher expression of IL-3.

In the second intron of mouse IL-3, there is a unique direct repeat

TABLE I

EXPRESSION OF IL-3 GENE IN STABLE
TRANSFORMANTS OF L CELLS

	IL-3 Activity (U/ml)
Mock transfected cell	<100
Stable transformant	
Clone 1	6217
Clone 2	608
Clone 3	3503
Clone 4	286
Clone 5	1991
Clone 6	416
Clone 7	1991
Clone 8	4517
Clone 9	2218
Clone 10	2400
Clone 11	91
Clone 12	10240
COS-supernatant transfected	
with pcD-IL-3	30720

which shares homology with repeats of the 20-bp sequence found in the human genome that has enhancer activity (see Section II,A). To investigate whether this repeat in IL-3 has enhancer activity, we introduced the repeated sequence into a plasmid carrying the SV40 early promoter which lacks an enhancer element. Preliminary results indicate that the repeat in the IL-3 gene has enhancer activity in mouse L cells.

C. TRANSCRIPTION OF THE IL-3 GENE in Vitro

Transcription by RNA polymerase II is efficiently initiated at the putative mouse IL-3 cap site in HeLa whole cell extracts prepared according to Manley *et al.* (1980). pMIL-3, a plasmid containing the mouse IL-3 5′ flanking regions and about one hundred nucleotides of coding sequence, was linearized at a site 330 nucleotides downstream from the cap site. When this linearized plasmid was used as a template in the presence of a HeLa whole cell extract, a transcript of approximately 330 nucleotides was observed (Fig. 8, lane 1). This transcript was sensitive to 0.5 μg/ml α-amanitin (Fig. 8, lane 2).

S1 nuclease mapping data are also consistent with *in vitro* initiation at the IL-3 cap site predicted from S1 mapping of *in vivo*-synthesized messenger RNA. Unlabeled *in vitro*-synthesized RNA was hybridized to a 5′ end-labeled probe at a site 115 bases downstream from the cap site. An

S1 nuclease digestion product of 112–115 bases was observed following polyacrylamide gel electrophoresis (Fig. 8, lane 3). This product was not observed when 0.5 μg/ml α-amanitin was included in the transcription reaction (Fig. 8, lane 4). Similar results were obtained when an extract prepared from the T cell hybridoma FS614.13 was used as a source of transcription enzymes (Fig. 8, lanes 5 and 6).

Since IL-3 may not be naturally expressed in cells other than activated T cells at high level, these results may indicate that the transcription of

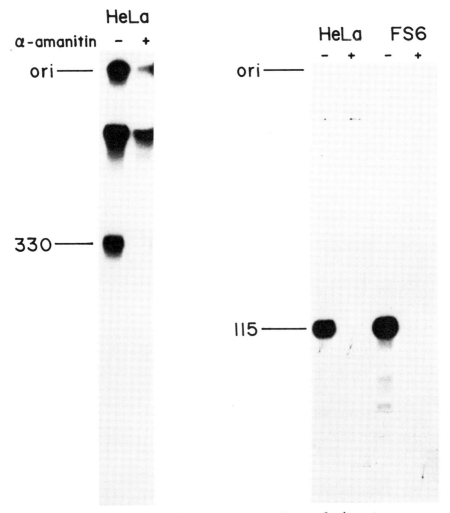

FIG. 8. Transcription of IL-3 gene *in vitro*. See text for discussion.

IL-3 in L cell stable transformants, and cell extracts prepared as described above, are not regulated. In order to further study the regulation of lymphokine genes during T cell activation, the establishment of improved experimental systems will be required. These include a method for introducing the genes into T cell clones and the preparation of T cell transcription extracts after activation.

IV. Role of T Cell-Derived CSFs in Hematopoiesis

Blood cells are produced and destroyed continuously under precise control mechanisms in bone marrow. Evidence indicates that the bone marrow stromal cells have a major role in normal, constitutive hematopoiesis (Dexter *et al.*, 1985). In helper T cells, the production of GM-CSF and IL-3 increases rapidly in response to activation by antigen or lectin, whereas no activity can be detected without activation. We have shown that induction of GM-CSF and IL-3 in helper T cells involves a transcriptional process. Inducible production of CSFs by T cells under immune stress may affect hematopoiesis in the bone marrow. Although the exact role of T cell-induced CSFs in normal hematopoiesis remains to be determined, abnormal (high, low, or constitutive) production of CSFs by T cells may contribute to the etiology of some hematopoietic disorders. This possibility could directly be tested at the mRNA level by use of cloned lymphokine gene probes. Hematopoietic diseases may also be caused by abnormal expression of CSFs by stromal cells, abnormal expression of CSFs and their receptors in hematopoietic progenitor cells, or alteration of the intracellular signal transduction pathways which regulate the proliferation and differentiation of hematopoietic progenitor cells. Studies on the regulation of expression of hematopoietic growth factor genes should shed light on the role of these factors in both normal and abnormal hematopoiesis.

REFERENCES

Benoist, C., O'Hare, K., Breathnach, R., and Chambon, P. (1980). *Nucleic Acids Res.* 8, 127–142.
Breathnach, R., Benoist, C., O'Hare, K., Gannon, F., and Chambon, P. (1978). *Proc. Natl. Acad. Sci. U.S.A.* 75, 4853–4857.
Dexter, T. M., Heyworth, C., and Whetton, A. D. (1985). *BioEssays 2*, 154–158.
Dierks, P., Van Ooyen, A., Cochran, M. D., Dobkin, C., Reiser, J., and Weissmann, C. (1983). *Cell 32*, 695–706.
Dynan, W. S., and Tijan, P. (1983). *Cell 32*, 669–680.
Fromm, M., and Berg, P. (1982). *J. Mol. Appl. Genet.* 1, 457–481.
Fujita, T., Takaoka, C., Matsui, H., and Taniguchi, T. (1983). *Proc. Natl. Acad. Sci. U.S.A.* 80, 7437–7441.
Fuse, A., Fujita, T., Yasumitsu, H., Kashima, N., Hasegawa, K., and Taniguchi, T. (1984). *Nucleic Acids Res.* 12, 9323–9331.

Gough, N. M., Gough, J., Metcalf, D., Kelso, A., Grail, D., Nicola, N. A., Burgess, A. W., and Dunn, A. R. (1984). *Nature (London)* **309**, 763–767.

Gray, P. W., and Goeddel, D. V. (1982). *Nature (London)* **298**, 859–863.

Gray, P. W., and Goeddel, D. V. (1983). *Proc. Natl. Acad. Sci. U.S.A.* **80**, 5842–5846.

Hamada, H., Seidman, M., Howard, B. H., and Gorman, C. M. (1984). *Mol. Cell. Biol.* **4**, 2622–2630.

Haniford, D. B., and Pulleyblank, D. E. (1983). *Nature (London)* **302**, 632–634.

Kaibuchi, K., Takai, Y., and Nishizuka, Y. (1985). *J. Biol. Chem.* **260**, 1366–1369.

Lee, F., Yokota, T., Otsuka, T., Gemmel, L., Larson, N., Luh, J., Arai, K., and Rennick, D. (1985). *Proc. Natl. Acad. Sci. U.S.A.* **82**, 4360–4364.

McKnight, S. L., Kingsbury, R. C., Spence, A., and Smith, M. (1984). *Cell* **37**, 253–262.

Manley, J. A., Fire, A., Cano, A., Sharp, P. A., and Gefter, M. (1980). *Proc. Natl. Acad. Sci. U.S.A* **77**, 3855–3859.

Miyatake, S., Yokota, T., Lee, F., and Arai, K. (1985). *Proc. Natl. Acad. Sci. U.S.A.* **82**, 316–320.

Nabel, G., Greenberger, J. S., Sakakeeny, M. A., and Cantor, H. (1981). *Proc. Natl. Acad. Sci. U.S.A.* **78**, 1157–1161.

Nishizuka, Y. (1984). *Nature (London)* **308**, 693–697.

Nordheim, A., and Rich, A. (1983a). *Nature (London)* **303**, 674–679.

Nordheim, A., and Rich, A. (1983b). *Proc. Natl. Acad. Sci. U.S.A.* **80**, 1821–1825.

Orkin, S. H., Kazazian, H. H., Antonarakis, S. E., Goff, S. C., Boehm, C. D., Sexton, J. P., Waber, P. G., and Giardina, P. J. V. (1982). *Nature (London)* **296**, 627–631.

Prystowsky, M. B., Ely, J. M., Beller, D. I., Eisenbert, L., Goldman, J., Remold, H., Vogel, S. N., and Fitch, F. W. (1982). *J. Immunol.* **129**, 2337–2344.

Rosenthal, N., Kress, M., Gruss, P., and Khoury, D. (1983). *Science* **222**, 749–755.

Treisman, R., Orkin, S. H., and Maniatis, T. (1983). *Nature (London)* **302**, 591–596.

Wang, A. H.-J., Quigley, G. J., Kolpack, F. J., Crawford, J. L., Van Boom, J. H., Van der Marel, G., and Rich, A. (1979). *Nature (London)* **282**, 680–686.

Weiher, H., Konig, M., and Gruss, P. (1983). *Science* **219**, 626–631.

Weiss, A., Imboden, J., Shobck, D., Stobo, J. (1984). *Proc. Natl. Acad. Sci. U.S.A.* **81**, 4169–4173.

Ymer, S., Tucker, W. Q. J., Sanderson, C. J., Hapel, A. J., Campbell, H. D., and Young, I. G. (1985). *Nature (London)* **317**, 255–258.

Yokota, T., Lee, F., Rennick, D., Hall, C., Arai, N., Mosmann, T., Nabel, G., Cantor, H., and Arai, K. (1984). *Proc. Natl. Acad. Sci. U.S.A.* **81**, 1070–1074.

Yokota, T., Arai, N., Lee, F., Rennick, D., Mosmann, T., and Arai, K. (1985). *Proc. Natl. Acad. Sci. U.S.A.* **82**, 68–72.

Glucocorticoid Regulation of Lymphokine Production by Murine T Lymphocytes

JANICE CULPEPPER AND FRANK LEE

DNAX Research Institute of Molecular and Cellular Biology, Palo Alto, California 94304

I. Introduction

Glucocorticoid hormones have a wide variety of effects on both lymphoid and nonlymphoid cells. These hormones, produced by the adrenal cortex, have predominantly catabolic effects on tissues such as muscle, bone, and lymphoid tissue, while the effects are primarily anabolic in the liver. Their action results in a general inhibition of protein synthesis in many tissues leading to a flow of amino acids to the liver where they are utilized for gluconeogenesis. While it is well known that many glucocorticoids can have potent antiinflammatory effects as well as immunosuppressive properties, the precise molecular mechanisms underlying these effects have been obscure. In this article, we will be primarily concerned with the specific effects glucocorticoids have on T lymphocytes. Other aspects of glucocorticoid effects on inflammation and immunoregulation have been covered in recent reviews (Crupps and Fauci, 1982; Fahey *et al.*, 1981).

A. GENERAL FEATURES OF STEROID HORMONE ACTION

A large body of experimental evidence now exists which provides a molecular basis for the action of steroid hormones including the glucocorticoids. These results substantiate many of the aspects of the general model first proposed by Jensen and co-workers nearly 20 years ago (1968). Unlike polypeptide hormones, which in general interact with specific cell surface receptors, steroids enter cells through passive diffusion. Once in the cytoplasm of a hormone-responsive cell, steroids are bound with high affinity by soluble receptor proteins which have specificity for particular classes of steroid molecules. The binding of the steroid appears to lead to "activation" of the receptor–steroid complex, generally thought to involve a conformational change in the protein. The steroid bound receptor molecules then accumulate within the nucleus by an unknown mechanism (Yamamoto and Alberts, 1976; Higgins and Gehring, 1978). In the nucleus the activated steroid receptors act as specific transcriptional regulators to induce and/or repress the transcription of certain target genes.

275

B. REGULATION OF GENE EXPRESSION
BY GLUCOCORTICOID HORMONES

A number of specific genes in divergent cells and tissues has been shown to be positively regulated by glucocorticoid hormones. In general, the addition of hormone leads to a rapid increase in the rate of transcription of the gene. In some cases, there is good evidence that the steroid hormone acts directly to induce transcription of the gene. Experiments performed in the presence of protein synthesis inhibitors have demonstrated that some hormone effects do not require the prior production of other proteins. For example, the induction of tyrosine aminotransferase mRNA in rat hepatoma cells or of mouse mammary tumor virus mRNA in mouse cells is unaffected by inhibitors of protein synthesis (Peterkofsky and Tomkins, 1967; Ringold et al., 1983). Other notable examples of specific gene activation mediated by glucocorticoids include the induction of metallothionein genes in mouse liver, as well as in a variety of cultured cells, and the induction of the growth hormone gene in pituitary cells (Mayo and Palmiter, 1985).

One characteristic of glucocorticoid regulation of transcription is its selectivity. Typically, very few genes are affected in the target cell, the precise genes varying from one cell type to another according to the physiological function of that cell. In the case of rat hepatoma cells, two dimensional protein gel analysis suggests that 0.5–1% of the detectable cellular proteins are inducible by glucocorticoids (Ivarie and O'Farrell, 1978). It is likely that many hormone-responsive cells exhibit a similar limited response to hormone. The factors operating within each cell to limit the hormone response to particular genes are presently unknown, but chromatin structure is postulated to play a role.

While the best-characterized cases of glucocorticoid regulation of gene expression involve induction of the target genes, there is also evidence that these hormones can down-regulate certain genes. Less than 0.5% of cellular proteins in rat hepatoma cells appears to be repressed by glucocorticoids (Ivarie and O'Farrell, 1978). Specific examples of down-regulation include transcription of the rat α-fetoprotein gene, the rat and mouse pro-opiomelanocortin genes, and ribosomal RNA presursors in mouse lymphoma cells (Turcotte et all, 1985; Nakanishi et al., 1977; Cavanaugh and Thompson, 1983). In the case of the α-fetoprotein gene, glucocorticoids can prevent initiation of transcription of the gene, even in the presence of protein synthesis inhibitors. These findings suggest that hormone-receptor complexes can interact directly with target genes to inhibit transcription.

C. MOLECULAR BASIS OF STEROID RECEPTOR ACTION

Recent advances in two areas have led to a molecular view of how steroid receptors may function to regulate specific gene expression. First, the biochemical purification of the glucocorticoid receptor has allowed both an initial characterization of the protein and a functional evaluation of its DNA binding properties. Second, mutational studies combined with gene transfer experiments on specific hormone responsive genes have defined *cis* acting regulatory sequences required for hormonal regulation.

Both of these approaches have been combined in studies of two glucocorticoid inducible systems, the human metallothionein gene and mouse mammary tumor virus. The glucocorticoid receptor has been purified to near homogeneity from rat liver and has a monomer molecular weight of approximately 90,000 (Wrange *et al.*, 1979; Geisse *et al.*, 1982). DNase footprinting studies with purified receptor show that there are two or three binding sites in the mouse mammary tumor virus promoter region (Scheidereit and Beato, 1984; Payvar *et al.*, 1983). These sites overlap those sites identified by mutational studies (Hynes *et al.*, 1983; Majors and Varmus, 1983; Buetti and Diggelman, 1983; Lee *et al.*, 1984). Studies using purified rat glucocorticoid receptor with the human metallothionein gene have led to similar conclusions.

Footprinting studies suggest the presence of at least two binding sites for the receptor protein in the region upstream of the transcription initiation site (Karin *et al.*, 1984). The location of these sites is similar to the analogous sites in the mouse mammary tumor virus promoter. Furthermore, there are short (6 base pair) sequence homologies shared between the mouse mammary tumor virus and the metallothionein receptor binding sites (Scheidereit and Beato, 1984). These sequences have been proposed to constitute the core of a receptor recognition sequence.

In addition to the identification of receptor binding sequences, other studies suggest possible mechanisms for the transcriptional activation process. The sequences which bind to the receptor and which are responsible for hormonal regulation can be separated from the MMTV promoter and can be fused to a heterologous promoter such as the Herpes thymidine kinase promoter, rendering the hybrid promoter hormonally responsive (Majors and Varmus, 1983; Chanlder *et al.*, 1983). These results indicate that the receptor binding sequences can function as an independent regulatory element distinct from the promoter. Hormonal induction is also maintained when either the orientation or location of the MMTV regulatory element is altered relative to other promoters (Chandler *et al.*, 1983; Ponta *et al.*, 1985). These properties are similar to those of viral or cellular enhancers, but the precise mechanism by which the receptor activates specific transcription has yet to be established.

II. Glucocorticoid Effects on T Lymphocytes

A. LYMPHOKINES PRODUCED BY ACTIVATED T CELLS

T cells activated either by lectins, such as Con A, or specifically by antigen produce a variety of soluble mediators. Until recently, the biochemical nature of many of these factors, as well as their precise biological properties, could not be established. The combined approaches of protein purification and molecular cloning have provided sufficient quantities of purified material for biological characterization.

Several of the soluble factors produced by activated T cells are involved in amplifying immune or inflammatory reactions. IL-2 is a growth factor produced by many activated T cells. Its role is stimulating the proliferation of T cells is well established, and there are recent reports that it is involved in stimulating B cells as well. Interferon-γ (IFN-γ), another product of activated T cells, which may also be involved in stimulating B cells, activates macrophages as well. Murine T cells also produce two colony stimulating factors. One of these, IL-3, also known as multi-CSF, is capable of stimulating the growth of multiple lineages of hematopoietic cells from progenitor cells originating in bone marrow. A second colony stimulating factor, GM-CSF, is more restricted in its action and stimulates the proliferation of only granulocytes and macrophages. Each of these proteins has been purified either from T cell conditioned medium or from expression of the cloned gene in microorganisms. In addition to these factors, there are others, less well characterized, which appear to act specifically on B cells, in stimulating either proliferation or differentiation.

Through the work of a number of laboratories including our own, cDNA clones have been isolated for murine IL-2, IL-3, GM-CSF, and IFN-γ (Yokota *et al.*, 1984, 1985; Fung *et al.*, 1984; Gough *et al.*, 1984; Gray and Goeddel, 1983). We have used these cDNA probes, as described below, to analyze the expression of lymphokines in cloned T cell lines exposed to glucocorticoids.

B. Glucocorticoid Effects on Mixed Lymphocyte Populations

Initial studies of Gillis *et al.* (1979) suggested that glucocorticoids prevent the clonal expansion of stimulated T lymphocytes. They went on to show that the antiproliferative effects of the synthetic glucocorticoid, dexamethasone, on cytotoxic T cells could be reversed by the addition of supernatants containing T cell growth factor (IL-2). This result suggested that in the presence of dexamethasone the cells did not produce suffi- cient IL-2 to promote proliferation. Based on this finding it was proposed that dexamethasone inhibits the production of IL-2 by stimulated T lymphocytes. Arya *et al.* (1984) confirmed this interpretation when they demonstrated, using an IL-2 cDNA probe, that dexamethasone prevents the accumulation of IL-2 mRNA in mitogen-stimulated human pe- ripheral blood lymphocytes. They also found that dexamethasone inhib- its the accumulation of the mRNA encoding IFN-γ, suggesting that dex- amethasone can inhibit the production of other lymphokines. However, the possibility that IFN-γ production was reduced as a consequence of decreased IL-2 levels could not be ruled out. Moreover, from these studies on mixed cell populations, it was not possible to ascertain if dexamethasone acts directly or indirectly on T lymphocytes to inhibit the production of IL-2.

C. Glucocorticoid Regulation of Cloned T Helper Cell Lines

To determine if glucocorticoids act directly on T lymphocytes, and to determine the spectrum of T cell genes regulated by glucocorticoids, we used a murine helper T cell clone designated $C1.Ly1^{+}2^{-}/9$ (Nabel *et al.*, 1981). This clone can be induced to secrete several lymphokines (see Table I). One of these is IL-3, which can be detected by its mast cell

TABLE I
INDUCIBLE GENE EXPRESSION IN CLONED T CELL LINES

	$C1.Ly1^{+}2^{-}/9$	GK15-1
IL-3	+	+
GM-CSF	+	+
IL-2	−	+
γ-IFN	−	+
Preproenkephalin	+	+

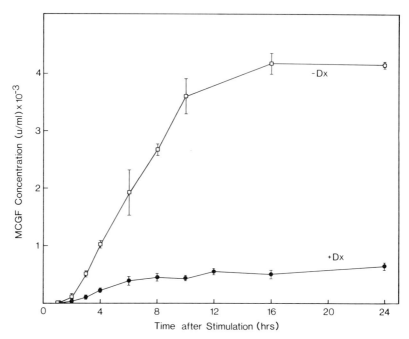

Fig. 1. Time course of MCGF production by Con A-stimulated Cl.Ly1$^+$2$^-$/9 cells in the presence (+) or absence (−) of dexamethasone (Dx). Cl.Ly1$^+$2$^-$/9 cells at 5 × 10^5/ml were incubated in the presence or absence of 10^{-6} M dexamethasone for 1 hr prior to the addition of 4 μg/ml Con A. At the indicated times after Con A addition, the supernatants were collected, dialyzed, and assayed for MCGF activity. Each value is the mean ± SD of triplicated assays. (From Culpepper and Lee, 1985, with permission.)

growth factor (MCGF) activity in the cell supernatants (Rennick *et al.*, 1985). To study the effect of dexamethasone on the induction of IL-3, Cl.Ly1$^+$2$^-$/9 was incubated with or without 10^{-6} M dexamethasone for 1 hr prior to the addition of Con A, then supernatants were collected at various times and assayed for MCGF activity. As shown in Fig. 1, in the absence of dexamethasone MCGF activity accumulates rapidly in the supernatants reaching a plateau after 16 hr. However, the accumulation of MCGF activity in supernatants of dexamethasone-treated cells was inhibited from the earliest time point and throughout the 24 hr of the experiment. Overall, the induction of MCGF activity by Con A was 7-fold less in the hormone-treated cells than in the control cells.

As shown in Fig. 2, incubation of Cl.Ly1$^+$2$^-$/9 cells for 1 hr with varying concentrations of dexamethasone prior to Con A stimulation produced a dose-dependent decrease in the levels of MCGF activity in the supernatants. Half-maximal inhibition was achieved between 10^{-8} and 10^{-9} M dexamethasone, and concentrations greater than 10^{-7} M produced maximal inhibition. This finding is consistent with the hypothesis that the inhibition of MCGF production is a glucocorticoid receptor-mediated process. Thus, dexamethasone inhibits the induction of IL-3 by Con A in C1.Ly1^{+}2^{-}/9 cells; this inhibition is rapid, and a maximal effect is achieved even if dexamethasone is added simultaneously with Con A. Significant levels of inhibition were also seen when dexamethasone was added after Con A, suggesting that dexamethasone inhibits an ongoing process such as transcription or translation.

To examine the effect of dexamethasone on the accumulation of IL-3 mRNA, C1.Ly1^{+}2^{-}/9 cells were incubated in the presence or absence of dexamethasone for 1 hr stimulated with Con A for 5 or 10 hr then harvested and poly(A)$^{+}$ RNA prepared. A Northern blot of this mRNA probed with ^{32}P-labeled IL-3 cDNA is shown in Fig. 3. Cells stimulated

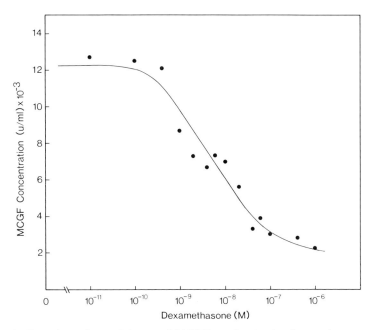

FIG. 2. Dose-dependent inhibition of MCGF production by dexamethasone-treated Con A stimulated C1.Ly1^{+}2^{-}/9 cells. C1.Ly1^{+}2^{-}/9 cells at 5 × 10^5/ml were incubated with varying concentrations of dexamethasone for 1 hr prior to the addition of 4 μg/ml Con A. Sixteen hours after the addition of Con A, the supernatants were collected, dialyzed, and assayed for MCGF activity.

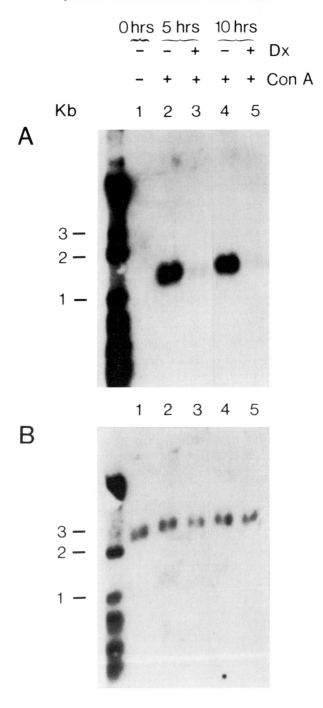

with Con A accumulate high levels of IL-3 mRNA; however, in cells stimulated in the presence of dexamethasone, the levels of IL-3 mRNA are considerably lower. There is 18-fold less IL-3 mRNA in cells 5 hr after stimulation and 30-fold less in cells 10 hr after stimulation. These differences in IL-3 mRNA accumulation in the presence and absence of dexamethasone are sufficient to account for the differences seen in the amounts of MCGF activity in the supernatants. The levels of mRNA encoding Thy-1, a constitutively expressed cell surface marker, are un- affected by dexamethasone treatment, as are several other parameters of cell metabolism such as total RNA or protein synthesis (Culpepper and Lee, 1985). Additional experiments demonstrated that dexamethasone does not affect the stability of IL-3 mRNA and does not cause an ac- cumulation of precursor mRNA in either the cytoplasm or nucleus of hormone-treated cells. The combined data strongly suggest that dex- amethasone selectively inhibits the transcription of the IL-3 gene.

The mRNAs encoding granulocyte–macrophage colony stimulating factor (GM-CSF) and TY5, a gene of unknown function, are also induced by Con A in C1.Ly1^{+}2^{-}/9 cells. The accumulation of both of these mRNAs is also inhibited in the presence of dexamethasone (Culpepper and Lee, 1985). However, the inhibition of TY5 was only several-fold, with significant amounts of TY5 mRNA still being produced in the pres- ence of hormone.

The finding that dexamethasone can regulate the expression of several lymphokines by a mitogen-stimulated helper T cell clone establishes that dexamethasone acts directly on T cells. It is also clear from these results that dexamethasone can regulate the expression of lymphokines such as IL-3 and GM-CSF in cells that do not produce IL-2, demonstrating that the expression and regulation of these lymphokines can occur indepen- dent of IL-2 production.

To investigate glucocorticoid effects on the expression of other T cell genes, we used a murine helper T cell clone that makes a broader range of lymphokines (Table I). This clone, GK15-1, produces IL-2, IL-3, GM- CSF, and IFN-γ in response to the mitogen Con A or following activa- tion by its specific antigen (Giedlin et al., 1985). Poly(A)$^{+}$ mRNA was prepared from GK15-1 cells stimulated either with Con A or with anti-

---

FIG. 3. RNA blot analysis of mRNA obtained from C1.Ly1^{+}2^{-}/9 cells incubated with or without dexamethasone prior to Con A stimulation. Poly(A)$^{+}$ RNA (3 μg) isolated from C1.Ly1^{+}2^{-}/9 cells [uninduced (lane 1), 5 hr Con A stimulation (lane 2), 1 hr 10^{-6} M dexamethasone preincubation and 5 hr Con A stimulation (lane 3), 10 hr Con A stimula- tion (lane 4), and 1 hr 10^{-6} M dexamethasone preincubation and 10 hr Con A stimulation (lane 5)] were analyzed using cDNA probes encoding IL-3 (top) and Thy-1 (bottom). (From Culpepper and Lee, 1985, with permission.)

gen for 4 hr in the presence or absence of 10^{-6} M dexamethasone. The results of Northern blots analyzed with several different cDNA probes are shown in Fig. 4. GK15-1 cells stimulated with Con A accumulated significant levels of IL-3 mRNA; in the presence of dexamethasone the levels of IL-3 mRNA were reduced. However, in contrast to the 15- to 30-fold inhibition of IL-3 mRNA seen with Con A-stimulated C1.-Ly1^{+}2^{-}/9 cells, a 4- to 5-fold reduction is observed with these cells. These results are also consistent with the levels of MCGF activity present in the supernatants from these cells. Probing of the mRNA with the cDNA encoding GM-CSF revealed a similar 4- to 5-fold inhibition by dexamethasone (Fig. 4).

Compared to stimulation with Con A, activation of GK15-1 cells with antigen generally results in lower levels of both IL-3 and GM-CSF mRNA (Fig. 4). Significantly, the treatment of antigen-stimulated cells with dexamethasone results in decreased levels of both IL-3 and GM-CSF mRNA. These findings suggest that glucocorticoids can regulate the expression of lymphokines induced under physiological conditions. The same RNA samples were also probed with cDNAs encoding IFN-γ or IL-2. As seen with IL-3 and GM-CSF mRNA, FN-γ and IL-2 mRNA levels were greatly increased by Con A stimulation, and in the presence of hormone the levels were reduced 2- and 4-fold, respectively (Fig. 4 and date not shown).

The RNAs were also analyzed with cDNA probes for preproenkephlin, IL-2 receptor, β chain of the T cell receptor, and Thy-1 (Miller *et al.*, 1985; Chien *et al.*, 1984; Hiraki *et al.*, 1986). The results obtained with these probes are summarized in Table II. Preproenkephelin mRNA has recently been identified as being highly expressed in two Con A-stimulated helper T cell clones, but not in uninduced cells (Zurawski *et al.*, 1986). When mRNA from Con A-stimulated GK15-1 cells was probed with the cDNA encoding preproenkephlin, the mRNA was found to be induced. However, unlike the lymphokines discussed above, the mRNA from cells stimulated with Con A in the presence of dexamethasone had

FIG. 4. Effect of dexamethasone on the expression of lymphokine mRNAs in mitogen- and antigen-stimulated GK15-1 cells. GK15-1 cells at 1×10^6/ml were stimulated in the presence or absence of 10^{-6} M dexamethasone with 4 μg/ml Con A, or with 0.04% v/v chicken red blood cells (antigen) in the presence of 5×10^6 presenting cells/ml as described in Giedlin *et al.* (1985). Poly(A)$^+$ mRNA (5 μg) isolated from GK15-1 cells [uninduced (lane 1), 4 hr Con A stimulation (lane 2), 2 hr dexamethasone preincubation and 4 hr Con A stimulation (lane 3), 4 hr antigen stimulation (lane 4), 2 hr dexamethasone preincubation and 4 hr antigen stimulation (lane 5)] were electrophoresed in a denaturing gel, blotted onto nitrocellulose, and hybridized with ^{32}P-labeled cDNA probes encoding IL-3 (A), GM-CSF (B), and IFN-γ (C).

A

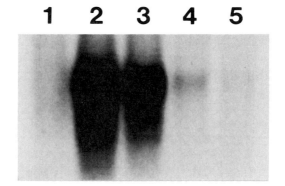

B

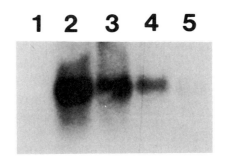

C

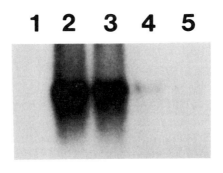

TABLE II
GLUCOCORTICOID REGULATION OF T CELL GENES

Gene	Induction	Glucocorticoid regulation
Class I[a]	Mitogen and antigen	Repressed
Class II[b]	Mitogen and antigen	No effect
Class III[c]	Constitutive	No effect

[a] IL-2, IL-3, GM-CSF, IFN-γ.
[b] Preproenkephalin.
[c] IL-2 receptor, β chain T cell receptor, Thy-1.

the same level of preproenkephalin as the mRNA from the cells stimulated in the absence of hormone. At present this is the only example of an inducible gene which is not regulated by glucocorticoids.

As found in the case of the C1.Ly1$+2^-$/9 cells, the constitutive expression of Thy-1 mRNA is unaffected by either Con A stimulation or dexamethasone treatment. mRNAs encoding both the β chain of the T cell receptor and the IL-2 receptor are constitutively expressed at low levels by GK15-1 cells, and stimulation of the cells with Con A increases this expression less than 2-fold. This small enhancement is unaffected by the presence of dexamethasone.

Based on the results presented here, T lymphocyte genes can be grouped into 3 classes on the basis of their induction properties and their response to hormone. In the first class are the mitogen- and antigen-inducible genes whose expression is inhibited by glucocorticoid exposure during the stimulation. This class includes the lymphokines IL-2, IL-3, GM-CSF, and IFN-γ. The second class has only one member thus far, preproenkephalin. This gene is inducible, but is not regulated by glucocorticoids. The last class contains the genes which are constitutively expressed, Thy-1, β chain of the T cell receptor, and the IL-2 receptor. The expression of these genes is unaffected by glucocorticoids.

III. Conclusion

It has become clear from recent studies that T cell lymphokines constitute an important set of soluble regulatory molecules which mediate cell growth and differentiation. The genes encoding these proteins are under strict regulation. They are essentially "off" in unactivated or resting T cells, but their mRNAs can exceed 1% of the activated T cell's total mRNA. Activation of T cells involves a complex interaction of an antigen with its specific receptor on the surface of the T cell, leading through unknown mechanisms to activation of specific transcription of genes, including lymphokine genes. Glucocorticoid hormones are a second external signal which can modulate lymphokine gene expression. These hormones appear to function through their cellular receptors to repress lymphokine gene transcription.

The DNA binding properties of steroid-receptor complexes suggest two models for the negative regulation by glucocorticoids. The steroid-receptor complex might bind to the regulatory region of a lymphokine gene and simply block transcription initiation by RNA polymerase. Alternatively, the steroid–receptor complex might prevent the interaction of other cellular proteins, required for the induction process, with their target sites. Either model would predict the existence of sites for the glucocorticoid receptor in the lymphokine gene or its flanking sequences. This prediction can now be tested experimentally. Another piece of information presently lacking is whether *de novo* protein synthesis is required either for induction of transcription or for glucocorticoid-mediated repression. When this issue is resolved, one can be more certain about the direct or indirect role of steroids in regulating lymphokine expression.

In our studies two different helper clones have been used to examine glucocorticoid effects. These two clones were representative of two subclasses of helper cells distinguished on the basis of their lymphokine expression. One class produces IL-3 and GM-CSF but does not produce IL-2 or IFN-γ, while the other class produces all four lymphokines (Mosmann *et al.*, 1986). These two classes appear to differ somewhat in their glucocorticoid responses as well. The first class appears to respond strongly to glucocorticoids by down-regulating lymphokine production to less than 10% of the fully induced levels. Glucocorticoids also modulate lymphokine expression downward in the second class of T cell, but substantial levels continue to be made even in the presence of hormone. How the differential response to hormone treatment correlates with true functional differences of these cell types remains to be determined. While lymphokine production by cytotoxic T cells has not been as well characterized, Kelso and Munck (1984) have documented both the production of certain lymphokines by cytotoxic T cell lines and their inhibition by glucocorticoids.

It is obvious that additional studies will be required to elucidate the mechanism by which glucocorticoids regulate the expression of inducible genes in T cells. The availability of molecular clones for many of the known lymphokines combined with the availability of a variety of cloned hormone-responsive T cell lines will facilitate further work. It is hoped

that an understanding of how these hormones function in T cell regulation will lead to general insights into the role of T cells in inflammation
and regulation of immune responses.

ACKNOWLEDGMENTS

We would like to thank Dr. G. Nabel for stimulating an initial interest in steroid
regulation of lymphokines, and Dr. M. Giedlin for providing the GK15-1 cell line and
helpful advice on the growth of T cell clones. We thank J. Zahner and G. Burget for their
help in preparing the manuscript.

REFERENCES

Arya, S. K., Wong-Staal, F., and Gallo, R. C. (1984). *J. Immunol.* **133**, 273–276.
Buetti, E., and Diggelmann, H. (1983). *EMBO J.* **2**, 1423–1429.
Cavanaugh, A. H., and Thompson, E. A. (1983). *J. Biol. Chem.* **258**, 9768–9773.
Chandler, V. L., Maler, B. A., and Yamamoto, K. R. (1983). *Cell* **33**, 489–499.
Chien, Y.-H., Gascoigne, N. R. J., Kavaler, J., Lee, N. E., and Davis, M. M. (1984).
    Nature (London) **309**, 322–326.
Crupps, T. R., and Fauci, A. S. (1982). *Immunol. Rev.* **65**, 133–155.
Culpepper, J., and Lee, F. (1985). *J. Immunol.* **135**, 3191–3197.
Fahey, J. V., Guyre, P. M., and Munck, A. (1981). *Adv. Inflammation Res.* **2**, 21–51.
Fung, M. C., Hapel, A. J., Ymer, S., Cohen, D. R., Johnson, R. A., Campbell, H. D.,
    and Young, I. G. (1984). *Nature (London)* **307**, 233–237.
Geisse, S., Scheidereit, C., Westphal, H. M., Hynes, N. E., Groner, B., and Beato, M.
    (1982). *EMBO J.* **1**, 1613–1619.
Giedlin, M. A., Longenecker, B. M., and Mosmann, T. R. (1986). *Cell. Immunol.* **97**,
    357–370.
Gillis, S., Crabtree, G. R., and Smith, K. A. (1979). *J. Immunol.* **123**, 1624–1631.
Gough, N. M., Gough, J., Metcalf, D., Kelso, A., Grail, D., Nicola, N. A., Burgess, A.
    W., and Dunn, A. R. (1984). *Nature (London)* **309**, 763–767.
Gray, P. W., and Goeddel, D. V. (1983). *Proc. Natl. Acad. Sci. U.S.A.* **80**, 5842–5846.
Higgins, S. J., and Gehring, U. (1978). *Adv. Cancer Res.* **28**, 313–197.
Hiraki, D. D., Nomura, D., Yokota, T., Arai, K., and Coffman, R. L. (1986). Submitted.
Hynes, N., van Ooyen, A. J. J., Kennedy, N., Herrlich, P., Ponta, H., and Groner, B.
    (1983). *Proc. Natl. Acad. Sci. U.S.A.* **80**, 3637–3641.
Ivarie, R. D., and O'Farrell, P. H. (1978). *Cell* **13**, 41–55.
Jensen, E. V., Suzuki, T., Kawashima, T., Strumpf, W. E., Jungblut, P. W., and De-
    Sombre, E. R. (1968). *Proc. Natl. Acad. Sci. U.S.A.* **59**, 632–638.
Karin, M., Haslinger, A., Holtgreve, H., Richards, R. I., Krauter, P., Westphal, H. M.,
    and Beato, M. (1984). *Nature (London)* **308**, 513–519.
Kelso, A., and Munck, A. (1984). *J. Immunol.* **133**, 784–791.
Lee, F., Hall, C. V., Ringold, G. M., Dobson, D. E., Luh, J., and Jacob, P. E. (1984).
    Nucleic Acids Res. **12**, 4191–4206.
Majors, J., and Varmus, H. E. (1983). *Proc. Natl. Acad. Sci. U.S.A.* **80**, 5866–5870.
Mayo, K. E., and Palmiter, R. D. (1985). *Biochem. Actions Horm.* **12**, 69–88.
Miller, J., Malek, T. R., Leonard, W. J., Greene, W. C., Shevach, E. M., and Germain,
    R. N. (1985). *J. Immunol.* **134**, 4212–4217.
Mosmann, T. R., Cherwinski, H., Bond, M. W., Giedlin, M. A., and Coffman, R. L.
    (1986). *J. Immunol.* **136**, 2348–2357.

Nabel, G., Greenberger, J. S., Sakakeeney, M. A., and Cantor, H. (1981). *Proc. Natl. Acad. Sci. U.S.A.* **78**, 1157–1161.

Nakanishi, S., Kita, T., Taii, S., Imura, H., and Numa, S. (1977). *Proc. Natl. Acad. Sci. U.S.A.* **74**, 3283–3286.

Payvar, F., DeFranco, D., Firestone, G. L., Edgar, B., Wrange, O., Okret, S., Gustafsson, J.-A., and Yamamoto, K. R. (1983). *Cell* **35**, 381–392.

Peterkofsky, B., and Tomkins, G. M. (1967). *Proc. Natl. Acad. Sci. U.S.A.* **60**, 222–228.

Ponta, H., Kennedy, N., Skroch, P., Hynes, N. E., and Groner, B. (1985). *Proc. Natl. Acad. Sci. U.S.A.* **82**, 1020–1024.

Rennick, D. M., Lee, F. D., Yokota, T., Arai, K., Cantor, H., and Nabel, G. J. (1985). *J. Immunol.* **134**, 910–914.

Ringold, G. M., Dobson, D. E., Grove, J. R., Hall, C. V., Lee, F., and Vannice, J. L. (1983). *Recent Prog. Horm. Res.* **39**, 387–424.

Scheidereit, C., and Beato, M. (1984). *Proc. Natl. Acad. Sci. U.S.A.* **81**, 3029 3033.

Turcotte, B., Guertin, M., Chevrette, M., and Belanger, L. (1985). *Nucleic Acids Res.* **13**, 2387–2398.

Wrange, O., Carlstedt-Duke, J., and Gustafsson, J.-A. (1979). *J. Biol. Chem.* **254**, 9284–9290.

Yamamoto, K., and Alberts, B. (1976). *Annu. Rev. Biochem.* **45**, 721–746.

Yokota, T., Lee, F., Rennick, D., Hall, C., Arai, N., Mosmann, T., Nabel, G., Cantor, H., and Arai, H. (1984) *Proc. Natl. Acad. Sci. U.S.A.* **81**, 1070–1074.

Yokota, T., Arai, N., Lee, F., Rennick, D., Mosmann, T., and Arai, K. (1985). *Proc. Natl. Acad. Sci. U.S.A.* **82**, 68–72.

Zurawski, G., Benedik, M., Kamb, B. J., Abrams, J. S., Zurawski, F. M., and Lee F. D. (1986). *Science* **232**, 772–775.

And Now for Something Completely Differential

C. G. LOBE, V. H. PAETKAU, AND R. C. BLEACKLEY

Department of Biochemistry, University of Alberta, Edmonton, Alberta, Canada T6G 2H7

I. Introduction

A. STRATEGY

Most of the articles in this book focus on molecular genetic approaches to the study lymphokine and lymphokine receptor genes and the regulation of their expression. The experiments described in this contribution address the question of what subsequently happens when a lymphokine interacts with its receptor to stimulate a T cell along a particular differentiative pathway. The approach is again one of molecular genetics and could be generally applied to any T cell subset.

The strategy used is based upon the hypothesis of Hastie and Bishop (1976). They postulated that each cell type possesses a small number of high-abundance mRNAs which are expressed at a very low level, if at all, in other cell types. Furthermore, these mRNAs would encode the proteins necessary to carry out that cell's specialized functions. Thus, if these characteristic mRNAs could be isolated, they would provide extremely useful tools to study how a cell performs its unique functions at the molecular level. With the advent of recombinant DNA technology it is now possible to identify this subset of mRNAs through the isolation of their corresponding cDNAs.

We decided to test whether this hypothesis could be extended to closely related T cells which have either differentiated along alternate routes or differ in their state of activation. This article will focus on the molecules induced upon T lymphocyte stimulation, in particular molecules which are expressed in activated cytotoxic T lymphocytes (CTL). CTL must express a number of cytotoxicity-related proteins and the corresponding mRNAs. In order to identify such molecules we used the differential hybridization method to isolate cDNAs which are characteristic of activated cytotoxic T cells. This approach has been extremely rewarding in a number of different systems, including the isolation of several myoblast-specific genes (Hastings and Emerson, 1982), brain-specific sequences (Milner and Sutcliffe, 1983), five cell-cycle specific genes (Hirschhorn *et al.*, 1984), platelet-derived growth factor-induced genes (Cochran *et al.*, 1983), and, most spectacularly, in the cloning of the genes encoding the T cell antigen receptors (Hedrick *et al.*, 1984; Yanagi *et al.*, 1984).

291

B. T Cell Activation

The development of a cellular immune response is a complex process in which the interaction of several cells, directly and via intercellular signal molecules, results in the generation of a CTL capable of lysing a target cell. Most T cells are in an inactive or precursor state. The dual signal of antigen and a lymphokine triggers them to synthesize new RNAs and proteins, increase in size (blast transformation), and eventually proliferate. These activated cells are of two classes: regulatory cells [helper (Th) and suppressor (Ts) T cells] and effector cells [cytotoxic T cells (Tc or CTL)]. The sequence of events required for T cell activation are fairly well defined (Fig. 1). Foreign antigens from the surface of a stimulator cell are recognized in association with class II major histocompatibility complex (MHC) antigens via the antigen receptor of the Th cell. Syngeneic antigen presenting cells (APC) produce interleukin (IL-1) when they encounter antigen. The dual signals of antigen and IL-1 induce the Th cell to synthesize and secrete a variety of lymphokines. These factors are generally glycoproteins which stimulate growth and differentiation of many types of hematopoietic cells and include colony stimulating factors for granulocytes and macrophages (CSF-GM), interleukin 3 (IL-3), interferon-gamma, interleukin 2 (IL-2), and a variety of B cell growth and differentiation factors. Concurrently, antigen plus

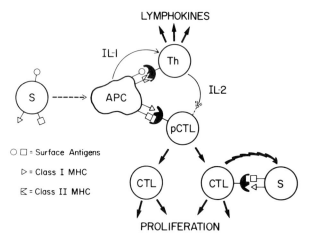

Fig. 1. Cellular interactions involved in the generation of a cytotoxic T cell response. Surface antigens from a stimulator cell (S) are processed by an antigen presenting cell (APC) and recognized by the antigen receptors on helper T lymphocytes (Th) and precursor cytotoxic T lymphocytes (pCTL). The resultant CTL is capable of lysing any antigen bearing target cell which it then encounters. See text for explanation of signaling events.

type I MHC-specified molecules are recognized, again via the T cell antigen receptor, by a precursor cytotoxic T cell (pCTL).

When the pCTL is initially stimulated with antigen, there is a transient burst of transcription and a subsequent synthesis of new proteins, including the IL-2 receptor, transferrin receptor, c-*myc*, and MHC molecules (Kronke *et al.*, 1985; Neckers and Cossman, 1983; Kelly *et al.*, 1983; Cotner *et al.*, 1983). Up-regulation of the transferrin receptor is necessary since transferrin is a universal requirement for long-term growth of all mammalian cell types (Cotner *et al.*, 1983). The protooncogene c-*myc* is a nuclear DNA binding protein which seems to be involved in the transit of cells from the G_0 to the G_1 phase of the cell cycle (Persson and Leder, 1984). Expression of IL-2 receptors on the pCTL allows binding of the lymphokine, produced by the neighboring Th, and progression to the second stage of cell activation in which DNA synthesis takes place and the cells proliferate into a clonal population of cytotoxic cells expressing the same specific T cell antigen receptor (Lowenthal *et al.*, 1985). These cells are now competent to bind and lyse target cells.

C. Mechanism of CTL-Induced Lysis

The essential changes a pCTL undergoes to become a killer cell and the mechanism by which it then lyses its target are not known in any molecular detail. Studies using metabolic inhibitors, antibodies against cell surface proteins, and observations of morphological changes as the CTL caries out its function enable some general deductions to be made about the mechanism of lysis (Berke, 1983; Nabholz and MacDonald, 1983). The lytic reaction requires direct target contact and is unidirectional—the effector cell comes away uninjured, and in fact can kill more than one target cell (Zagury *et al.*, 1975). Binding of target cells is Mg^{2+}-dependent and requires energy. The cells come into close proximity and the plasma membranes interdigitate at the contact region. Initial Ca^{2+}-independent steps occur upon target conjugation, which can be blocked by inhibitors of methylation or compounds which alkylate cell-surface thiol groups. This is followed by Ca^{2+}-dependent steps, in which serine proteases may play a role (Redelman and Hudig, 1983).

Within 30 min after binding, the microtubule-organizing center (MTOC) and Golgi apparatus (GA) of the effector cell are reoriented proximal to the contact area (Kupfer and Dennert, 1984). This observation suggests a delivery of cytotoxic substances from secretory vesicles of the GA, since membrane-inserted and -secreted cell products are processed and packaged in that organelle. The possible effector molecules of lysis were originally discovered by electron microscopy of CTL and lysed target membranes (Dennert and Podack, 1983). Lytically active CTL contain characteristic dense granules. Upon stimulation with antigen or Con A, proteins which appear to originate in these granules polymerize to form two types of tubular structures distinguished by their diameters (160 and 70 Å), designated poly(P)$_1$ and poly(P)$_2$. These "polyperforins" are transferred to the membrane of the target cell, resulting in trans-membrane channel formation similar, but different in size, to comple-ment lesions. In fact, Podack and Konigsberg (1984) demonstrated that isolated CTL granules are capable of Ca^{2+}-dependent cytolysis with comparable or higher activity than, but without the target specificity of, the cells they were isolated from. When analyzed on SDS–PAGE, six major protein bands are characteristic of cytolytic granules. Membranes of target cells lysed by granules show the characteristic donut-shaped lesions of the same dimensions as poly(P)$_1$ and poly(P)$_2$. This is analogous to the final event in complement-mediated cytolysis, in which C9 poly-merizes to form disulfide-linked tubular structures which lyse targets by membrane insertion and channel formation.

Although the studies to date have defined the stages involved in killer T cell activation and function and the nature of some of the essential components in this process, one is left with many questions regarding the precise molecular identity of the individual components involved. Assuming killer T cells possess a characteristic set of proteins to carry out their specialized function, these must be encoded by mRNA transcripts which are CTL specific. Our approach to identifying molecules which are necessary for killer cell function has been to generate a cDNA library from a cloned cytotoxic T cell line and use differential hybridization analysis to identify recombinants which represent mRNAs transcribed in mouse cytotoxic T cells and not in helper cells or thymocytes.

II. Results and Discussion

A. cDNA LIBRARY CONSTRUCTION AND SCREENING

Messenger RNA from an IL-2-dependent cytotoxic T cell clone (MTL2.8.2; Bleackley et al., 1982) was used as a template to synthesize double-stranded cDNA (Gubler and Hoffman, 1983). After size selection (> 500 bp) and addition of EcoRI linkers, the cDNA was ligated to pUC13 vector and used to transfect Escherichia coli JM83 competent cells (Maniatis et al., 1982). Four thousand recombinants were picked into individual wells of microtiter plates and replicated onto nitro-cellulose filters for screening. Details of the experimental methods used have been published elsewhere (Lobe et al., 1986a).

In order to identify cDNA clones which represent mRNAs expressed in activated killer T cells and not in other cell types, the ordered library was screened by differential hybridization. Single-stranded cDNA probe was synthesized from mRNA of three different types of cells: the killer T cell line used to generate the library, an antigen-specific helper T cell clone (which represents T cells that have differentiated along an alternate route to a functionally distinct cell type), and thymocytes (which represent a heterogeneous population of precursor cells). By identifying recombinants which hybridized only with probe from the CTL line and not with the helper T cells or thymocytes, we hoped to identify mRNAs which encode proteins vitally important in the function of cytotoxic T cells. Potentially interesting clones were rescreened, and 36 recombinants were clearly expressed at a high level in cytotoxic cells and at vastly lower levels in the helper cells and thymocytes (Fig. 2). Two clones were chosen for more extensive analysis: clone B10 because it appeared to be the most abundant in the library, cross-hybridizing strongly with eight other inserts, and clone C11 because it weakly cross-hybridized with B10 but not with all B10-related clones (one other C11-related sequence was found) (Fig. 3). Subsequently a cDNA library from the cytotoxic T cell clone AR1, which had been size-selected for cDNAs >1000 bp (kindly provided by H. Gershenfeld), was screened and a full-length C11 clone identified.

B. CLONES B10 AND C11 ARE CTL-SPECIFIC

The expression of B10 and C11 in a variety of cells and tissues was monitored by cytodot analysis (White and Bancroft, 1982) (Fig. 4). The results with B10 and C11 were the same, namely that they are expressed in cytotoxic T cells and not in other lymphoid or nonlymphoid tissue. The highest signal was detected with MTL2.8.2, the killer cell line which was used to generate the cDNA library. A weaker but positive signal was seen with MTLIII, a variant of MTL2.8.2 which has a lower cytotoxic activity and has become IL-2 independent. A similar level of expression was observed in a fetal thymus-derived T cell clone which is still being characterized (Teh *et al.*, 1985). To date, B10 and C11 expression has been detected in 7/7 CTL and 0/3 helper cell clones. The other cell types tested, including murine brain, liver, thymus, and lyopolysaccharide (LPS)-activated B cells and human CTL, gave no signal.

Interestingly, in a long-term mixed lymphocyte reaction (MLR) culture restimulated with IL-2 18 days after the initial antigen stimulation, there was an increase in expression of both B10 and C11 after 2 days. Cytotoxicity in these cells increased 10-fold by the third day following IL-2 addition. Control samples with addition of fresh media alone did not exhibit this induction. Also, the two cDNA clones do not represent

A. CTL cDNA

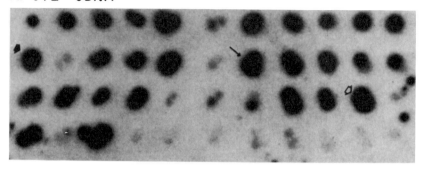

B. HELPER cDNA

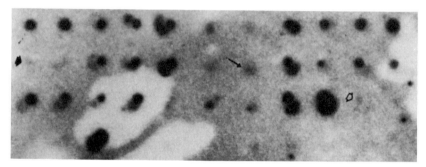

C. THYMUS cDNA

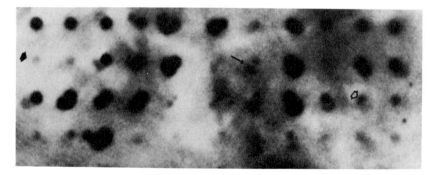

FIG. 2. Screening for CTL-specific cDNAs by differential hybridization. An ordered array of cDNA clones, generated from a cloned killer cell, were lysed and baked on nitrocellulose. After prehybridization the same filter was hybridized in turn with single-stranded cDNA probe synthesized from various cells: A, cloned T killer cells; B, cloned T helper cells; C, mouse thymocytes. Arrows indicate some examples of potential CTL-specific cDNAs.

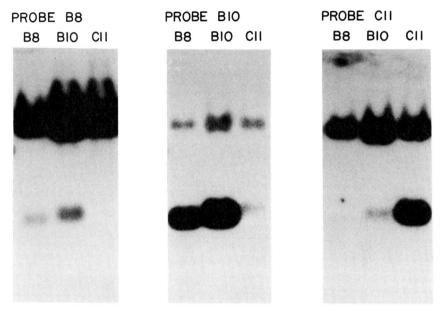

FIG. 3. Cross-hybrization of CTL-specific clones. Plasmid DNA from a number of relevant clones was digested with *Eco*RI to cut out the insert and fractionated by agarose gel electrophoresis. The fragments were transferred to nitrocellulose and hybridized with nick-translated plasmid. The probes used (B8, B10, and C11) are indicated. The high-molecular-weight band hybridizing in all lanes is vector DNA.

sequences expressed generally in activated lymphocytes, since a spleen population enriched for B cells and stimulated with LPS does not express either of the sequences, whereas μ heavy chain mRNA is greatly increased (data not shown).

C. Northern Blot Analysis with B10 and C11

Analysis on Northern blots confirmed the tissue specificity results of the cytodot data. Both clones hybridized to mRNA from two cytotoxic T cell lines including MTL2.8.2 (Fig. 5), as well as five other CTL clones for which the data are not shown. No bands were seen for thymocytes, an antigen-specific helper cell (CH1; Lobe *et al.*, 1986a), or the murine T lymphoma line EL-4 (Farrar *et al.*, 1980). RNA from murine liver and brain, LPS-stimulated B cells, and the myeloma S194 were also analyzed by Northern blot and showed no hybridization to B10 or C11.

The two clones showed an interesting difference in hybridization patterns; B10 hybridized to a single mRNA species of approximately 1000

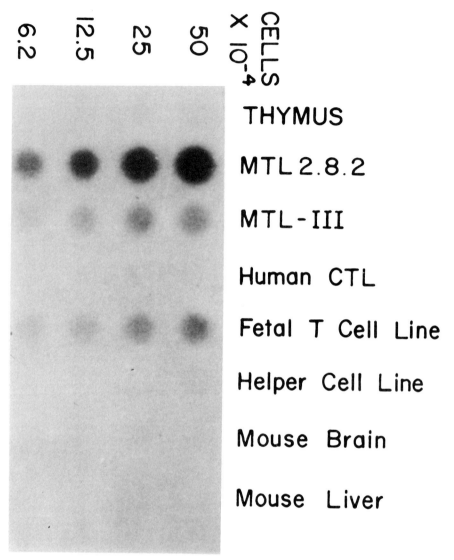

FIG. 4. Expression of B10 in various cell types. Cytoplasmic dot blots were prepared from murine thymus, brain and liver tissues, a cloned murine killer T cell (MTL2.8.2), an IL-2-independent subclone of MTL2.8.2, a fetally derived T cell clone and an antigen-dependent cloned helper T cell, and hybridized with nick-translated B10. Clone C11 gave identical results.

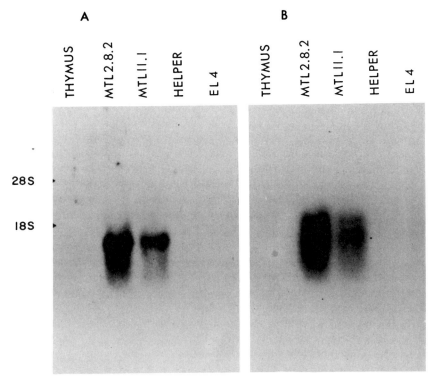

FIG. 5. Northern blot analysis of B10 and C11 transcripts. Poly(A)$^+$ RNA from the cell types indicated was fractionated on a formaldehyde–agarose gel, transferred to nitrocellulose, and hybridized with nick-translated probes B10(A) and C11(B).

bases, whereas C11 hybridized to two mRNAs of 1000 and 1400 bases. The relationship between these three bands is uncertain at present. The 1400 nucleotide mRNA probably corresponds to the full-length C11 clone we have sequenced. The shorter 1000 nucleotide band detected by C11 may arise from the same gene by differential RNA processing or by alternative exon usage, perhaps yielding membrane and secreted forms of the protein encoded. The 420-bp B10 insert and 1400-bp C11 insert have been sequenced (Sanger *et al.*, 1980), and comparison has revealed an 80% homology between them over 380 base pairs, suggesting the mRNAs are transcribed from two different but related genes (Lobe *et al.*, 1986b). We are presently screening for other full-length C11 clones and a full-length B10 clone, as well as genomic clones, to address the question of the identity and relation of the transcripts.

D. B10 AND C11 ARE INDUCED DURING CTL ACTIVATION

A primary objective for isolating mRNAs characteristic of lytically active CTL was to identify proteins which play a role in either activation or the lytic mechanism itself. Transcripts which encode these proteins would be expected to be induced following antigen stimulation but preceding the actual increase in cytotoxic activity. To monitor the level of B10 and C11 expression during a cytotoxic response, CBA/J spleen cells were stimulated with either mitomycin C-treated EL-4 cells (which do not express B10 or C11) or Con A. On each of the 6 days following antigen stimulation, the level of cytoxicity was measured in a chromium release assay (Shaw *et al.*, 1978), and cytodots were prepared and hybridized with nick-translated B10 or C11. Relative mRNA levels were determined by scanning densitometry of the cytodot autoradiogram on an ELISA plate reader.

In the allo-specific response, the level of cytotoxicity peaked at day 4, and both B10 and C11 mRNA increased from no detectable expression at day 1 to a strong signal peaking at days 3 and 4 (Fig. 6). With Con A stimulation, killing activity again peaked at day 4, but the peak of mRNA expression occurred on day 3. In both experiments, the mRNA expression returned to background levels by day 6, whereas there were still significant levels of killing activity. Similar observations were made when long-term MLR cultures were restimulated with IL-2, as mentioned above, where expression was induced by day 2 and the lytic activity peaked at day 3. In each case, an increase in transcription precedes phenotypic expression by approximately 24 hr. Therefore, it appears that B10 and C11 gene expression is induced upon cell activation prior to measurable cytotoxic activity. Thus, the mRNAs detected by B10 and C11 fulfill the primary criteria for molecules which encode proteins involved in cell activation and/or cytolysis.

E. B10 AND C11 ENCODE SERINE PROTEASES

The inserts of B10 (420 bp) and the full-length C11 clone (1400 bp) were sequenced (Sanger *et al.*, 1980) and open-reading frames identified

---

FIG. 6. Expression of CTL-specific genes during an allogeneic cytotoxic response. Spleen cells from CBA/J mice were stimulated with mitomycin C-treated EL-4 cells. On days 1–6 after stimulation, the level of specific (αEL-4), cross-reacting (αS194), and syngeneic (αRI) cytotoxicity was measured in a chromium release assay. Concurrently, the relative levels of B10 and C11 expression were monitored by hybridization to cytodots prepared from cells on the same days. The lower panel shows the cytodot data, while the upper panel shows the level of cytotoxity and the relative mRNA expression quantitated from the cytodots by densitometric scanning.

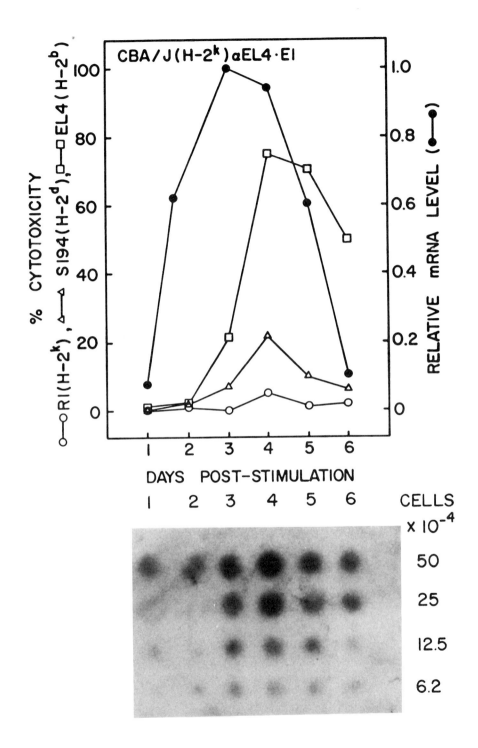

(Lobe *et al.*, 1986b). As mentioned, when B10 and C11 are compared they show 80% homology over 380 nucleotides. The B10 sequence includes a 110 nucleotide 3' untranslated region and a poly(A) tract. The C11 clone contains a much longer 3' untranslated sequence (582 nucleotides). The putative start codon of C11 is preceded by a potential ribosome binding site, CCUUCCG (Hagenbuchle *et al.*, 1978), and polyadenylation signals for both clones occur just upstream of the poly(A) tract. Of the first 12 amino acids predicted by the C11 sequence, 10 are hydrophobic and the second residue (Lys) is basic, suggesting this could be a signal sequence to direct secretion or intracellular organelle location. We have named the predicted products *c*ytotoxic *c*ell *p*roteins (CCP). The proteins encoded by C11 and B10 will be referred to as CCPI and CCPII, respectively.

An exciting finding regarding the nature of the B10- and C11-encoded proteins was made when the sequences were compared with others in the National Biomedical Research Foundation (NBRF) protein sequence data bank. The predicted protein sequences bear a striking resemblance to a number of serine proteases, ranging from 30 to 40% when optimally aligned using the Dayhoff algorithm (Lobe *et al.*, 1986b; Dayhoff, 1979). This is particularly evident for C11 as the entire coding sequence has been determined. The amino acid residues which comprise the catalytic triad forming the charge–transfer relay system in serine proteases (His-57, Asp-102, and Ser-195 in chymotrypsin) (Neurath, 1984) are all found in the C11-encoded protein (Fig. 7). The sequences around these residues, which are highly conserved in serine proteases, are also conserved in the C11 gene product.

The protein which displayed the greatest homology with CCPI was rat mast cell protease type II (RMCPII, also known as group-specific protease), where out of 215 amino acids encoded by C11, 109 were identical, giving a match per length of 51% (Fig. 7). RMCPII was thought to be unique among serine proteases, as it displayed a number of very unusual structural characteristics which affect substrate binding (Woodbury *et al.*, 1978, 1980). The protein predicted by C11, CCPI, shares all of these differences with RMCPII, except one (Lobe *et al.*, 1986b).

F. POSSIBLE FUNCTIONS OF CCPI AND CCPII

The kinetics of the induction of these genes would suggest that they play a key role in activation and/or lysis. As discussed in the introduction, there appear to be two stages of CTL activation between target conjugation and the actual lysis event. These can be distinguished by adding inhibitors with various specificities to target/effector cell mix-

CCPI	1	IleIleGlyGlyHisGluValLysProHisSerArgProTyrMetAlaLeuLeuSerIleLysAspGlnGlnProGlu AlaIleCysGlyGlyPheLeuIle ArgGluAspPhe
RMCPII	1	IleIleGlyGlyValGluSerIleProHisSerArgProTyrMetAlaHisLeuAspIleValThrGluLysGlyLeuArgValIleCysGlyGlyPheLeuIleSerArgGln Phe
CCPI	39	ValLeuThrAlaAlaHisCysGluGlySerIleIleAsnValThrLeuGlyAlaHisAsnIleLeuLysGluGlnGlnValIleProMetValLysCysIleProHisPro
RMCPII	40	ValLeuThrAlaAlaHisCysLysLysGlyLysArgGluIleThrValIleLeuGlyAlaHisAspValSerArgLysGluSerThrGlnGlnLysIleLysValGlnIleIleGlnIleIleHisGlu
CCPI	79	AspTyrAsnProLysThrPheSerSerAsnAspIleMetLeuLeuLysLeuLysSerAlaAlaLysSerAlaLysThrArgAlaValAlaArgProLeuAsnLeuProArgArgAsnValLysPro
RMCPII	80	SerTyrAsnSerValProAsnLeuHisAspIleMetLeuLeuLysLeuGluLysLysValGluLeuThrProAlaValAsnValAsnValProLeuProSerProAspPheIleHisPro
CCPI	119	GlyAlaAspValCysTyrValAlaAlaGlyTrpGlyArgMetAlaProMetGlyLysTyrSerAsn ThrLeuGlnGluValGluLeuThrValGlnLysAspArgGluCysGluSerTyr
RMCPII	120	GlyAlaMetCysTrpAlaAlaGlyTrpGlyLysThrGlyValArgAspPro ThrSerTyrThrLeuArgGluValGluLeuArgIleMetAspGluLysLysAlaCysValAspTyrArg
CCPI	157	PheLysAsnArgTyrAsnLysThrAsnGlnIleCysAlaGlyAspProLysThrLysArgAlaSerPheArgGlyAspSerGlyGlyProLeuValCysLysLysValAlaAlaAlaGlyIleIle
RMCPII	159	TyrTyrGlu Tyr LysPhe GlnValCysValGlySerProThrThrLeuArgAlaAlaPheMetGlyAspSerGlyGlyProLeuLeuCysAlaGlyValAlaAlaHisGlyIle
CCPI	197	ValSerTyrGlyTyrLysAspGlySerProProArgAlaPheThrLysValSerSerPheLeuSerTrpIleLysLysThrMetLysSerSer
RMCPII	196	ValSerTyrGlyHisProAspAlaLysProProAlaIlePheThrArgValSerSerThrTyrValPro ThrIleAsnAlaValIleAsn

FIG. 7. The protein sequence of CCPI compared with RMCPII. The DNA sequence of full-length C11 was determined and an open-reading frame identified. The predicted protein sequence (CCPI) was found to be homologous to a variety of serine proteases. The highest homology was found with RMCPII, residues which form the characteristic catalytic triad of serine proteases are marked (*). The overall homology is 51%. The numbers at the start of and this comparison is shown above. Vertical lines represent amino acid identity; the numbers at the start of each line refer to the amino acid residue at that position, and these are based on the published sequence of RMCPII.

tures, either before or after a Ca^{2+} pulse (Golstein and Smith, 1976). Although conjugate formation can occur in the absence of Ca^{2+}, the cation must be present for lysis to proceed. Inhibitors of methylation or compounds which alkylate cell-surface thiol groups are most effective at blocking the killer cell's ability to mediate cytolysis if added before Ca^{2+} addition. Therefore thiol- and methylation-dependent steps probably occur concurrently with or shortly after the initial effector–target interaction (Redelman and Hudig, 1983). Indirect evidence suggests the involvement of serine proteases in the later Ca^{2+}-dependent activation stage since CTL-mediated killing can be inhibited by substrates of both trypsin- and chymotrypsin-like proteases, as well as protease inhibitors such as diisopropylfluorophosphate (DFP), α-$_1$-antitrypsin, and α-$_1$-antichymotrypsin, if added as late as the Ca^{2+} addition (Redelman and Hudig, 1983). Macromolecular, irreversible protease inhibitors block killing activity but only when included in the killing assay, not if the cells are pretreated. Because these antiproteases cannot penetrate the cell efficiently, the proteases involved are likely to be cell surface or secreted products (CCPI leader sequence?). The fact that pretreatment with inhibitors failed to block lysis indicates the serine proteases are synthesized or activated after target conjugation. We have shown that upon antigen stimulation, the genes encoding CCPI and II become transcriptionally active. The sequence of C11 indicates that CCPI, like RMCPII, is not produced as a zymogen as most serine proteases are, so it would not need to be activated by proteolytic cleavage.

Inhibitors of chymotrypsin-like serine proteases have a minimal effect on target binding, even at concentrations which block 90% of the cytolytic activity, but they can block cytolysis when added as late as the Ca^{2+} addition (Redelman and Hudig, 1983). This indicates that one or more serine-dependent proteases with an aromatic amino acid cleavage specificity (i.e., chymotrypsin-like) take part in the Ca^{2+}-dependent events. Since lysis is not blocked if the inhibitors are added after the Ca^{2+} addition, it is unlikely that they are involved in the final lytic reaction.

Pasternack and Eisen (1985) demonstrated that a trypsin-like esterase is also activated in CTL and Con A-stimulated thymocytes. Because trypsin substrates do not have a linear effect of inhibition and the protein can be labeled with [^{3}H]DFP more intensely in cell lysates than intact CTL, they suggested that this esterase is intracellular or in a zymogen form. Another CTL-specific clone, AR10, has been isolated by Gershenfeld and Weissman (1986) and encodes a trypsin-like esterase which is produced in a zymogen form.

The involvement of serine proteases has led to speculation that CTL lysis may be mediated via a cascade mechanism of activation similar to the complement cascade (Mayer *et al.*, 1978; Redelman and Hudig, 1980). In such a system, a series of proteases would be involved, each one converting the next in the series from a zymogen to an active form. There is no direct evidence that the complement proteins themselves are involved; antibodies against complement components do not abrogate CTL lysis (Henney and Mayer, 1971). Certainly the proteins encoded by B10 and C11 show only limited homology with any components of the complement system. It is also unlikely that serine proteases are responsible for the final lytic event, as serine protease inhibitors do not reduce the efficiency of CTL at lysing their targets but effectively reduce the number of active cells (Redelman and Hudig, 1980). Instead, as for complement, they may well play a role in assembly of a membrane penetrating complex, the polyperforins which have been observed by electron microscopy. They may also be involved in release of cytotoxic granules, since it has been suggested that the protein to which CCPI shows a striking homology, RMCPII, is involved in degranulation of atypical mast cells (Woodbury and Neurath, 1980).

III. Summary

The results of this study demonstrate that CTL, pCTL, and Th cells differ sufficiently to allow cloning of moderate to high abundance subset- or activation-specific cDNAs by differential hybridization. Although we have so far restricted ourselves to CTL, we have preliminary evidence to suggest that the same methods could be used to clone Th- or thymocyte-specific genes and could, by inference, be used to clone genes characteristic of any T cell subset. In addition, less abundant subset-specific genes could be isolated using the elegant subtractive methods developed by Mark Davis.

The two CTL-specific genes which we have so far characterized appear to encode serine proteases. For the first time our results demonstrate unequivocally that chymotrypsin-like proteases are expressed in activated CTL. Furthermore, in all of our experiments to date, expression of CCPI and II correlates with phenotypic development of cytotoxicity. The fact that CCPI and II are serine proteases suggests a protease cascade type mechanism operative in CTL somewhat analogous to the action of complement in B lymphocytes. This type of mechanism offers a tremendous advantage to the cell for control and amplification of enzyme function.

The genes which we have cloned will undoubtedly be useful as probes to study the intracellular mechanisms which control expression of CCPI and II during T cell differentiation. Furthermore, a detailed knowledge of the molecular events in CTL activation and lysis could well lead to the development of rational and innovative forms of immunotherapy.

ACKNOWLEDGMENTS

The authors gratefully acknowledge Dr. C. Havele, who provided cells and performed the chromium release assays, B. Finlay, who carried out most of the sequencing, H. Gershenfeld and Dr. I. Weissman, who provided us with the AR1 library and communicated their data prior to publication, and R. Bradley, who prepared the figures. The work described was funded by the Mecical Research Council of Canada. R.C.B. is supported by the National Cancer Institute of Canada through the Terry Fox Special Initiatives Program, and C.G.L. is the recipient of a studentship from the Alberta Heritage Foundation for Medical Research.

REFERENCES

Berke, G. (1983). *Immunol. Rev.* **72**, 5–42.

Bleackley, R. C., Havele, C., and Paetkau, V. (1982). *J. Immunol.* **128**, 758–767.

Cochran, B. H., Reffel, A. C., and Stiles, C. D. (1983). *Cell* **33**, 939–947.

Cotner, T., Williams, J. M., Christenson, L., Shapiro, H. M., Strom, T. B., and Strominger, J. (1983). *J. Exp. Med.* **157**, 461–472.

Dayhoff, M. O. (1979). *In* "Atlas of Protein Sequence and Structure" (M. O. Dayhoff, ed.), Vol. 5, Suppl. 3, p. 1. National Biomedical Research Foundation, Washington, D.C.

Dennert, G., and Podack, E. R. (1983). *J. Exp. Med.* **157**, 1483–1495.

Farrar, J. J., Fuller-Farrar, J., Simon, P. L., Hilfiker, M. L., Stadler, B. M., and Farrar, W. L. (1980). *J. Immunol.* **125**, 2555–2558.

Gershenfeld, H., and Weissman, I. (1986). *Science* **232**, 854–858.

Golstein, P., and Smith, E. T. (1976). *Eur. J. Immunol.* **6**, 31–37.

Gubler, U., and Hoffman, B. J. (1983). *Gene* **25**, 263–269.

Hagenbuchle, O., Santer, M., and Steitz, J. A. (1978). *Cell* **13**, 551–563.

Hastie, N. D., and Bishop, J. O. (1976). *Cell* **9**, 761–774.

Hastings, K. E. M., and Emerson, C. P. Jr. (1982). *Proc. Natl. Acad. Sci. U.S.A.* **79**, 1553–1557.

Hedrick, S. M., Nielson, E. A., Kavaler, J., Cohen, D. I., and Davis, M. M. (1984). *Nature (London)* **308**, 153–158.

Henney, C. J., and Mayer, M. M. (1971). *Cell. Immunol.* **2**, 702–705.

Hirschhorn, R. R., Aller, P., Yuan, Z. A., Gibson, C. W., and Baserga, R. (1984). *Proc. Natl. Acad. Sci. U.S.A.* **81**, 6004–6008.

Kelly, K., Cochran, B. H., Stiles, C. D., and Leder, P. (1983). *Cell* **35**, 603–610.

Kronke, M., Leonard, W. J., Depper, J. M., and Greene, W. C. (1985). *J. Exp. Med.* **161**, 1593–1598.

Kupfer, A., and Dennert, G. (1984). *J. Immunol.* **133**, 2762–2766.

Lobe, C. G., Havele, C., and Bleackley, R. C. (1986a). *Proc. Natl. Acad. Sci. U.S.A.* **83**, 1448–1452.

Lobe, C. G., Finlay, B. B., Paranchych, W., Paetkau, V. H., and Bleackley, R. C. (1986b). *Science* **232**, 858–861.

Lowenthal, J. W., Tougne, C., MacDonald, H. R., Smith, K. A., and Nabholz, M. (1985). *J. Immunol.* **134**, 931–939.

Maniatis, T., Fritsch, E. F., and Sambrook, J. (1982. "Molecular Cloning: A Laboratory Manual." Cold Spring Harbor Laboratory, Cold Spring Harbor, New York.

Mayer, M. M., Hammer, C. H., Michaels, D. W., and Shin, M. L. (1978). *Immunochemistry* **15**, 813–831.

Milner, R. J., and Sutcliffe, J. G. (1983). *Nucleic Acids Res.* **11**, 5497–5520.

Nabholz, M., and MacDonald, H. R. (1983). *Annu. Rev. Immunol.* **1**, 273–306.

Neckers, L. M., and Cossman, J. (1983). *Proc. Natl. Acad. Sci. U.S.A.* **80**, 3494–3498.

Neurath, H. (1984). *Science* **224**, 350–357.

Pasternack, M. S., and Eisen, H. N. (1985). *Nature (London)* **314**, 743–745.

Persson, H., and Leder, P. (1984). *Science* **225**, 718–721.

Podack, E. R., and Konigsberg, P. J. (1984). *J. Exp. Med.* **160**, 695–710.

Redelman, D., and Hudig, D. (1980). *J. Immunol.* **124**, 870–878.

Redelman, D., and Hudig, D. (1983). *Cell. Immunol.* **81**, 9–21.

Sanger, F., Coulson, A. R., Barrell, B. G., Smith, A. J. H., and Roe, B. A. (1980). *J. Mol. Biol.* **143**, 161–178.

Shaw, J., Monticone, V., Mills, G., and Paetkau, V. (1978). *J. Immunol.* **120**, 1974–1980.

Teh, H. S., Ho, M., and McMaster, W. R. (1985). *J. Immunol.* **135**, 1582–1588.

White, B. A., and Bancroft, F. C. (1982). *J. Biol. Chem.* **257**, 8569–8572.

Woodbury, R. G., and Neurath, H. (1980). *FEBS Lett.* **114**, 189–196.

Woodbury, R. G., Katunuma, N., Kobayashi, K., Titani, K., and Neurath, H. (1978). *Biochemistry* **17**, 811–819.

Yanagi, Y., Yoshikai, Y., Leggett, K., Clark, S. P., Aleksander, I., and Mak, T. W. (1984). *Nature (London)* **308**, 145–149.

Zagury, D., Bernard, J., Theirness, N., Feldman, M., and Berke, G. (1975). *Eur. J. Immunol.* **5**, 818–822.

Subject Index

A

Actinomycin D, synergism with TNF *in vitro*, 196
Adipocytes, cachectin binding, 195
Amino acid sequences
  CTL-specific serine proteases, 302–303
  GM-CSF,
    human, 7, 10
    murine, 7, 10, 212, 215
  IFN-γ
    bovine, rat, 158
    human, 29–30, 152–153, 158
    murine, 156–158
  IL-1,
    murine, 140–141, 147
    rabbit, 145–146, 147
  IL-1α, human, 144, 147
  IL-1β, human, 142–143, 147
  IL-2, human
    deduced from cDNA sequence, 7, 9, 29–30
    from leukemic Jurkat cells, 38–39
    from normal T cells, 38
  IL-2, murine, 7, 9
  IL-2 receptor,
    human, 97, 104–105, 113–115, 124–125
    murine, 114, 124–125
  IL-3, murine, 4–6, 241–242
  IL-4, human, murine, 9–11
  LT, human, 201
    homology with TNF, 168, 203–204
  Multi-CSF, murine, 212, 215
  TNF,
    human, 165–168, 172, 190–192
      homology with LT, 168, 203–204
    murine, 170–172, 184–185, 190–192

B

Bovine papilloma virus (BPV), vector for
  human IL-2 receptor cDNA, 113–115
  murine IL-3 cDNA, 13

C

Cachectin, murine
  binding by adipocytes, 195
  identity with TNF, 195
Cell lines
  AP8 (monkey), expression of
    human IFN-β, 24, 26
    human IFN-γ, 26, 28–29
  C127 (murine mammary epithelium), expression of
    human IL-2 receptor, 110–112, 114–118
    number per cell, 117, 118
    IL-3 cDNA, 13
    murine IL-2 receptor, 111
  CHO (Chinese hamster ovary), expression of
    human IFN-γ, 31
    human TNF, 192
  COS (monkey kidney), expression of
    human IFN-γ, 152
    human TNF, 192
    lymphokines, 3–5, 7–10, 12
    murine IL-3, 248–249
  EL4 (murine T-lymphoma), induction of
    IL-2 mRNA, 80, 82–86
    MMTV mRNA, 88–91
  FDC-P1–IL-3 (infected with retrovirus-containing plasmids)
    IL-3 secretion, 251
    lack of detectable virus, 251
    leukemogenicity, 251–252
  HL-60 (human promyelocytic leukemia)
    TNF
      induction by PMA, 164–165
      isolation and purification from, 165
    TNF mRNA isolation, 165
  HT-2 (IL-2-dependent murine T cells),
    IL-2 receptor, 125–126
  Jurkat, leukemic, human *see* Jurkat cells
  L (murine fibroblasts), expression of
    IL-2 receptor, 124–126
    IL-3, 13, 268–270